Advances in Gynaecological Pathology

For Churchill Livingstone

Publisher: Timothy Horne
Project Editor: Dilys Jones
Editorial Co-ordination: Editorial Resources Unit
   Copy Editor: Alison Whitehouse
   Indexer: Laurence Errington
Production: Ian Hunter
Design: Design Resources Unit
Sales Promotion Executive: Hilary Brown

Advances in Gynaecological Pathology

Edited by

David Lowe MD MIBiol MRCPath
Senior Lecturer, Department of Histopathology, St Bartholomew's Hospital Medical College, London, UK

Harold Fox MD FRCPath FRCOG
Professor of Reproductive Pathology, University of Manchester; Honorary Consultant Pathologist, St Mary's Hospital, Manchester, UK

CHURCHILL LIVINGSTONE
EDINBURGH LONDON MADRID MELBOURNE NEW YORK AND TOKYO 1992

CHURCHILL LIVINGSTONE
Medical Division of Longman Group UK Limited

Distributed in the United States of America by Churchill
Livingstone Inc., 650 Avenue of the Americas, New York,
N.Y. 10011, and by associated companies, branches and
representatives throughout the world.

First published 1992

ISBN 0-443-04377-9

British Library Cataloguing in Publication Data
A catalogue record for this book is available from the
British Library.

Library of Congress Cataloging in Publication Data
A catalog record for this book is available from the Library of
Congress.

The
publisher's
policy is to use
**paper manufactured
from sustainable forests**

Produced by Longman Singapore Publishers Pte Ltd
Printed in Singapore

Preface

The idea for a collection of articles on the changes in the last few years in the theory and practice of gynaecological pathology stemmed from a symposium on ovarian pathology at the Royal College of Pathologists in London. The enthusiasm for the subject was obvious, and was equally evident at a subsequent joint symposium held by the Royal College of Obstetricians and Gynaecologists and the Royal College of Pathologists. We have asked many of the speakers at these symposia to develop their themes in this book, and also invited contributions from continental Europe, North America and Australia.

It is impossible in a book of this size to cover all new aspects of gynaecological pathology. We have tried to include topics on disease classifications that are under discussion and modification, and on diagnostic features of diseases that are confusing or poorly understood. We have also provided information on recent technological advances that are useful in diagnosis and research.

There is an increasing awareness of the importance of pathology in clinical obstetrics and gynaecology. We hope that this book will be of interest to clinicians as well as pathologists, and encourage the growing interest in the subject.

London and
Manchester, 1992

D. G. L.
H. F.

Contributors

Jan P. A. Baak MD PhD FRCPath
Professor of Pathology, Free University Hospital, Amsterdam,
The Netherlands

Elizabeth Benjamin MB BS MRCPath
Senior Lecturer and Honorary Consultant Pathologist, Department of
Histopathology, University College and Middlesex School of Medicine,
London, UK

Christine Bergeron MD
Pathologist, Institut de Pathologie et Cytologie Appliquées, Paris, France

Lawrence J. R. Brown BSc MB BS MRCPath
Consultant Histopathologist, Leicester Royal Infirmary, Leicester, UK

C. Hilary Buckley MD FRCPath
Senior Lecturer in Gynaecological Pathology, University of Manchester;
Honorary Consultant Histopathologist, St Mary's Hospital, Manchester,
UK

Marigold Curling MB BS MRCP LRCS
Consultant Cytopathologist, St Bartholomew's Hospital, London, UK

Annabelle Farnsworth MB BS FRCPA
Director of Anatomical Pathology, Prince Alfred Hospital, Camperdown,
Sydney, New South Wales, Australia

Alex Ferenczy MD
Professor of Pathology and Obstetrics and Gynecology, Sir Mortimer B.
Davis–Jewish General Hospital and McGill University, Montreal,
Quebec, Canada

Harold Fox MD FRCPath FRCCOG
Professor of Reproductive Pathology, University of Manchester;
Honorary Consultant Pathologist, St Mary's Hospital, Manchester, UK

M. Anna Kelsey MRCPath
Consultant Histopathologist, Royal Manchester Children's Hospital, Manchester, UK

Sally A. Lane MB ChB
Registrar, Department of Pathology, University of Leeds, Leeds, UK

Robin Leake MA DPhil
Reader, Department of Biochemistry, University of Glasgow, Glasgow, UK

David Lowe MD MIBiol MRCPath
Senior Lecturer, Department of Histopathology, St Bartholomew's Hospital Medical College, London, UK

Melanie J. Newbould BSc MB BS MRCPath
Senior Registrar in Paediatric Pathology, Royal Manchester Children's Hospital, Manchester, UK

Philip Quirke BM PhD MRCPath
Senior Lecturer and Honorary Consultant, Department of Pathology, University of Leeds, Leeds, UK

Terence P. Rollason BSc MB ChB MRCPath
Senior Lecturer, Department of Pathology, University of Birmingham, Birmingham, UK

Peter Russell MB BS BSc(Med) FRCPA
Senior Histopathologist, King George V and Royal Prince Alfred Hospitals, Sydney; Clinical Lecturer in Pathology, University of Sydney, Sydney, New South Wales, Australia

Robert E. Scully MD
Professor of Pathology, Harvard Medical School, Boston; Pathologist, Massachusetts General Hospital, Boston, Massachusetts, USA

Brian L. Sheppard DPhil MRCPath
Associate Professor of Human Reproduction, Trinity College Department of Obstetrics and Gynaecology, University of Dublin, St James's Hospital, Dublin, Eire

Graham R. Taylor PhD
Principal Molecular Geneticist, Yorkshire Regional DNA Laboratory, Leeds General Infirmary, Leeds, UK

P. J. van Diest MD PhD
Pathologist, Department of Pathology, Free University Hospital, Amsterdam, The Netherlands

James V. Watson MB BS MSc FRCR
MRC Senior Clinical Scientist and Consultant Oncologist, MRC Clinical

Oncology Unit, The Medical School, University of Cambridge, Cambridge, UK

Michael Wells BSc(Hons) MD MRCPath
Senior Lecturer in Pathology, University of Leeds; Honorary Consultant Pathologist, Leeds General Infirmary, Leeds, UK

Robert H. Young MD MRCPath
Associate Professor of Pathology, Harvard Medical School, Boston; Associate Pathologist, Massachusetts General Hospital, Boston, Massachusetts, USA

Contents

1. Hormone receptors in normal tissues and neoplasms of the female genital system

Robin Leake

INTRODUCTION

It has been established for many years that various tissues of the genital tract are sensitive to specific hormones. Each of these hormones acts through its own specific receptor. Peptide hormones are charged molecules and so cannot cross the cell membrane; in these cases the receptor is a component of the plasma membrane, with the ligand (hormone) binding site of the receptor sticking out from the cell (the so-called extracellular domain). Steroid hormones are, on the other hand, all synthesized from cholesterol and so are relatively soluble in the cell membrane. Not surprisingly, therefore, steroid hormone receptors are found inside the target cell. Much of the function of the ovary is regulated by peptide hormones, but growth and differentiation of most of the genital tract is under the control of steroid hormones. This chapter will concentrate on the receptors for steroid hormones and, in particular, on receptors for oestradiol and progesterone.

Before assessing the significance of the presence, or absence, of oestrogen and progesterone receptors in normal and abnormal gynaecological tissues, it is useful to summarize the sites of receptor in intact cells, and to comment on the sensitivity and selectivity of the various assay methods.

INTRACELLULAR LOCATION OF RECEPTORS

Steroid receptors were first identified after the development of radiolabelled ligands (Jensen & Jacobson 1960). Initial studies involved homogenization of tissue in hypotonic buffers and ultracentrifugation. Such treatment led to the recovery of steroid receptors in both the soluble and pellet fractions. Not unreasonably, this led to the assumption that receptors with no steroid attached (empty receptor) are in the soluble fraction and steroid-bound (activated) receptors are tightly bound to the chromatin. In 1984, two separate sets of experiments suggested that such an interpretation was incorrect. Greene and his colleagues developed various monoclonal antibodies against the oestrogen receptor and showed that staining could be detected only in the nuclear fraction of target cells (King & Greene 1984). At the same time, Gorski's group (Welshons et al 1984) used techniques to

1

separate intact 'nucleoplasts' and 'cytoplasts' and also found that virtually all oestrogen receptor, whether activated or not, was located in the nucleoplast.

Concurrent work from several laboratories (Baulieu 1987) showed that empty oestrogen receptor is associated with heat-shock protein-90. The current concept (see Fig. 1.1) is that each oestrogen receptor molecule is synthesized from the appropriate mRNA on a polysome in the cytoplasm. However, immediately after synthesis it dimerizes with another oestrogen receptor molecule and the dimer is then bound by a dimer of heat-shock protein-90 (there may also be another small molecule involved). The heat-shock protein/oestrogen receptor complex then goes immediately into the nucleus—one role of the heat-shock protein may be to guide the oestrogen receptor dimer through the nuclear membrane. The complex remains inactive until free oestradiol molecules reach the nucleus. One oestradiol molecule binds each receptor molecule causing the heat-shock protein dimer to dissociate. The oestradiol/receptor complex (still a dimer) then binds to and activates the target genes in the chromatin. The process of progesterone receptor activation is very similar except that the progesterone/heat-shock protein complex only contains a single progesterone receptor molecule.

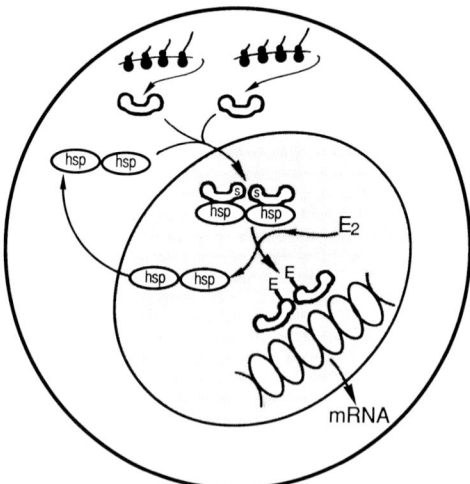

Fig. 1.1 A diagrammatic representation of oestrogen receptor distribution and function in the cell. Each receptor molecule is synthesized as a monomer but, immediately on release from the polysome, it forms a mirror-image dimer with another newly synthesized monomer. This receptor dimer forms a complex with a dimer of heat-shock protein 90 (hsp) and the complex goes straight into the nucleus where it remains until activated by the binding of oestradiol to the steroid binding site in the receptor (s). The activated receptor dimer then interacts with specific structural genes whilst the heat-shock protein 90 dimer is recycled into the cytoplasm.

RECEPTOR DETECTION

Various biochemical methods have been tried for the determination of the concentration and specificity of steroid receptors. However, much the most common method used was the dextran-coated charcoal or ligand-binding assay. This assay has been described in detail (Leake & Habib 1987). It was the favoured biochemical assay for a variety of reasons. Firstly, it assessed receptor concentration and binding affinity. Additionally, it could be used on relatively small amounts of tissue and was least likely to mistake non-specific binding for specific binding. There were various computer programs available for analysis of the data. Perhaps the two most compelling reasons for using this method were (1) most of the clinical data were reported using this method; (2) external quality assessment was easiest for laboratories using this method (Koenders & Thorpe 1983). Data are reported on soluble fractions from tissue homogenates for receptor concentrations as low as 2 fmol/mg protein. Quality assessment, however, shows that laboratories have difficulty in reproducibly measuring receptor content below 10 fmol/mg protein. Recently assays have also been carried out on tissue homogenates using enzyme immunoassays incorporating antibodies against either the oestrogen receptor or the progesterone receptor. These correlate well, qualitatively, with the dextran-coated charcoal assays; for example, Ferno et al (1989) quote a correlation of $r_s = 0.77$ for endometrial cancer tissue and 0.91 for normal tissue for progesterone receptor assayed by the dextran-coated charcoal method and the enzyme immunoassay. However, enzyme immunoassays give higher absolute values and so clinical cut-off levels (usually established using the dextran-coated charcoal method) may have to be altered.

The main disadvantage of biochemical methods is that they use a tissue homogenate and so lose the advantage that intact tissue provides of getting specific information on the cell types that contain receptor. Equally, they cannot show whether receptor is evenly distributed in a particular cell type or whether there is some heterogeneity (which might have clinical implications). The development of immunohistochemical kits (oestrogen receptor immunocytochemical assay and progesterone receptor immunocytochemical assay) has now permitted the staining of tissue sections for steroid receptors. The initial kits worked only on frozen sections (McCarty et al 1985), though they gave good qualitative agreement with the biochemically determined receptor status. More recent developments have allowed some degree of semi-quantitation (McCarty et al 1986) and even use in paraffin-embedded material (Jackson et al 1989), though these latter methods are still dependent on the initial method of fixation (the time and temperature of exposure to fixative and the nature of the fixative). Of course, immunohisto-chemical methods cannot give the same quantitative values as biochemical assays and use of both methods is still recommended where possible. These antibody kits (oestrogen receptor immunocytochemical assay and progesterone receptor immunocytochemical assay) also give good results on fine-needle aspirates (Masood 1988). As would be expected from the cellular distribution of oestrogen receptor (shown in Fig. 1.1) staining of oestrogen receptor and progesterone receptor is confined principally to the nucleus.

RECEPTORS IN THE ENDOMETRIUM

Normal tissue

Normal endometrial epithelial cells are perhaps the most commonly studied normal target cells for ovarian steroids. In the premenopausal uterus, the loss of much of the epithelial lining during menstruation is followed by extensive DNA synthesis and cell division induced by oestradiol. The postovulatory rise in plasma progesterone, however, is accompanied by a rapid fall in DNA synthesis and a switch to secretory behaviour, typified by the rapid increase in Golgi apparatus (Fenoglio et al 1982). Perhaps the most significant observation is that the plasma level of oestradiol is the same on day 21 of a 28-day cycle, when DNA synthesis is minimal, as on day 9, when maximum DNA synthesis is taking place. Evidence has been presented that progesterone can directly inhibit oestrogen-induced DNA synthesis in endometrial epithelial cells and also suppress synthesis of oestrogen receptor (Clark & Peck 1979).

The endometrial stroma also contains steroid receptors (Press & Green 1984). Stromal changes induced by oestrogens include increased synthesis of collagen, the production of reversible gaps between the endothelial cells of capillaries, and the hypertrophy and hyperplasia of capillary endothelium. Progesterone, in the postovulatory phase, induces decidual transformation. When assessing steroid receptor levels in endometrial tissue, it is important to remember that the stromal contribution to total receptor numbers can be very considerable. Another possible complication in assessing steroid receptor numbers is that, in synchronized cells, the levels of oestrogen receptor can vary by seven-fold in different stages of the cell cycle (Nishiya et al 1988). Additionally, a decrease in soluble oestrogen receptor and progesterone receptor content along the length of the uterus from fundus to cervix has been reported (Tsibris et al 1981, Robel et al 1981), though Bayard et al (1978) claim that there is no systematic variation down the uterus. Nevertheless, biopsies should, where possible, be confined to the mid-region of the uterine cavity.

Steroid receptors and the ovarian cycle

Since oestrogen action induces progesterone receptor synthesis, whereas progesterone action results in a fall in oestrogen receptor, it is not surprising that both oestrogen receptor and progesterone receptor levels change during the ovarian cycle. Given the difficulties in defining the day of the cycle precisely, most authors simply group data into early and late proliferative phases and early and late secretory phases. Using assays to calculate the sum of occupied and unfilled soluble receptors, one can show that the level of oestrogen receptor reaches a peak in late proliferative phase, then falls during the secretory phase (Bayard et al 1978, Levy et al 1980, van der Walt et al 1986). This is true for both Caucasian and Japanese women, though the absolute level of oestrogen receptor is much lower in the Japanese (Punnonen et al 1984). Nuclear (tightly bound) oestrogen receptor has also been shown to rise in early and late proliferative phases but fall thereafter (Soutter et al 1979, Levy et al 1980).

Soluble progesterone receptor shows a peak in late proliferative phase (Bayard et al 1978, Levy et al 1980), whereas nuclear progesterone receptor reaches a peak in early secretory phase (Robel et al 1981). The difference in behaviour of soluble and nuclear progesterone receptor presumably reflects the fact that it becomes activated and able to tightly bind chromatin only once it has bound to progesterone, and this becomes available only in the early secretory phase. More recent studies have used the immunohisto-chemical kits; with these, the staining is confined almost entirely to the nucleus. In one study (Clark et al 1987), in the proliferative phase uterus it was shown that the intensity of staining for progesterone receptor was greatest in the endometrial gland nuclei, slightly less in the myometrial cell nuclei and much less, though usually still positive, in the stromal cell nuclei. The greatest differences in oestrogen receptor content during the menstrual cycle are seen in the glandular elements (Thornton & Wells 1987).

Endometrial hyperplasia

Steroid receptor levels in endometrial hyperplasia have been said to be elevated (Castagnetta et al 1983). In a careful study using immunohisto-chemistry, Bergeron et al (1988) have shown, however, that progesterone receptor levels are elevated only in hyperplasia without cytological atypia and are low in epithelium of endometrial intraepithelial neoplasia (hyper-plasia with cytological atypia).

Endometrial cancer

Relation to stage and grade

In endometrial cancer, there is general agreement that the presence of oestrogen receptor and progesterone receptor correlate well with both stage (Billiet et al 1982, Genton & Buchi 1982, Castagnetta et al 1983, Kaupilla et al 1986) and grade (Bonte et al 1981, Ehrlich et al 1981, Castagnetta et al 1983, Kaupilla et al 1986). Composite figures for grade in relation to soluble oestrogen receptor or soluble progesterone receptor are given in Table 1.1,

Table 1.1   Incidence of soluble oestrogen receptor and soluble progesterone receptor in endometrial cancer in relation to histological grade

Histological grade	Soluble oestrogen receptor %	Soluble progesterone receptor(%)
I	90	83
II	75	61
III	55	22
Metastatic	49	29

The figures represent a composite from data in the papers cited in the text.

and incidence in relation to the combined presence of oestrogen receptor and progesterone receptor in Table 1.2. The importance of the presence of both oestrogen receptor and progesterone receptor stems from the fact that, in endometrium, progesterone receptor synthesis is induced by active oestrogen receptor and, therefore, the presence of both receptors shows that the hormone-sensitivity mechanism is intact. This should, therefore, make the combined index a better predictor of response to hormone therapy (Castagnetta et al 1983). Indeed, Deligdisch & Holinka (1987) have gone so far as to suggest that endometrial cancer should be split into two separate diseases, one which is hormone-sensitive, better differentiated and less aggressive, and one which is hormone-independent, less differentiated and should, perhaps, be treated more aggressively.

Intratumoural variation

Receptor status can be different when assayed in different areas of an endometrial cancer (Castagnetta et al 1983). This 'macroheterogeneity' reflects prognosis (Castagnetta et al 1987). Microheterogeneity is also seen when immunohistochemical methods are used (Zaino et al 1988), though the relationship of this heterogeneity to prognosis is yet to be established.

Prognosis

In one study, univariate analysis showed that longer survival of patients with endometrial cancer is associated with the presence of either oestrogen receptor or progesterone receptor (Borazjani et al 1989) though multivariate analysis showed that progesterone receptor status, grade of tumour and site of metastasis were the three most valuable parameters. Sutton et al (1989) showed that grade $(P=0.0002)$, peritoneal cytology $(P=0.0002)$ and progesterone receptor status $(P=0.004)$ were the three variables most closely associated with disease-free survival. De Cicco-Nardone et al (1989) showed that the combined presence of oestrogen receptor and progesterone receptor was associated with better survival, and Castagnetta et al (1987)

Table 1.2 Incidence of both soluble oestrogen receptor and soluble progesterone receptor in relation to histological grade

Histological grade	Oestrogen receptor and progesterone receptor	Incidence (%)
I	93/135	69
II	114/213	54
III	9/78	12

showed that presence of soluble and nuclear oestrogen receptor in three separate areas of tumour indicated better survival. Taking a combination of oestrogen receptor status with ploidy is said to increase the prognostic discriminance (Iversen et al 1988, Lindahl et al 1989). Ingram et al (1989) point out the value of measuring concentration of progesterone receptor, rather than simply progesterone receptor status: patients with more than 100 fmol/mg cytosol protein have a 3-year survival of 93% compared with only 36% for those with less than 100 fmol/mg ($P < 0.0001$). Chambers et al (1988) looked even more closely at concentration ranges of both oestrogen receptor and progesterone receptor and showed that if concentration is included then oestrogen receptor can be an even better predictor than grade. The importance of measuring both quantitatively is also stressed by Palmer et al (1988) who suggested that long-term survival requires oestrogen receptor concentrates of more than 70 and progesterone receptor concentrates of more than 30 fmol/mg protein. In his review of almost 20 years of steroid receptor assays in endometrial cancer, Kauppila (1989) concluded that progesterone receptor content was more strongly correlated with prognosis than any of the conventional clinico-pathological parameters. He concluded that oestrogen receptor and progesterone receptor content should both be assessed before selecting adjuvant therapy, a view previously expressed by Liao et al (1986).

Response to therapy

No index of biological function is justified if it does not play a useful role in predicting either the course of the disease or the response to a particular type of therapy. In theory, steroid receptor content should be a good index of response to endocrine therapy. In practice, in endometrial cancer oestrogen receptor status seems to be of little value but progesterone receptor status is a very good index of potential response to progestin. Earlier data on this have been reviewed by Ehrlich et al (1981) and Kaupilla (1984), and more recent data from Ehrlich's group (Ehrlich et al 1988) confirms it. By combining the data, a table of response to progestin in relation to progesterone receptor status can be constructed (see Table 1.3). The demonstration of sustained response in 72/79 patients whose advanced or metastatic disease was progesterone receptor positive indicates a high

Table 1.3 Response rates to progestin, in advanced endometrial cancer, in relation to progesterone receptor status

Progesterone receptor positive		Progesterone receptor negative	
Resp.	Non-resp.	Resp.	Non-resp.
72	7	14	96

Resp. = sustained response to progestin therapy (minimum length of response varies from one author to another); Non-resp. = no sustained response to progestin.

degree of accuracy. However, 14/110 progesterone receptor negative patients also responded to progestin therapy. Such patients should not be deprived of a chance of endocrine therapy. One possible explanation for this apparent discrepancy is that some endocrine factors can suppress receptor synthesis or mask receptor detection. Longterm progestin therapy is known to suppress progesterone receptor levels and, if these patients had received any pre-operative progestin, for example, this could have induced a 'false-negative' result in the progesterone receptor assay. Short-term tamoxifen, on the other hand, induces progesterone receptor synthesis, and advantage of this has been taken to develop sequences of tamoxifen and progestin so that progesterone receptor levels are maintained for a longer period (Bonte et al 1986, Iacobelli et al 1986).

RECEPTORS IN THE CERVIX

Normal tissue

Although cervical cancer is not normally considered likely to be hormone-sensitive, the proliferation of the squamous cells of the cervix (and also of the vagina) is modulated by steroid hormones during the menstrual cycle. The growth of cervical stroma, seen at puberty and during pregnancy, is caused by oestrogens. The mucous secretions of the columnar epithelium are also induced by steroids. The hormone sensitivity of the squamous epithelium is clearly demonstrated during hormone replacement therapy. The basal cells become active and the thin, inactive squamous epithelium responds by adopting the normal, premenopausal state.

In a recent study, using immunohistochemical techniques Mosny et al (1989) have shown that the oestrogen receptor content of the squamous epithelium varies during the menstrual cycle. In the early proliferative phase, cells of all layers were negative for oestrogen receptor staining. In the mid-phase of proliferation, the basal and parabasal layers became positive and, in the secretory phase, positively stained nuclei were found in the superficial layers. In this study, no progesterone receptor was found in any squamous cells. In an earlier study using biochemical assays, Sanborn et al (1978) demonstrated both soluble oestrogen receptor and progesterone receptor but suggested that oestrogen receptor did not fluctuate during the menstrual cycle. They did, however, see a small loss of progesterone receptor during the luteal phase. Soutter et al (1981, 1983) found both soluble and nuclear oestrogen receptor in normal cervix, with the nuclear oestrogen receptor being present at levels similar to those in the endometrium. However, Toppila et al (1983) found receptors in only a very small proportion of normal tissues assayed. Confirmation of the presence of oestrogen receptor and progesterone receptor in normal cervix came from Sadan et al (1989) who suggested that progesterone receptor levels may decrease as tissue becomes pre-invasive. Further support for the presence of functional steroid receptors in the normal cervix comes from Ciocca et al (1986) who have studied changes in an oestrogen-responsive protein throughout the cervix during the menstrual cycle.

Cervical cancer

Incidence

Because normal cervix can contain oestrogen receptor and progesterone receptor, it is important that, in carrying out assays on tumour tissue, histological checks are made to ensure that most of the tissue being assayed is, in fact, tumour tissue. The literature certainly shows a wide variation in the incidence of oestrogen receptor in cervical cancer. Soutter et al (1983) found 71% oestrogen receptor positive in a study in which careful histological checks were included. Peyrat et al (1983) found a similar number (75%) oestrogen receptor positive, whereas Martin et al (1982) found only 33% oestrogen receptor positive. Various small studies have ranged from 12% (Toppila et al 1983) to 100% (Syrjala et al 1978). This large variation can be partly explained in terms of different tissue handling and assay methodology, but it certainly confirms that studies should be considered only if there are reasonably large numbers of patients involved.

The incidence of progesterone receptor has been less well studied but the overall conclusion is that progesterone receptor incidence is lower than oestrogen receptor. Some of the existing data are summarized in Table 1.4.

Because evidence of functionality of receptor has been used to give better discrimination of hormone dependence in breast cancer (see Soutter & Leake 1987 for review), it may be relevant to look at indices of receptor function in cervical cancer. The usual indices are (1) presence of nuclear, tightly bound receptors, and (2) presence of progesterone receptor (supposedly oestrogen-induced). When one of these two criteria is applied to cervical cancer, then the proportion of patients who might be expected to have hormone-sensitive cancer is reduced to about 20% (see Table 1.5).

Table 1.4   Incidence of soluble progesterone receptor in cervical cancer

Reference	No. of patients	No. progesterone receptor positive	% progesterone receptor positive
Ford et al (1983)	24	5	21
Gibbons & O'Brien (1983)	30	8	27
Toppila et al (1983)	17	6	35
Peyrat et al (1983)	32	13	42
Gao et al (1983)	19	10	53
Hunter et al (1987)	56	18	30
Harding et al (1990a)	95	38	40

The cut-off point for progesterone receptor positivity differed amongst the studies.

Table 1.5   'Functional' oestrogen receptors in squamous cervical cancer

Reference	Definition of 'functional'	No. of patients	No. 'functional'	% 'functional'
Soutter et al (1983)	ER_c/ER_n	58	11	19
Toppila (1983)	ER/PR	17	2	12
Ford et al (1983)	ER/PR	24	5	21
Peyrat et al (1983)	ER/PR	32	12	37
Hunter et al (1987)	ER/PR	56	16	29
Harding et al (1990a)	ER/PR	80	19	24

ER = oestrogen receptor; PR = progesterone receptor; ER_c = soluble receptor; ER_n = nuclear receptor.

Table 1.6   'Functional' oestrogen receptors in adenocarcinoma of cervix

Reference	Definition of 'functional'	No. of patients	No. 'functional'	% 'functional'
Ford et al (1983)	ER/PR	6	3	50
Peyrat et al (1983)	ER/PR	9	6	67
Toppila (1983)	ER/PR	6	4	67
Harding et al (1990)	ER/PR	13	8	62

ER = oestrogen receptor; PR = progesterone receptor.

However, there is a clear suggestion that adenocarcinoma might have a higher incidence of functional receptor and so be more suitable for endocrine therapy (Table 1.6).

Prognosis

Martin et al (1986) studied 246 women with primary carcinoma of the cervix. The mean survival time of those who died was 15 months and the survivors were followed for an average of 34 months. The survival curves showed no difference between the oestrogen receptor positive and negative groups, nor between the progesterone receptor positive and negative groups. Hunter et al (1987) studied 70 cases and found oestrogen receptor level of > 3 fmol/mg protein in 41% of cases but progesterone receptor level of > 3 fmol/mg protein in only 30%. Oestrogen receptor and progesterone receptor were both present in 28%. A weak correlation ($P = 0.063$) was found between progesterone receptor and survival but there was no correlation between presence of oestrogen receptor and survival. Twiggs et al (1987) identified a possible prognostic role for oestrogen receptors specifically in Stage 1B cervical cancer. Additional prognostic information has been provided by Fujimoto et al (1989) who conclude that there was no relationship between the presence of progesterone receptor, or androgen receptor, and prognosis but that patients whose tumours contained in excess of 5 fmol/µg DNA (surprisingly oestrogen receptor-rich, in our experience) tended to have a longer survival than those with less. A recent study from our own group (Harding et al 1990a) of 102 cervical carcinomas showed a correlation among oestrogen receptor negativity, poorer differentiation and larger tumours. However, this study showed no overall difference in the progression-free survival of the oestrogen receptor positive and negative groups. Thus, the overall conclusion must be that steroid receptor status is not a good prognostic discriminant in cervical cancer.

In addition to the biochemical studies, the presence of oestrogen receptor and progesterone receptor in cervical cancer has been sought using the immunohistochemical assay. Mosny et al (1989) stated categorically that no oestrogen receptor or progesterone receptor was detectable in neoplastic cells. In view of the foregoing biochemical data, this observation is surprising and further immunohistochemical studies are awaited with interest.

Endocrine therapy in cervical cancer

Given the low incidence of 'functional' steroid receptors in cervical squamous cancer, a relatively low response rate to endocrine therapy would be predicted. Thus even if this subgroup of patients did have hormone-sensitive disease, an appropriate response rate would be detected only in a large study. Unfortunately, the early studies were all on small groups of patients who were often additionally suffering from very advanced disease (Varga & Henriksen 1964, Van Exter & Pauls 1972, Malkasian et al 1974). Not surprisingly, all these studies reported only marginal effects of endocrine therapy.

A study by Sugimori et al (1976) showed that additional oestrogen could give a marked improvement to 5-year survival after radiotherapy. A more recent study (Twiggs et al 1987) showed no response to tamoxifen but, again, the patients had already proved refractory to chemotherapy. A study should perhaps be mounted of first-line endocrine therapy in patients whose biological markers suggest likely response to such therapy.

STEROID RECEPTORS IN THE OVARY

Given the complex nature of ovarian pathology and the limited number of reports available, this review is confined to steroid receptors in ovarian epithelial cells.

Normal tissue

In most normal epithelial cells of the reproductive system, evidence suggests that synthesis of progesterone receptor is induced through gene activation by oestrogen receptor. The normal ovary is different in that 84% of cells contain progesterone receptor, whereas only 35% contain oestrogen receptor (combined figures from Vihko et al 1983, Willcocks et al 1983, Lantta 1984). Furthermore, oestrogen receptor is present at only low concentrations (5–15 fmol/mg cytosol protein) whereas progesterone receptor is present at the same range found in hormone-sensitive breast cancer (50–950 fmol/mg protein).

Ovarian cancer

Progesterone receptor incidence is a little lower in benign disease than in normal tissue but much lower in cancer. Oestrogen receptor is much higher in cancer. In the recent study from our laboratory of 89 untreated ovarian cancer patients (Harding et al 1990b) 53% were oestrogen receptor positive, 40% progesterone receptor positive, but only 33% positive for both oestrogen receptor and progesterone receptor; 40% were oestrogen receptor/progesterone receptor negative. A similar figure of 27% for incidence of oestrogen receptor/progesterone receptor positivity was reported by Friedlander et al (1989) in a study of 92 patients. A study by Sutton et al (1986a) of 44 patients gave 69% oestrogen receptor positive and 35% progesterone receptor positive. Anderl et al (1988) studied 62 patients and found 63% to be oestrogen receptor negative, with 35% progesterone receptor negative. Masood et al (1989) reported 68% oestrogen receptor positive and 49% progesterone receptor positive. Thus, although the cut-off values used in different studies varied over a considerable range (5–50 fmol/mg cytosol protein—see Harding et al 1990b for discussion), there is general agreement that around 30% of untreated ovarian epithelial cancers will contain functional receptors, using the definition of presence of both oestrogen receptor and progesterone receptor.

Use of the immunohistochemical assay in place of the biochemical assay gives similar results. Masood (1988) showed that the dextran-coated charcoal and immunohistochemical assays were concordant in 91% of cases. He also reported success in staining fine-needle aspirates taken from distant metastases. Nardelli et al (1987) used the enzyme immunoassay method and also reported good agreement with the dextran-coated charcoal assay, confirming the work of Holt & Bolanos (1986).

In those studies where oestrogen receptor and progesterone receptor status have been related to histological subtypes, serous and endometrioid tumours most frequently contain both receptors (Toppila et al 1986, Sutton et al 1986a), though not all studies agree with this [see Harding et al (1990b) in whose study only serous tumours had a significantly higher incidence of oestrogen receptor and progesterone receptor].

Some studies have examined the correlation of oestrogen receptor and progesterone receptor with ploidy. Iversen et al (1988) found oestrogen receptor more commonly in diploid than aneuploid tumours, whereas Jakobsen et al (1988) found no correlation between the two parameters. In a study of 92 patients with ovarian cancer, Friedlander et al (1989) found 11% of tumours were both oestrogen receptor and progesterone receptor rich. These tumours comprised 23% of the diploid and 5% of the aneuploid ($P<0.01$). Receptor negative tumours had a median S phase of 18.8% compared with 12% for the receptor positive tumours ($P<0.02$). These results imply that there might be a prognostic advantage for patients with oestrogen receptor/progesterone receptor positive tumours.

Prognosis and therapy

Because of the prognostic value of oestrogen receptor and/or progesterone receptor in other gynaecological tissues, various authors have investigated their prognostic role in ovarian epithelial cancer. Bizzi et al (1988) applied multivariate analysis and concluded that the main determinants for good prognosis were low residual tumour, serous histological type and oestrogen receptor positivity. In contrast, Anderl et al (1988) found no significant survival advantage in the group with higher oestrogen receptor and progesterone receptor content; significantly, perhaps, they were also unable to show any advantage in adding anti-oestrogen therapy into their treatment regimen. Iversen et al (1986), in a study of only 31 patients, found the median survival for patients with progesterone receptor positive or oestrogen receptor/progesterone receptor positive tumours was 30 and 31.5 months respectively, whilst that for receptor negative tumours was only 10 and 9 months. This would suggest that a combination of oestrogen receptor and progesterone receptor is the best discriminant, a conclusion borne out by the larger study of Harding et al (1990b). Slotman et al (1989) also found a survival advantage ($P<0.05$) for patients with progesterone receptor-rich tumours.

Studies on the effects of endocrine therapy on ovarian cancer have been small. Weiner et al (1987) entered 37 patients into a trial of tamoxifen. Median survival was 7 months for non-responders versus 16 months for responders (complete plus partial response plus static). There was no correlation between response and oestrogen receptor or progesterone receptor status. However, all patients had been heavily pre-treated with multiple chemotherapy and, as this can markedly alter receptor content, this was not a fair test. In studies of endocrine therapy on unselected patients, the best results suggest an overall response of around 15% (Mangioni et al 1981, Freedman et al 1986). This would fit in with the levels cited for oestrogen receptor-rich/progesterone receptor-rich tumours (Friedlander et al 1989, Harding et al 1990b), although no study has yet been carried out in which objective response of ovarian epithelial cancer to endocrine therapy has been correlated with good receptor estimation in cases not complicated by prior therapies.

RECEPTORS IN OTHER GYNAECOLOGICAL CANCERS

Various studies have reported receptor status in small groups of patients with 'unusual' gynaecological tumours, though in most cases the groups are too small for serious analysis. Before discussing these, it should be remembered that as many as one in five women may have uterine leiomyomas (fibroids) at some point in their reproductive life. Since oestrogens are thought to play a significant role in their development, several studies have investigated the occurrence of both oestrogen receptor and progesterone receptor in leiomyomas. In a study by Navarro et al (1989), oestrogen receptor was found in 84% of leiomyomas and progesterone receptor in 80%. The concentration range for progesterone receptor (805–2000 fmol/mg protein) was relatively high compared with normal myometrium. Marelli et al (1989) showed that oestrogen receptor and progesterone receptor concentration in leiomyomas was similar in the uterine fundus, body and isthmus and, further, was constant across large leiomyomas. The increased level in leiomyomas, compared with normal myometrium, was confirmed by Lumsden et al (1989) who also showed that treatment with luteinizing hormone releasing hormone agonists can influence receptor levels (oestrogen receptor showing a rise, and progesterone receptor a fall).

Sutton et al (1986b) reported low receptor levels (10–16 fmol/mg protein) in uterine sarcomas, with an incidence of around 50%. Levels were not influenced by stage, grade or mitotic count. Progesterone receptor was higher in patients under 50 years of age. Endometrial stromal sarcomas had higher oestrogen receptor and progesterone receptor levels than other histological types. Low-grade endometrial stromal sarcoma had higher oestrogen receptor levels and better survival than their high-grade counterparts. For all types of stromal sarcoma, oestrogen receptor seems to be an index of good prognosis, though objective response to endocrine therapy was observed in only one endometrial stromal sarcoma. This suggestion was later supported by Tosi et al (1989) who showed that those sarcomas containing very high numbers of mitoses were oestrogen receptor negative. Tseng et al (1986) have suggested that endocrine therapy might be recommended for those sarcomas showing high levels of progesterone receptor.

Auerbach et al (1988) report on ovarian ependymoma, concluding that, although pure neuroectodermal ovarian tumours were rare, they might contain oestrogen receptor and progesterone receptor, since tumours of the central nervous system of similar histology do so. They report one case with both oestrogen receptor (17 fmol/mg) and progesterone receptor (80 fmol/mg). No endocrine therapy was tried but the case was made for its consideration for use in such tumours.

GENERAL DISCUSSION

Steroid receptors are found in varying degrees and at varying concentrations in all gynaecological malignancies. In endometrial cancer, progesterone receptor status is a very good discriminant for selecting endocrine therapy for advanced disease. In ovarian cancer, the presence of both oestrogen receptor and progesterone receptor selects out a small group with better prognosis, though no adequate studies have yet revealed whether this group would benefit from early endocrine therapy. The prognostic value of oestrogen receptor and progesterone receptor in cervical cancer is probably too small to justify their measurement. Further studies on oestrogen receptor and progesterone receptor in unusual malignancies, and exploration of endocrine therapy on oestrogen receptor/progesterone receptor positive tumours, seem worthwhile.

Immunohistochemical studies now allow analysis of the distribution of receptors. This is particularly valuable where both epithelial and stromal tissues can be receptor positive. However, in many cancers, concentration of receptor is important before clinical decisions are made. Ideally, therefore, both biochemical and immunohistochemical information should be sought.

ACKNOWLEDGEMENTS

I am very grateful to all my colleagues, both within the research group and in the hospitals, who have contributed to our own research in this area. I am most grateful to ICI Pharmaceuticals (Dr Ian Jackson) for continued support and encouragement of our gynaecological cancer work.

REFERENCES

Anderl P, Fuith L C, Daxenbichler G, Marth C, Dapunt O 1988 Correlation between steroid hormone receptors, histological and clinical parameters in ovarian carcinoma. Gynecological and Obstetrical Investigation 25: 135–140

Auerbach R, Mittal K, Schwartz P E 1988 Estrogen and progestin receptors in an ovarian ependymoma. Obstetrics and Gynecology 71: 1043–1045

Baulieu E-E 1987 Steroid hormone antagonists at the receptor level: a role for heat shock protein MW 90,000 (hsp 90). Journal of Cell Biochemistry 35: 161–174

Bayard F, Damilano S, Robel P, Baulieu E-E 1978 Cytoplasmic and nuclear oestradiol and progesterone receptors in human endometrium. Journal of Clinical Endocrinology and Metabolism 46: 635–648

Bergeron C, Ferenczy A, Shyamala G 1988 Distribution of estrogen receptors in various cell types of normal, hyperplastic and neoplastic human endometrial tissues. Laboratory Investigation 58: 338–345

Billiet G, De Hertogh R, Bonte J, Ide P, Vlaemynck G 1982 Estrogen receptors in human uterine adenocarcinoma: correlation with tissue differentiation, vaginal karyopyknotic index, and effect of progestogen or anti-oestrogen treatment. Gynecologic Oncology 14: 33–39

Bizzi A, Codegoni A M, Landoni F et al 1988 Steroid receptors in epithelial ovarian carcinoma: relation to clinical parameters and survival. Cancer Research 48: 6222–6226

Bonte J, Ide P, Billiet G, Wyants P 1981 Tamoxifen as a possible chemotherapeutic agent in endometrial adenocarcinoma. Gynecologic Oncology 11: 140–161

Bonte J, Janssens J P, Ide P 1986 Modalities and results of a combined anti-estrogenic therapy by means of tamoxifen and medroxyprogesterone in gynecologic cancerology. European Journal of Gynaecological Oncology 7: 45–50

Borazjani G, Twiggs L B, Leung B S, Prem K A, Adcock L L, Carson L F 1989 Prognostic significance of steroid receptors measured in primary metastatic and recurrent endometrial carcinoma. American Journal of Obstetrics and Gynecology 161: 1253–1257

Castagnetta L, LoCasto M, Mercadante T, Polito L, Cowan S, Leake R E 1983 Intra-tumoural variation of oestrogen receptor status in endometrial cancer. British Journal of Cancer 47: 261–267

Castagnetta L, LoCasto M, Granata O M, Calabro M, Ciaccio M, Leake R E 1987 Soluble and nuclear oestrogen receptor status of advanced endometrial cancer in relation to subsequent prognosis. British Journal of Cancer 55: 543–546

Chambers J T, MacLusky N, Eisenfield A, Kohorn E I, Lawrence R, Schwartz P E 1988 Estrogen and progestin receptor levels as prognosticators for survival in endometrial cancer. Gynecologic Oncology 31: 65–81

Ciocca D R, Puy L A, Lo Castro G 1986 Localization of an estrogen-responsive protein in the human cervix during menstrual cycle, pregnancy, and menopause and in abnormal cervical epithelia without atypia. American Journal of Obstetrics and Gynecology 155: 1090–1096

Ciocca D R, Puy L A, Fasoli L C 1989 Study of estrogen receptor, progesterone receptor, and the estrogen-regulated Mr 24,000 protein in patients with carcinomas of the endometrium and cervix. Cancer Research 49: 4298–4304

Clark J H, Peck E J Jr 1979 Female sex steroids: receptors and function. Monographs in endocrinology. Springer-Verlag, Berlin, vol 14

Clarke C L, Zaino R J, Feil P D et al 1987 Monoclonal antibodies to human progesterone receptor: characterization by biochemical and immunohistochemical techniques. Endocrinology 121: 1123–1132

De Cicco Nardone F, Benedetto M T, Rossiello F et al 1989 Hormone receptor status in human endometrial adenocarcinoma. Cancer 64: 2572–2578

Deligdisch L, Holinka C F 1987 Endometrial carcinoma: two diseases? Cancer Detection and Prevention 10: 237–246

Ehrlich C E, Young P C M, Clearly R E 1981 Cytoplasmic progesterone and oestradiol receptors in normal, hyperplastic and carcinomatous endometria: therapeutic implications. American Journal of Obstetrics and Gynecology 141: 539–546

Ehrlich C E, Young P C, Stehman F B, Sutton G P, Alford W M 1988 Steroid receptors and clinical outcome in patients with adenocarcinoma of the endometrium. American Journal of Obstetrics and Gynecology 158: 796–807

Fenoglio C M, Crum C P, Ferenczy A 1982 Endometrial hyperplasia and carcinoma: are ultrastructural, biochemical and immunocytochemical studies useful in distinguishing between them? Pathology Research and Practice 174: 257–284

Ferno M, Borg A, Horvath G, Lindahl B 1989 Enzyme immunoassay of progesterone receptor in cancerous and normal endometrial tissue. A comparison with the dextran-coated charcoal method. Anticancer Research 9: 1681–1683

Ford L C, Berek J S, Lagasse L D, Hacker N F, Heins Y L, DeLange R J 1983 Estrogen and progesterone receptor sites in malignancies of the uterine cervix. Gynecologic Oncology 15: 27–31

Freedman R S, Saul P B, Edwards C L et al 1986 Ethinyl estradiol and medroxyprogesterone acetate in patients with epithelial ovarian cancer: a Phase II study. Cancer Treatment Reports 70: 369–373

Friedlander M L, Quinn M A, Fortune D et al 1989 The relationship of steroid receptor expression to nuclear DNA distribution and clinicopathological characteristics in epithelial ovarian tumors. Gynecologic Oncology 32: 184–190

Fujimoto J, Fujita H, Hosoda S, Okada H, Tamaya T 1989 Prognosis of cervical cancers with reference to steroid receptors. Nippon Gan Chiryo Gakkai Shi 24: 21–31

Gao Y L, Twiggs L B, Leung B S et al 1983 Cytoplasmic estrogen and progesterone receptor in primary cervical carcinoma: clinical and histopathologic correlates. American Journal of Obstetrics and Gynecology 146: 299–306

Genton C Y, Buchi K 1982 Are the histological and ultrastructural features of endometrial carcinoma reliable indicators of their steroid receptor content? Gynecological and Obstetrical Investigation 13: 213–225

Gibbons W E, O'Brien T J 1983 Basis for hormone manipulation of gynecological tumours. In: Morrow C P, Bonnar J, O'Brien T J, Gibbons W E (eds) Recent clinical developments in gynecologic oncology. Raven Press, New York, p 99–106

Harding M, McIntosh J, Paul J et al 1990a Oestrogen and progesterone receptors in carcinoma of the cervix. Clinical Oncology 2: 313–317

Harding M, Cowan S, Hole D et al 1990b Estrogen and progesterone receptors in ovarian cancer. Cancer 65: 486–491

Holt J A, Bolanos J 1986 Enzyme-linked immunochemical measurement of estrogen receptor in gynecologic tumours, and an overview of steroid receptors in ovarian carcinoma. Clinical Chemistry 32: 1836–1843

Hunter R E, Longcope C, Keough P 1987 Steroid hormone receptors in carcinoma of the cervix. Cancer 60: 392–396

Iacobelli S, Scambia G, Atlante G, Landoni F, Sismondi P, Vecchio F 1986 Effect of tamoxifen on steroid hormone receptors and creatine kinase activity in human endometrial carcinoma. European Journal of Cancer and Clinical Oncology 22: 105–110

Ingram S S, Rosenman J, Heath R, Morgan T M, Moore D, Varia M 1989 The predictive value of progesterone receptor levels in endometrial cancer. International Journal of Radiation Oncology and Biological Physics 17: 21–27

Iversen O E, Skaarland E, Utaaker E 1986 Steroid receptor content in human ovarian tumors: survival of patients with ovarian carcinoma related to steroid receptor content. Gynecologic Oncology 23: 65–76

Iversen O E, Utaaker E, Skaarland E 1988 DNA ploidy and steroid receptors as predictors of disease course in patients with endometrial carcinoma. Acta Obstetrica Gynecologica Scandinavia 67: 531–537

Jackson P, Teasdale J, Cowen P N 1989 Development and validation of a sensitive immunohistochemical oestrogen receptor assay for use on archival breast cancer tissue. Histochemistry 92: 149–152

Jakobsen A, Hansen V, Poulsen H S 1988 DNA profile and steroid receptor content of human ovarian cancer. European Journal of Gynaecological Oncology 9: 461–463

Jensen E V, Jacobson H T 1960 In: Pincus G, Vollmer E P (eds) Activity of steroids in relation to cancer. Academic Press, New York, p 161–183

Kaupilla A 1984 Progestin therapy of endometrial, breast and ovarian carcinoma. Acta Gynecologica Scandinavia 63: 441–450

Kaupilla A 1989 Oestrogen and progestin receptors as prognostic indicators in endometrial cancer. A review of the literature. Acta Oncologica 28: 561–566

Kauppila A J, Isotalo H E, Kivinen S T, Vihko R K 1986 Prediction of clinical outcome with estrogen and progestin receptor concentrations and their relationship to clinical and histopathological variables in endometrial cancer. Cancer Research 46: 5380–5384

King W J, Greene G L 1984 Monoclonal antibodies localise oestrogen receptor in the nuclei of target cells. Nature 307: 745–747

Koenders T, Thorpe S M 1983 Standardisation of steroid receptor assays in human breast cancer I. Reproducibility of estradiol and progesterone receptor assays. European Journal of Cancer and Clinical Oncology 19: 1221–1229

Lantta M 1984 Estradiol and progesterone receptors in normal ovary and ovarian tumours. Acta Obstetrica Gynecologica Scandinavia 63: 497–503

Leake R E, Habib F 1987 Steroid hormone receptors: assay and characterisation. In: Green B, Leake R E (eds) Steroid hormones: a practical approach. IRL, Oxford, p 67–92

Levy C, Robel P, Gautray J P et al 1980 Estradiol and progesterone receptors in human endometrium: normal and abnormal menstrual cycles and early pregnancy. American Journal of Obstetrics and Gynecology 136: 646–651

Liao B S, Twiggs L B, Leung B S, Yu W C, Potish R A, Prem K A 1986 Cytoplasmic estrogen and progesterone receptors as prognostic parameters in primary endometrial carcinoma. Obstetrics and Gynecology 67: 463–467

Lindahl B, Alm P, Ferno M et al 1989 Prognostic value of steroid receptor concentration and flow cytometrical DNA measurements in stage I–II endometrial carcinoma. Acta Oncologica 28: 595–599

Lumsden M A, West C P, Hawkins R A, Bramley T A, Rumgay L, Baird D T 1989 The binding of steroids to myometrium and leiomyomata (fibroids) in women treated with the gonadotrophin-releasing hormone agonist Zoladex (ICI 118630). Journal of Endocrinology 121: 389–396

McCarty K S Jr, Miller L S, Cox E B, Conratt J, McCarty K S Sn 1985 Estrogen receptor analyses: Correlation of biochemical and immunohistochemical methods using monoclonal anti-receptor antibodies. Archives of Pathology and Laboratory Medicine 109: 716–721

McCarty K S, Szabo E, Flowers J L 1986 Use of a monoclonal anti-oestrogen receptor antibody in the immunohistochemical evaluation of human tumours. Cancer Research 46: 4244s–4248s

Malkasian G D, Decker D G, Jorgensen E O, Webb M J 1974 Evaluation of 6,17α-dimethyl-6-dehydroprogesterone for treatment of recurrent and metastatic gynecologic malignancy. American Journal of Obstetrics and Gynecology 118: 461–465

Mangioni C, Franceschi S, La Vecchia C, D'Incalci M 1981 High dose medroxyprogesterone acetate (MPA) in advanced epithelial ovarian cancer resistant to first- or second-line chemotherapy. Gynecologic Oncology 12: 314–318

Marelli G, Codegoni A M, Bizzi A 1989 Estrogen and progesterone receptors in leiomyomas and normal uterine tissues during reproductive life. Acta Europa Fertility 20: 19–22

Martin J D, Hahnel R, McCartney A J, Woodings T 1982 Prognostic value of estrogen receptors in cancer of the uterine cervix. New England Journal of Medicine 306: 485–491

Martin J D, Hahnel R, McCartney A J, Woodings T L 1983 The effect of estrogen receptor status on survival in patients with endometrial cancer. American Journal of Obstetrics and Gynecology 147: 322–324

Martin J D, Hahnel R, McCartney A J, De Klerk N 1986 The influence of estrogen and progesterone receptors on survival in patients with carcinoma of the uterine cervix. Gynecologic Oncology 23: 329–335

Masood S 1988 Use of monoclonal antibodies in immunohistochemical localization of estrogen receptors in ovarian cancer. Cancer Detection and Prevention 12: 283–290

Masood S, Heitmann J, Nuss R C, Benrubi G I 1989 Clinical correlation of hormone receptor status in epithelial ovarian cancer. Gynecologic Oncology 34: 57–60

Mosny D S, Herholz J, Degen W, Bender H G 1989 Immunohistochemical investigations of steroid receptors in normal and neoplastic squamous epithelium of the uterine cervix. Gynecologic Oncology 35: 373–377

Nardelli, G B, Lamaina V, Dal Pozzo M, Onnis G L 1987 Determination of ER in ovarian cancer using monoclonal antibody technology. Clinical Experiments in Obstetrics and Gynecology 14: 185–187

Navarro D, Cabrera J-J, Falcon O et al 1989 Monoclonal antibody characterization of progesterone receptors, estrogen receptors and the stress-responsive protein 27 kDa (SRP27) in human uterine leiomyoma. Journal of Steroid Biochemistry 34: 491–498

Nishiya I, Kagabu T, Saito S, Fujimoto J, Okada H 1988 Relationship between changes of the steroid receptor and synchronization in human endometrial adenocarcinoma cells *in vitro*. Cytometry 9: 588–593

Palmer D C, Muir I M, Alexander A I, Cauchi M, Bennett R C, Quinn M A 1988 The prognostic importance of steroid receptors in endometrial carcinoma. Obstetrics and Gynecology 72: 388–393

Peyrat J P, Vandewalle B, Gougeon E et al 1983 Second International Congress on Hormones and Cancer. Journal of Steroid Biochemistry 19: 74S

Punnonen R, Lukola A, Kudo R 1984 Cytoplasmic estrogen receptor concentrations in the endometrium of Finnish and Japanese women. European Journal of Obstetrics, Gynaecology and Reproductive Biology 17: 321–325

Press M F, Greene G L 1984 Methods in laboratory investigation: an immunocytochemical method for demonstrating estrogen receptor in human uterus using monoclonal antibodies to human estrophilin. Laboratory Investigation 50: 480–486

Robel P, Mortel R, Baulieu E-E 1981 Estradiol and progesterone receptor in human endometrium. In: Litwack G (ed) Biochemical actions of hormones. Academic Press, New York, vol 8: 493–514

Sadan O, Frohlich R P, Driscoll J A, Apostoleris A, Savage N, Zakut H 1989 Is it safe to prescribe hormonal contraception and replacement therapy to patients with premalignant and malignant uterine cervices? Gynecologic Oncology 34: 159–163

Sanborn B M, Kuo H S, Held B 1978 Estrogen and progesterone binding concentrations in human endometrium and cervix throughout the menstrual cycle and in tissue from women taking oral contraceptives. Journal of Steroid Biochemistry 9: 951–955

Slotman B J, Kuhnel R, Rao B R, Dijkhuizen G H, De Graaff J, Stolk J G 1989 Importance of steroid receptors and aromatase activity in the prognosis of ovarian cancer: high tumor progesterone receptor levels correlate with longer survival. Gynecologic Oncology 33: 76–81

Soutter W P, Leake R E 1987 Steroid hormone receptors in gynaecological cancers. In: Bonnar J (ed) Recent advances in obstetrics and gynaecology. Churchill Livingstone, Edinburgh, vol 15: 175–194

Soutter W P, Hamilton K, Leake, R E 1979 High affinity binding of oestradiol 17β in the nuclei of human endometrial cells. Journal of Steroid Biochemistry 10: 529–534

Soutter W P, Pegoraro R J, Green-Thompson R W, Naidoo D V, Joubert S M, Philpott R H 1981 Nuclear and cytoplasmic oestrogen receptors in squamous carcinoma of the cervix. British Journal of Cancer 44: 154–159

Soutter W P, Pegoraro R J, Green-Thompson R W, Naidoo D V, Joubert S M, Philpott R H 1983 Nuclear and cytoplasmic oestrogen receptors in squamous carcinoma of the cervix. In: Morrow C P, Bonnar J, O'Brien T J, Gibbons W E (eds) Recent clinical developments in gynecologic oncology. Raven Press, New York, p 23

Sugimori H, Taki I, Koga K 1976 Adjuvant hormone therapy to radiation treatment for cervical cancer. Acta Obstetrica et Gynaecologica Japonica 23: 77–82

Sutton G P, Senior M B, Strauss J F, Mikuta J J 1986a Estrogen and progesterone receptors in epithelial ovarian malignancies. Gynecologic Oncology 23: 176–182

Sutton G P, Stehman F B, Michael H, Young P C, Ehrlich C E 1986b Estrogen and progesterone receptors in uterine sarcomas. Obstetrics and Gynecology 68: 709–714

Sutton G P, Geisler H E, Stehman F B, Young P C, Kimes T M, Ehrlich C E 1989 Features associated with survival and disease-free survival in early endometrial cancer. American Journal of Obstetrics and Gynecology 160: 1385–1391

Syrjala P, Kontula K, Janne O, Kauppila A, Vihko R 1978 Steroid receptors in normal and neoplastic human uterine tissue. In: Brush M G, King R J B, Taylor R (eds) Endometrial cancer. Ballière Tindall, London, p 242–251

Thornton J G, Wells M 1987 Oestrogen receptor in glands and stroma of normal and neoplastic human endometrium: a combined biochemical, immunohistochemical, and morphometric study. Journal of Clinical Pathology 40: 1437–1442

Toppila M, Willcocks D, Tyler J P P et al 1983 Sex steroid receptors in gynaecological malignancy. Journal of Obstetrics and Gynaecology 4: 53–59

Toppila M, Tyler J P, Fay R et al 1986 Steroid receptors in human ovarian malignancy. A review of four years tissue collection. British Journal of Obstetrics and Gynaecology 93: 986–992

Tosi P, Sforza V, Santopietro R 1989 Estrogen receptor content, immunohistochemically determined by monoclonal antibodies, in endometrial stromal sarcoma. Obstetrics and Gynecology 73: 75–78

Tsibris J C M, Fort F L, Cazenave C R et al 1981 The uneven distribution of estrogen and progesterone receptors in human endometrium. Journal of Steroid Biochemistry 14: 997–1000

Tseng L, Tseng J K, Mann W J et al 1986 Endocrine aspects of human uterine sarcoma: a preliminary study. American Journal of Obstetrics and Gynecology 155: 95–101

Twiggs L B, Potish R A, Leung B S et al 1987 Cytosolic estrogen and progesterone receptors as prognostic parameters in stage IB cervical carcinoma. Gynecologic Oncology 28: 156–160

van der Walt L A, Sanfilippo J S, Siegel J E, Wittliff J L 1986 Estrogen and progestin receptors in human uterus: reference ranges of clinical conditions. Clinical Physiology and Biochemistry 4: 217–228

Van Exter C, Pauls F 1972 Traitment des cancers avances du col par la medroxyprogesterone. Journal Gynecologie Obstetrique et Biologique Reproduction (Paris) 1 (5, suppl 2): 383–384

Varga A, Henriksen E 1964 Effect of 17α hydroxyprogesterone-17-*n*-caproate on various pelvic malignancies. Obstetrics and Gynecology 23: 51–62

Vihko R, Isotalo H, Kauppila A, Vierikko P 1983 Female sex steroid receptors in gynecological malignancies: clinical correlates. Journal of Steroid Biochemistry 19: 827–832

Weiner S A, Alberts D S, Surwit E A, Davis J, Grosso D 1987 Tamoxifen therapy in recurrent epithelial ovarian carcinoma. Gynecologic Oncology 27: 208–213

Welshons W V, Leiberman M E, Gorski J 1984 Nuclear localization of unoccupied oestrogen receptors. Nature 307: 747–749

Willcocks D, Toppila M, Hudson C N, Tyler J P P, Baird P J, Eastman C J 1983 Estrogen and progesterone receptors in human ovarian tumours. Gynecologic Oncology 16: 246–253

Zaino R J, Clarke C L, Mortel R, Satyaswaroop P G 1988 Heterogeneity of progesterone receptor distribution in human endometrial adenocarcinoma. Cancer Research 48: 1889–1895

2. Quantitation in gynaecological pathology

J. P. A. Baak   P. J. van Diest

INTRODUCTION

In tumours of the endometrium, ovary, cervix and vulva, histological typing and grading can be correlated both with their prognosis and with certain biochemical characteristics of the tumour. However, the difficulty in practice is that assessment of histological type and grade is subjective and not always reproducible. Quantitative microscopic analysis of cells and tissues can therefore be helpful, as it provides not only objective and measurable criteria but may also help to detect changes that may escape subjective assessment by the pathologist (Baak & Oort 1983, Oberholzer 1983, Hall & Fu 1985, Burger et al 1990).

As well as the conceptual background of quantitation in cancer pathology, this chapter will discuss some applications to endometrial malignancies and premalignant conditions as examples. Nearly all parts of the female genital tract have been subjected to quantitative cell and tissue analysis: a complete discussion would greatly exceed the available space here, and detailed descriptions can be found elsewhere (Baak 1991). Some aspects of automation will be considered and, finally, the possibility of assessing multidrug resistance will be discussed.

CONCEPTUAL BACKGROUND

Limitations of histological type

In spite of the evidence that microscopical features of primary gynaecological tumours have important prognostic value, the value of histological data in clinical decision making is restricted. Gynaecological oncologists do not always find the results of microscopical studies relevant enough or sufficiently reliable. Lack of agreement between pathologists can be one reason for this.

Two histological characteristics have been correlated with the prognosis of patients with gynaecological tumours: type and grade. It is indeed the case that in individual patients, the prognostic impact of certain rare subtypes is considerable and unambiguous. For example, FIGO Stage I endometrial carcinomas of papillary, adenosquamous, clear cell and glassy cell types are associated with a poor prognosis (typically about 35%, in contrast to 80–95% 5-year survival in the other types). Most cases are, however, of the usual endometroid type. For the same reasons, the prognostic value of typing in cancers of other sites is limited. Consequently, grading is probably more important in predicting the outcome in an individual patient. Assessment of grade, however, has implicit difficulties.

Difficulties of grading

As early as 1926, Broders (1926) proposed four grades for cancer. These depended on the percentage of 'undifferentiated' cells present in the tumour sections, as follows: grade 1, 1–25%; grade 2, 26–50%; grade 3, 51–75%; grade 4, 76–100%. Allen & Hertig (1949) proposed three grades (well-, moderately well-, and poorly-differentiated), based on the total histological appearance of the tumour. If accurately performed, the prognostic value of grading is evident from a number of studies (see for example Dembo et al 1982, Malkasian et al 1975, Sorbe et al 1982). In diagnostic practice, however, very few pathologists will actually perform a differential count of atypical nuclei, and in consequence the prognostic value of nuclear grade can vanish. Indeed, while studying patients treated with chemotherapy for advanced ovarian cancers, Neijt et al (1984) could not detect an effect of grade on prediction of survival.

In addition to this practical aspect of grading that diminishes its prognostic value, there is also a significant error due to the continuous nature of the histological features of different grades of malignant lesions (Langley et al 1983). It has been proved that with continuously variable lesions, reproducibility of assessments of the same slides by different pathologists can be embarassingly low (Baak & Oort 1991). Grade is a typical example of such a continuous variable because it ranges from very well differentiated to anaplastic with a number of classes in between (Fig. 2.1). The 'decision borders' between these classes are not always adequately defined, although for certain tumours the distinction criteria are

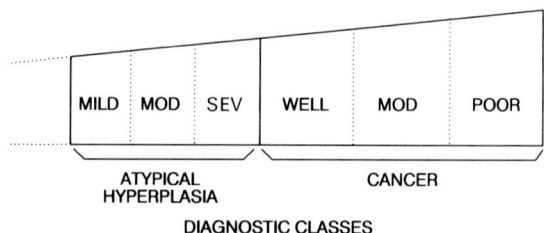

Fig. 2.1 Tumour grades form a continuous spectrum.

well established (such as for borderline and malignant ovarian tumours). Even then, the distinction cannot always be made with complete consistency, and the reproducibility among different observers is not very high (Baak et al 1986a). Considerable prognostic variability can therefore be expected in the same grade assessed by different pathologists. Indeed, in a multicentre evaluation of the same stage I endometrial cancers, the prognostic value of grades assessed by three pathologists varied considerably (Putten et al 1989). The same phenomenon was found in a multicentre evaluation of ovarian tumours (Baak et al 1986b). Nevertheless, a clear overall prognostic trend is usually evident: this means that the microscopical image of a primary tumour has important prognostic value, but reproducible methods must be applied to extract and make use of this.

It is not always fully realized that a particular grade bears a certain *prognostic probability*. A patient with a poorly-differentiated cancer is not committed to death but has a high probability of having aggressive metastases. On the other hand, a patient with a well-differentiated tumour is not necessarily 'out of the woods' as she still has a certain, although low, chance of dying from metastatic disease.

A final difficulty of grading is that usually three or four grades are diagnosable in both premalignant and malignant lesions: for example, mild, moderate and marked atypical hyperplasia, well-, moderately- and poorly-differentiated carcinoma. Such a three-class classification does not always adequately link up with clinical practice, which usually requires black-and-white decisions: hysterectomy or not? radiotherapy or not? Rather than asking 'is it a borderline or malignant tumour?' or 'is it well, moderately or poorly differentiated?' one should ask 'what is the chance of aggressive local disease or metastases in this particular case?' Instead of a three- or four-class system, we should try to develop a two-class system (Fig. 2.2). The quantitative pathological applications for gynaecological tumours are not yet ideal, but seem to approach this goal better than conventional grade and type. The applications so far developed for endometrial malignant and premalignant conditions will be described.

ENDOMETRIAL MALIGNANCIES AND PREMALIGNANCIES

Hyperplasia

Atypical hyperplasia of the endometrium is usually considered a precancerous lesion. Indeed, a considerable percentage of patients with this condition (10–20%) develop endometrial carcinoma (Gusberg & Kaplan 1963). Although the number of patients with atypical hyperplasia with progression to cancer is small, there were until recently no adequate criteria to predict the outcome in an individual case: when a diagnosis of atypical hyperplasia was made, hysterectomy was the usual treatment of choice. In addition, there is considerable disagreement between pathologists about the

HYPERPLASIAS

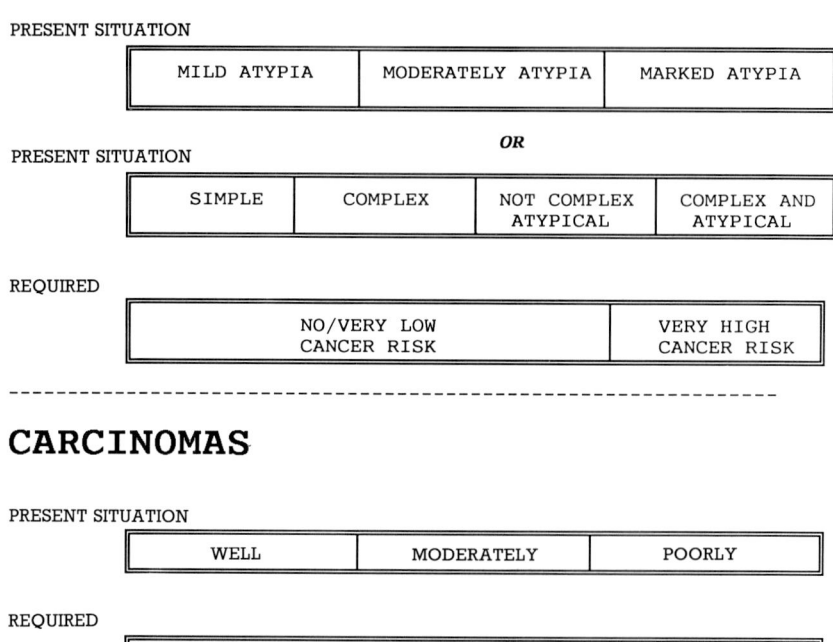

PRESENT SITUATION

MILD ATYPIA	MODERATELY ATYPIA	MARKED ATYPIA

OR

PRESENT SITUATION

SIMPLE	COMPLEX	NOT COMPLEX ATYPICAL	COMPLEX AND ATYPICAL

REQUIRED

NO/VERY LOW CANCER RISK	VERY HIGH CANCER RISK

CARCINOMAS

PRESENT SITUATION

WELL	MODERATELY	POORLY

REQUIRED

NO AGGRESSIVE METASTASES	AGGRESSIVE METASTASES

Fig. 2.2   The usual three- or four-class grading systems versus the two-class system.

criteria for differentiating between cases of 'adenomatous hyperplasia' and well- differentiated carcinoma (see also p. 207).

The use of morphometry in cases of endometrial atypical hyperplasia and well-differentiated carcinoma has shown that these conditions can be distinguished accurately by this technique (Baak et al 1978, 1980, 1981a, 1981b). Routine application of diagnostic morphometry over a longer period gave a considerable improvement over subjective routine evaluation (Baak et al 1982).

Colgan et al (1983) have further refined this approach. They described a morphometric classification rule that would predict the outcome of atypical hyperplasia. Using stepwise regression analysis and discriminant analysis, they found that two quantitative nuclear features were especially useful in predicting whether atypical hyperplasia will progress to cancer: the mean and standard deviation of the longest nuclear axis (parameters indicating the size and variation in size of the nuclei). Larger and more anisokaryotic nuclei were correlated with a higher risk of progression. In their prediction rule, the following decision scheme was used:

$$F = 7.13 + 1.24\,\overline{\text{MND}} - 3\,\text{S.D.(MND)},$$

where $\overline{\text{MND}}$ and S.D.(MND) are the mean and standard deviation, respectively, of the maximal nuclear diameter. Where the classification value, F, is less than zero no progression is predicted; where it is greater than zero, progression is predicted. In their study of 24 cases, one of the 16 patients with no progression had a classification score above zero, and three of the eight cases with progression had scores below zero: 83% of their cases were correctly predicted.

In another study, this predictive classification rule was tested in 42 cases of atypical hyperplasia obtained from a total of 2662 curettage specimens diagnosed as hyperplasia or carcinoma. Of these 42 cases, eight (17%) progressed to cancer, of whom seven scored above zero and one just below that value ($F = -0.3$). Although a considerable number of the cases without progression had values above zero, 11 (32%) scored below zero. Thus, in this independent 'test set' material, the nuclear morphometric classification rule described by Colgan et al (1983) proved to be accurate and useful in predicting the outcome of patients with atypical hyperplasia of the endometrium.

It is unlikely that nuclear morphometric features are the only morphological factors reflecting the outcome of the disease, and other quantitative parameters describing the architecture of the glands have also been studied for their potential value in identifying patients who will develop cancer. Using linear stepwise regression analysis and discriminant analysis, the percentage by volume of stroma to glands and the standard deviation of the *shortest* nuclear axis are the best discriminators (Fig. 2.3), although measurement of the outer surface density of the glands also adds to the discriminating power. The percentage by volume of stroma (which is obviously strongly negatively correlated to the percentage by volume of epithelium) is the best single prognostic variable and is highly reproducible. With the resulting linear function of three variables, a score (D) for each patient was computed as follows:

$$D = 0.6229 + 0.0439\,\text{PVS} - 0.3934\,\ln\text{S.D.(SNA)} - 0.1592\,\text{OSDG},$$

where PVS is the percentage by volume of stroma, S.D.(SNA) is the standard deviation of the shortest nuclear axis and OSDG is the outer surface density of the glands (see also p. 218).

In total, using these combined architectural and nuclear morphometric features with $D = 1.05$ as the decision threshold, 20 of the 32 cases without progression were separated from those who subsequently progressed (62.5%). In the other 19 cases with $D < 1.05$, seven progressed (37%) (Fig. 2.4). This is a considerable improvement over nuclear morphometric features alone. Compared with the qualitative classification rule described by Kurman et al (1985), a major advantage is that it is a two-group rather

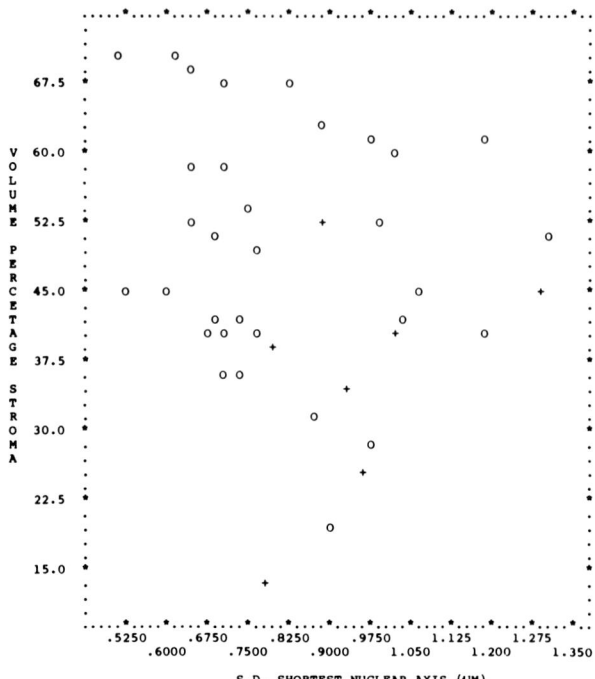

Fig. 2.3 Bivariate plot of the percentage by volume stroma in glands and the standard deviation of the shortest nuclear axis. ○, cases without progression to cancer; +, cases with progression. (Reproduced with permission from Baak et al 1988.)

than a four-group system. Further analyses of DNA ploidy, nuclear arrangement (stratification) and proliferation-associated features may improve these results and are currently under study.

Carcinoma

The incidence of endometrial carcinoma has increased in recent years and in some countries has become the second most frequent gynaecological tumour. Although a favourable outcome may be expected in about three-quarters of patients, a proportion of women with FIGO Stage I endometrial carcinomas will die as a result of their neoplasm within a few years of initial treatment. There are currently no accurate means of identifying those tumours that are likely to pursue a fatal course. Moreover, the death rate has not decreased and more precise predictors of outcome would be of considerable value to allow therapy to be individualized for each patient, which is essential to improve prognosis. In general, the stage, depth of myometrial invasion, nuclear and histological grade, and type have some predictive value as to the aggressiveness of the disease, but none of these

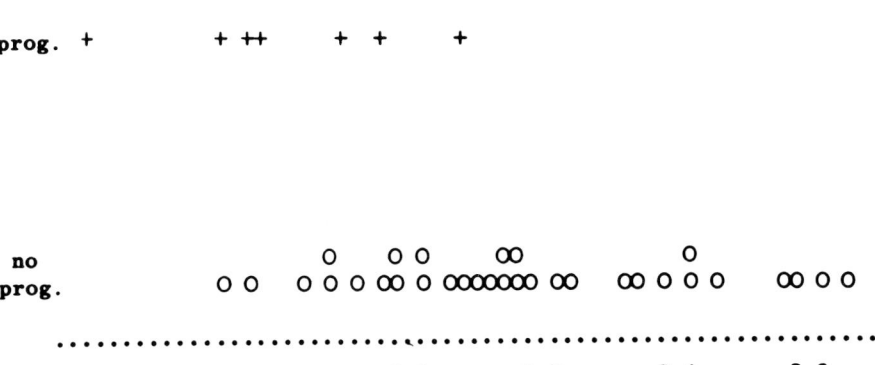

Fig. 2.4   Discriminant (D) scores of the 'progression' and 'no progression' patients.
(Reproduced with permission from Baak et al 1988.)

factors is a very accurate predictor. Moreover, for the reasons mentioned above, determination of the histological type is of limited value and grading of endometrial carcinoma is not always perfectly reproducible.

It also has been reported that the incidence of steroid hormone receptors has prognostic value (Creasman et al 1985), but not all authors could confirm this. Chromosomal instability leading to structural or numerical aberrations are recognized as an early feature of malignant transformation. Extensive cytogenetic studies have been carried out in a variety of tumours, but the procedure is laborious and not always available.

In the prospective study of van der Putten et al (1989) the mean shortest nuclear axis proved to discriminate significantly between surviving and non-surviving patients with Stage I disease. It appeared that the mean shortest nuclear axis was lower in the tumours of survivors compared with those of non-survivors. The mean nuclear area was smaller in the group of survivors compared with the group of non-survivors ($P<0.008$). The flow cytometrically assessed DNA ploidy, which was measured in 33 of the 38 patients, was highly discriminating ($P<0.01$) (Fig. 2.5). The latter confirmed the promising results of other studies (Atkins 1976, Moberger et al 1985).

Other single morphological features that discriminated significantly between surviving and dead patients were, in order of importance: depth of myometrial invasion of the tumour (significantly more often confined to the inner third in the surviving group than in the group of deceased patients, $P<0.01$); mean nuclear shape factor, which was lower in the surviving group ($P<0.03$); mean nuclear angle, which was larger in the surviving group ($P<0.03$); and mean nuclear axes ratio (higher in the group of survivors whose tumours had more elliptical nuclei). Using patients' status

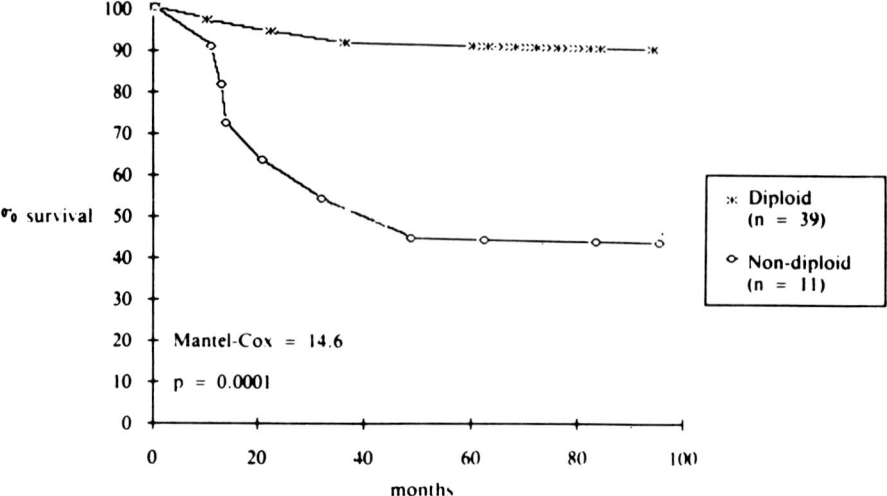

Fig. 2.5   Endometrial carcinoma Stage I: Kaplan-Meier survival curve of patients with diploid and non-diploid nuclear DNA content. Diploid tumours have a favourable outcome. Three of the 39 patients with diploid tumours died (Mantel-Cox = 14.6, P = 0.0001). (Reproduced with permission from Putten et al 1989.)

at 5-year follow-up as the decision threshold, the smallest but strongest set of independent parameters that discriminated best between survivors and non-survivors in Stage I carcinomas was found with multivariate stepwise linear regression analysis: this combination consisted of, in order of importance: mean shortest axis of the nucleus, DNA ploidy, and depth of myometrial invasion (R^2 = 0.78, P < 0.00001).

The combination of these three prognostic features resulted in an endometrial carcinoma Stage I prognostic index (ECPI-1), formulated as follows:

$$\text{ECPI-1} = 0.6494 \, \overline{\text{SNA}} + 0.639 (\text{DNA code}) + 0.2398 \, \text{MI} - 5.7283,$$

in which the mean shortest nuclear axis is expressed in micrometres to one decimal place; the DNA code is 1 for diploid, 2 for peritetraploid, 3 for aneuploid; and myometrial invasion, MI, is 1 for $\leqslant 1/3$, 2 for $> 1/3$. ECPI-1 < 0.87 = survivor and ECPI-1 $\geqslant$ 0.87 = non-survivor was taken as a classification rule.

The prognostic value of the combination of these features overshadowed the value of all other features investigated. The overriding prognostic value of this highly reproducible rule was clear from the complete separation of 27 survivors and six non-survivors in the 'learning' set of 33 patients. In an independent test set, all three non-survivors and 13 of the 14 survivors were correctly classified, thus confirming the accuracy and reliability of the rule in predicting the outcome for future patients with Stage I endometrial

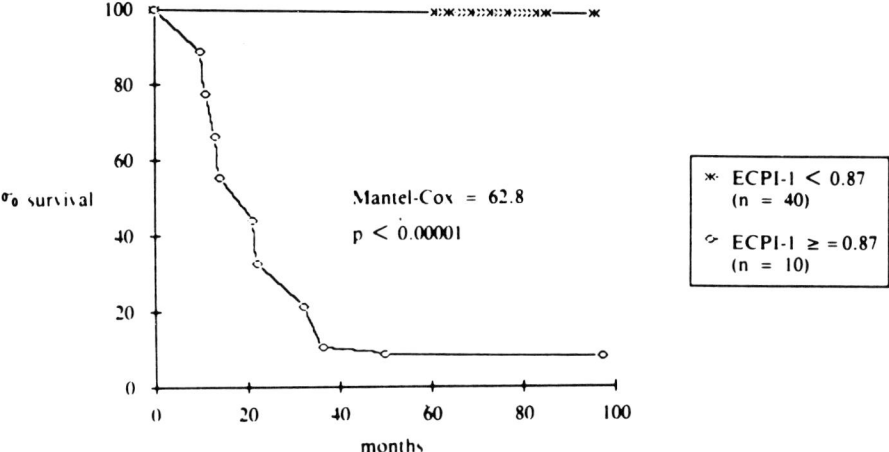

Fig. 2.6 Endometrial carcinoma Stage I: Kaplan-Meier survival curve of patients according to (<0.87) and high ($\geqslant0.87$) ECPI-1 scores. The former have a favourable outcome (Mantel-Cox$=62.8$, $P<0.00001$). (Reproduced with permission from Putten et al 1989.)

adenocarcinoma (Fig. 2.6). Technical difficulties with selection of nuclei to be measured (Fleege et al 1990), and with false negative, diploid results with flow cytometry due to admixture of diploid stromal cells, require special attention in the application of the method.

AUTOMATION

As described above, objective criteria that describe cell and tissue characteristics of tumours include the cellular DNA content, the mitotic index and the percentage by volume of epithelium. One paper has described an image analysis technique for the counting of nuclei in mitosis in tissue sections (Kaman et al 1984). Five experienced pathologists scored mitoses in photographs of preselected areas of breast cancer tissue sections. Objects consistently labelled as mitotic cells by all five pathologists were in the analysis considered to be mitoses. In total in that study, 45 mitoses, 68 possible mitoses and 1172 non-mitotic nuclei were analysed with digital image processing. The image analysis procedure was designed to give priority to a low false-negative rate; that is, misclassification of mitoses. The procedure consists of three steps:

- Segmentation of the image
- Reduction of the number of non-mitotic nuclei by using feature values based on the brightness histogram of the objects
- Fully automatic classification of the remaining objects using contour features.

The objects remaining after the first two steps were visualized in a composite display for interactive evaluation.

By this automated procedure a number of mitotic nuclei were missed, and only 85% of the non-mitotic nuclei were correctly identified. Although the results of the fully automatic procedure described were rather disappointing, the method can be very helpful in making a preselection of 'candidate' structures in the section, thus making mitotic counts much more time-efficient. Further improvement of both the staining and image processing method may help to improve the results of fully automated analysis (Kaman et al 1984).

The percentage by volume of epithelium is especially important in malignant disease of the ovary (Baak et al 1985), cervix (Fu et al 1987) and endometrium (Baak et al 1981a,b). This can be measured from the percentage of the total area occupied by the area of epithelium in tissue slides using interactive stereology. Practical application in diagnostic pathology, however, requires accurate counting of points and can be a tedious and time-consuming task. A considerable number of microscopic tissue fields is required to reach sufficient accuracy and, although the counting procedure is reproducible, the means of selection of microscopic fields may introduce undesired subjectivity. Recently, image analysis techniques for automated measurement of the percentages of epithelium and stroma in tumour tissue were described for ovarian, endometrial and breast tumours (Schipper et al 1987, 1989). One image processing method is based on the fact that epithelial nuclei are generally more tightly packed than stromal nuclei; this method can be applied to standard paraffin wax sections stained with pararosanilin Feulgen and naphthol yellow. Another method used sections stained for keratin. The area percentages, as assessed with image processing, were strongly correlated with control percentages established by interactive morphometry. Immunoquantitation of monoclonal antibodies and probes directed against proliferation- or differentiation-associated nuclear or cytoplasmic antigens is another promising area (Bacus et al 1989) (see also Ch. 4).

MULTIDRUG RESISTANCE DETERMINATION

Multidrug resistance (determined by *mdr* genes) can be induced in cancer cells in vitro by exposure to a single agent such as actinomycin D (Biedler & Riehm 1970, Kessel et al 1984). It is currently believed that tumour cell resistance may be at least one of the causes of failure of chemotherapy in cancer patients (De Vita 1985). Molecular probes and techniques to detect and quantify the amount of *mdr1* mRNA or its protein product P-glycoprotein in tumour cells has now been established by a semiquantitative slot-blot procedure (Goldstein et al 1989). Also, monoclonal antibodies have been used to detect P-glycoprotein in patients' tumour cells (Dalton et al 1989, Ma et al 1987) and at least two studies have reported a correlation of *mdr1* mRNA (Kahehi et al 1988) or P-glycoprotein (Salmon et al 1989) with resistance of tumour cells to vinblastine and doxorubicin, using in vitro chemosensitivity assays. At present it is not known whether the probes available are sensitive enough to detect relevant levels of multidrug resistance nor is it known what level of *mdr1* expression makes a cell resistant to particular anticancer drugs or sensitive to resistance modifiers such as verapamil. Sensitive functional assays for the detection of the multidrug resistance phenotype in human tumour cells are needed (Broxterman et al 1990). Such methods should be quantitative, specific, capable of detecting heterogeneity, and able to discriminate between dead and viable cells and between tumour and normal cells in clinical samples.

Another possibility is to quantitate by flow cytometry the number of cells with a fluorescent cytostatic drug. However, using flow cytometry, non-tumour cells can be positive, which can give false-positive results. Furthermore, tumour cells that have a cytostatic drug confined to their cytoplasm can be resistant and still give a positive signal. Differentiation between tumour cells and non-tumour cells is essential, as is determination of cytoplasmic versus nuclear accumulation of the drug. We used a confocal laser scan microscope (Baak et al 1987) to determine ratios of doxorubicin fluorescence in nuclei and cytoplasm, and the effect of verapamil on this ratio. The fluorescence is measured interactively, as follows. First, the contours of the nucleus and cytoplasm of the cells in the transmitted light image are traced. Then fluorescence is measured in the incident light mode. Data are transferred on-line to a computer for further processing. The results so far show that nuclear/cytoplasmic fluorescence ratio is strongly correlated with the level of multidrug resistance (Schuurhuis et al 1989).

CONCLUSIONS

Nearly all parts of the gynaecological system have been subjected to quantitative cell and tissue analysis. This has the advantages of higher accuracy, reproducibility and objectivity than qualitative type and grade, the possibility to detect small changes and differences, and better compatibility with clinical requests (a two-class instead of a three- or four-class system). In endometrial malignancies, prediction of prognosis is currently at least as good, in hyperplasias, or better, in carcinomas, than with conventional, subjective methods. Further automation, including functional testing on multidrug resistance, is a promising area that may help further acceptance of quantitative methods in diagnostic pathology.

REFERENCES

Allen M J, Hertig A S 1949 Carcinoma of the ovary. Am J Obstet Gynecol 58: 640–653
Atkins N B 1976 Prognostic significance of ploidy level in human tumors: I. Carcinoma of the uterus. J Natl Cancer Inst 56: 909–910

Baak J P A 1991 A manual of diagnostic morphometry in cancer diagnosis and prognosis. Springer-Verlag, Heidelberg

Baak, J P A, Oort J 1983 A manual of diagnostic morphometry. Springer-Verlag, Heidelberg

Baak J P A, Diegenbach P C, Oort J et al 1978 Application of quantitative microscopy to gynecological cancer. In: Chermant J L (ed) Quantitative analysis of microstructures in medicine. Riederer, Stuttgart, p 367–373

Baak J P A, Diegenbach P C, Oort J et al 1980 An example of quantitative microscopy in individual patient care. Mikroskopie 37 (suppl): 305–307

Baak J P A, Kurver P H J, Diegenbach P C et al 1981a Discrimination of hyperplasia and carcinoma of the endometrium by quantitative microscopy—a feasibility study. Histopathology 5: 61–86

Baak J P A, Kurver P H J, Overdiep S H et al 1981b Quantitative, microscopial, computer-aided diagnosis of endometrial hyperplasia or carcinoma in individual patients. Histopathology 5: 689–695

Baak J P A, Kurver P H J, Boon M E 1982 Computer-aided application of quantitative microscopy in diagnostic pathology. Pathol Annu 2: 287–306

Baak J P A, Fox J, Langley F A, Buckley H 1985 The prognostic value of morphometry in ovarian epithelial tumors of borderline malignancy. Int J Gynecol Pathol 4: 186–191

Baak J P A, Langley F A, Talerman A, Delemarre J F M 1986a Interpathologist and intrapathologist disagreement in ovarian tumor grading and typing. An Quant Cytol Histol 8: 354–358

Baak J P A, Wisse-Brekelmans E C M, Langley F A, Talerman A, Delemarre J F M 1986b Morphometric data to FIGO stage and histological type and grade for prognosis of ovarian tumors. J Clin Pathol 39: 1340–1346

Baak J P A, Thunnissen F B J M, Oudejans C B M, Schipper N W 1987 Potential uses of laser scan microscopy. J Appl Optics 26: 3413–3416

Baak J P A, Nauta J J P, Wisse-Brekelmans E C M, Bezemer P D 1988 Architectural and nuclear morphometrical features together are more important prognosticators in endometrial hyperplasia than nuclear morphometrical features alone. J Pathol 154: 335–341

Bacus S S, Goldschmidt R, Cin D et al 1989 Biological grading of breast cancer using antibodies to proliferating cells and other markers. Am J Pathol 1354: 783–787

Biedler J L, Riehm H 1970 Cellular resistance to actinomycin D in Chinese hamster cells in vitro: cross-resistance, radioautographic and cytogenetic studies. Cancer Res 30: 1174–1184

Broders A C 1926 Carcinoma: grading and practical application. Arch Pathol 2: 376–381

Broxterman H J, Schuurhuis G J, Lankelma J et al 1990 Towards functional screening for multidrug resistant cells in human malignancies. In: Enrico Mihich (ed) Drug resistance mechanisms and reversal. John Libbey, Rome, CK, vol I, p 309–319

Burger G, Oberholzer M, Vooijs G P 1990 Advances in analytical cellular pathology. Amsterdam: Excerpta Medica

Colgan T J, Norris H J, Foster W et al 1983 Predicting the outcome of endometrial hyperplasia by quantitative analysis of nuclear features using a linear discrimination function. Int J Gynecol Pathol 1: 347–352

Creasman W T, Soper J T, McCarty K S Jr et al 1985 Influence of cytoplasmic steroid receptor content on prognosis of early stage endometrial carcinoma. Am J Obstet Gynecol 151: 922–932

Dalton W S, Grogan T M, Meltzer P S et al 1989 Drug-resistance in multiple myeloma and non-Hodgkin's lymphoma: detection of P-glycoprotein and potential circumvention by addition of verapamil to chemotherapy. J Clin Oncol 7: 415–424

Dembo A J, Brown T C, Busch R S 1982 Clinicopathological correlates in ovarian cancer. Bull Cancer (Paris) 69: 292–297

De Vita V T Jr 1985 Principles of chemotherapy. In de Vita V T, Hellman S, Rosenberg S A (eds) Cancer: principles and practice of oncology. J B Lippincott, Philadelphia, p 257–285

Fleege J C, Diest P J van, Baak J P A 1990 Computer assisted efficiency testing of different sampling methods for selective nuclear graphic tablet morphometry. Lab Invest 63: 270–275

Fu Y S, Hall T L, Berek J S et al 1987 Prognostic significance of DNA ploidy and morphometric analyses of adenocarcinoma of the uterine cervix. Ann Quant Cytol Histol 9: 17–24

Goldstein L J, Galski H, Fojo A et al 1989 Expression of multidrug resistance gene in human cancers. J Natl Cancer Inst 81: 116–124

Gusberg S B, Kaplan A L 1963 Precursors of corpus cancer. Am J Obstet Gynecol 87: 662–678

Hall T L, Fu Y S 1985 Applications of quantitative microscopy in tumor pathology. Lab Invest 53: 5–21

Kahehi Y, Kanamaru H, Yoskida O et al 1988 Measurement of multidrug resistance messenger RNA in urogenital cancers; elevated expression in renal cell carcinoma is associated with intrinsic drug resistance. J Urol 139: 862–865

Kaman E J, Smeulders A W M, Verbeek P W et al 1984 Image processing for mitoses in sections of breast cancer: a feasibility study. Cytometry 5: 244–249

Kessel, D, Bosmann, H B 1970 On the characteristics of actinomycin D resistance in L5178Y cells. Cancer Res 30: 2695–2701

Kurman R J, Kaminski P F, Norris H J 1985 The behavior of endometrial hyperplasia. A long-term study of "untreated" hyperplasia in 170 patients. Cancer 56: 403–412

Langley F A, Baak J P A, Oort J 1983 Diagnosis making: error sources. In: Baak J P A, Oort J (eds) A manual of morphometry in diagnostic pathology. Springer-Verlag, Berlin, p 6–14

Ma D D F, Davey R A, Harman D H et al 1987 Detection of a multidrug resistance phenotype in acute non-lymphoblastic leukaemia. Lancet 1: 135–137

Malkasian G D, Decker D G, Web M J 1975 Histology of epithelial tumors of the ovary: Clinical usefulness and prognostic significance of the histologic classification and grading. Sem Oncol 2: 191

Moberger B, Auer G, Forsslund G et al 1985 The prognostic significance of DNA measurements in endometrial carcinoma. Cytometry 5: 430–436

Neijt J P, Bokkel Huinink W W van, Burg M E L van der et al 1984 Randomised trial comparing two combination chemotherapy regimens (Hexa-CAF vs CHAP-05) in advanced ovarian carcinoma. Lancet ii: 594–600

Oberholzer M 1983 Morphometrie in der Klinischen Pathologie. Springer-Verlag, Heidelberg, p 69–70

Putten H W H M, Baak J P A, Koenders T J M et al 1989 Prognostic value of quantitative pathologic features and DNA content in individual patients with stage I endometrial adenocarcinoma. Cancer 63: 1378–1387

Salmon S E, Grogan T M, Miller T et al 1989 Prediction of doxorubicin resistance in vitro in myeloma, lymphoma, and breast cancer by P-glycoprotein staining. J Natl Cancer Inst 81: 696–701

Schipper N W, Smeulders A W M, Baak J P A 1987 Quantification of epithelial volume by image processing applied to ovarian tumors. Cytometry 8: 345–352

Schipper N W, Smeulders A W M, Lange J H M, Baak J P A 1989 Quantification of epithelial area by image processing applied to endometrial carcinomas. Hum Pathol 20: 1125–1132

Schuurhuis G J, Broxterman H J, Cervantes A et al 1989 Quantitative determination of factors contributing to doxorubicin resistance in MDR cells. J Natl Cancer Inst 81: 1887

Sorbe B, Frankendal B, Veress B 1982 Importance of histologic grading in the prognosis of epithelial ovarian carcinoma. Obstet Gynecol 59: 576–582

3. Immunohistochemical markers in gynaecological pathology

Elizabeth Benjamin

INTRODUCTION

The ability to detect antigens in tissue by immunohistochemistry has enabled pathologists to correlate morphology with functional and bio-chemical characteristics. Immunohistochemistry has therefore become a useful diagnostic tool and its range of application in gynaecological pathology continues to be widely investigated. It is in neoplastic disease, particularly ovarian neoplasms, that much of the work in this field has been concentrated. Interpretation of stains for immunohistochemical markers in gynaecological diseases requires an understanding of the expression of these markers in the normal tissues of the female genital system and an awareness of the limitations of the techniques and markers used.

APPLICATIONS OF IMMUNOHISTOCHEMISTRY IN GYNAECOLOGICAL PATHOLOGY

Most immunohistochemical studies in gynaecological pathology have been directed towards the diagnosis and differential diagnosis of tumours. Immunohistochemistry can provide evidence of differentiation, give clues to histogenesis and, by identification of tumour products such as enzymes and hormones, give information about the functional activity of the neoplasm. Some of these tumour products may be measurable in the patient's serum, and have formed the basis of the clinical monitoring of tumour markers. More recently, tumour antigens have been used as targets in antibody-directed irradiation for advanced ovarian cancer (Epenetos et al 1986) and in imaging techniques such as radioimmunoscintigraphy (Jobling et al 1990).

Antibodies have been commercially developed to demonstrate steroid hormone receptors, growth factors and oncogene products, and may be useful in the management and assessment of prognosis for patients with gynaecological cancer. Some aspects of these have been discussed in other chapters in this book.

IMMUNOHISTOCHEMICAL METHODS

Immunohistochemical techniques are described in detail elsewhere (Polak & van Noorden 1988), but a few points should be emphasized. Good fixation of tissue is essential for optimal preservation of antigens, and both inadequate fixation and prolonged fixation may lead to loss of antigenicity. Paraffin-wax embedded, fixed tissues are suitable for demonstration of many antigens and so permit the analysis of archival material. Some of the currently available monoclonal antibodies may, unfortunately, require the use of fresh tissue for optimal antigen detection.

Pretreatment of paraffin-wax embedded tissue with proteolytic enzymes such as trypsin and pronase may be necessary to unmask antigenic sites. This step is not needed for all antibodies, and its indiscriminate use can be a source of error (Ordonez et al 1988). All immunohistochemical procedures must incorporate controls to ensure that the results are valid.

The most commonly used techniques are:

- Indirect immunoperoxidase method
- Peroxidase antiperoxidase method (PAP method)
- Avidin biotin method.

LIMITATIONS OF IMMUNOHISTOCHEMISTRY

Discrepancies in reported immunohistochemical results occur for a variety of reasons. These include different conditions of fixation among laboratories, and varying inter-laboratory procedures. Tumour cell populations often exhibit considerable antigen heterogeneity (Breitenecker et al 1989) so that tissue sampling is important. Another important cause is the different specificity of the antibodies used. For example, different available antibodies to carcinoembryonic antigen (CEA) may not detect the same epitope, and this may lead to discrepancies in reported detection rates of this marker in the same tumour type. Problems in the interpretation of immunohistochemical results may arise from non-specific staining as well as from cross reactivity of antibodies. Immunohistochemistry must therefore be used as an adjunct to histopathological diagnosis on routine chromatic stains. To rely on a single antibody is dangerous, and, wherever possible, a panel of antigen markers should be used.

OVARY

Common epithelial tumours

Tumour-associated antigens

Ovarian cancer associated or tumour specific antigens have been widely investigated. To date, the search for a truly ovarian cancer specific antigen has proved frustrating but several antibodies raised against ovarian carcinoma tissue or cell lines have a role in diagnosis and management. Many of these antibodies have been investigated as diagnostic serum markers rather than primarily for histopathological diagnosis. A wide range of antibodies that recognize tumour-associated antigens has been described (Bhattacharya et al 1985, Smith & Teng 1987, Daunter 1990); Table 3.1 lists some that are currently being investigated in ovarian carcinoma.

It has been shown that one or more serum markers may be demonstrable in patients with ovarian cancer, and that the tumour may not always be the source of the raised serum concentration of the marker (Motoyama et al 1990). It follows that the immunohistochemical identification of a marker in tumour tissue is a prerequisite to its use as a clinical marker to monitor disease progression. Most cancer-associated antigens are expressed by more than one type of tumour, and sometimes by tumours of diverse histogenesis. Many are expressed in fetal tissues and can also be found in some normal adult tissues.

Cancer antigen 125 (CA125).   This tumour-associated antigen was derived from an ovarian serous carcinoma cell line (Bast et al 1981). It is at present the most widely used tumour marker for ovarian carcinoma. It is expressed by more than 80% of non-mucinous ovarian tumours (Kabawat et al 1983), including serous, endometrioid, clear cell and undifferentiated carcinomas. Its clinical use is, however, limited by the fact that it reacts with 22% of non-gynaecological cancers, including those of the breast and gastrointestinal tract, as well as benign gynaecological conditions (for a review, see Daunter 1990). Raised serum concentrations of CA125 may also occur in carcinoma of the Fallopian tube, cervix and endometrium. The antigen, probably a Müllerian differentiation antigen, is also present in normal endocervix, endometrium and Fallopian tube (Kabawat et al 1983). Table 3.2 summarizes the reported frequency of the immunohistochemical demonstration of CA125 and other tumour markers in common epithelial tumours.

The antibody OC133 has similar binding properties to CA125 but reacts with serous tumours only (Berkowitz et al 1983, Masuko et al 1984).

CA19/9. This antigen, originally described in colonic carcinoma (Atkinson et al 1982), is expressed by most mucinous ovarian carcinomas. It may also be expressed by many serous and other non-mucinous ovarian carcinomas (Table 3.2). It is commonly used, in combination with CA125, for clinical monitoring of patients with ovarian carcinoma.

Carcinoembryonic antigen.   This has been extensively investigated in ovarian carcinoma with polyclonal and monoclonal antibodies. It is expressed mostly by mucinous carcinomas. Charpin et al (1982) showed an increasing incidence of expression, from 15% in benign mucinous tumours to 100% in mucinous carcinoma. Other studies (Table 3.2) have confirmed a greater degree of expression in borderline and malignant mucinous tumours than in cystadenoma but CEA has also been demonstrated in some serous and other non-mucinous ovarian tumours. There is wide variation in

Table 3.1 Some tumour-associated antigens to ovarian carcinoma

Monoclonal antibody	Antigen	Source of immunogen	Ovarian tumour reactivity	Reactivity with other gynaecological cancer	Reference
OC125	CA125 glycoprotein	Ovarian serous carcinoma	Serous[1], endometrioid	Cervix, endometrium, Fallopian tube	Berkowitz et al (1983), Kabawat et al (1983)
OC133	80kD glycoprotein	Ovarian serous carcinoma	Serous	Endocervix, endometrium	Bast et al (1981)
MOV2	High mol.wt mucin/glycoprotein	Ovarian mucinous carcinoma	Mucinous[1], serous, endometrioid	—	Masuko et al (1984), Tagliabue et al (1985)
OVTL3	—	Ovarian endometrioid carcinoma	Serous[1], endometrioid, clear cell, mucinous	Endometrium	Poels et al (1986)
B72.3	Tumour-associated glycoprotein TAG 72	Breast carcinoma	Endometrioid, serous, mucinous	Cervix, endometrium	Thor et al (1986)
NB/70K	Glycoprotein subfraction OCA	Ovarian cancer	Serous, mucinous, endometrioid	Cervix, endometrium	Knauf & Urbach (1980)
1D3	High mol.wt mucin	Ovarian cancer	Mucinous		Bhattacharya et al (1982)
4C7	—	Ovarian mucinous carcinoma	Mucinous, endometrioid, clear cell	—	Tsuji et al (1985)
3C2	—	Ovarian serous carcinoma	Serous, endometrioid		Tsuji et al (1985)
NS19-9	CA 19-9	Colonic carcinoma	Mucinous[1], endometrioid, serous	—	Atkinson et al (1982)

[1]Main tumour reactivity.

Table 3.2 Immunohistochemical markers in ovarian common epithelial tumours[1]

Tumour (n)	CA125: (% positive)	CA19-9: (% positive)	CEA (% positive)	Placental alkaline phosphatase (% positive)
Serous				
Benign (15)	80	6	0	83
Borderline (8)	100	87	6	100
Malignant (59)	100	40	17	84
Mucinous				
Benign (49)	0	73	45	0
Borderline (8)	12.5	87	87	0
Malignant (38)	16	86	97	0
Endometrioid				
carcinoma (27)	66	64	25	66
Clear cell				
carcinoma (20)	75	70	15	0
Undifferentiated				
carcinoma (17)	82	52	23	57
Mixed Müllerian				
tumour (5)	80	80	40	33

[1]Data compiled from Nouwen et al (1987), Motoyama et al (1990), and Hamilton-Dutoit et al (1990).

the reported detection rates of CEA in gynaecological cancer, which is probably related to the different specificities of the CEA antibodies used (Wagener et al 1984). CEA is a complex molecule with a number of epitopes and also cross-reactive antigens. It is probable that these factors contribute to the differences in detection rates of the antigen.

Placental alkaline phosphatase (PLAP). Serum concentrations of PLAP are raised in 6–64% of patients with ovarian cancer (Vergote et al 1987). PLAP is expressed by serous and endometrioid carcinomas (Nouwen et al 1987, Hamilton-Dutoit et al 1990) but not by mucinous tumours. There are two groups of tumour-associated PLAP: the Regan isoenzyme, identical to term placental alkaline phosphatase, and the Nagao type, termed PLAP-like (Hamilton-Dutoit et al 1990). They can be distinguished immunohistochemically and both have been detected in serous carcinomas (Fig. 3.1).

Alpha amylase. This has been demonstrated in serous tumours of benign, borderline and malignant types (Bruns et al 1982) and in endometrioid adenocarcinomas. Recently the enzyme has also been demonstrated in some mucinous adenocarcinomas (Griffin & Wells 1990). The antigen is normally detected in Müllerian-derived epithelia, including Fallopian tube, endometrium and endocervix.

Intermediate filaments

Intermediate filaments are components of the cytoskeleton of cells and may

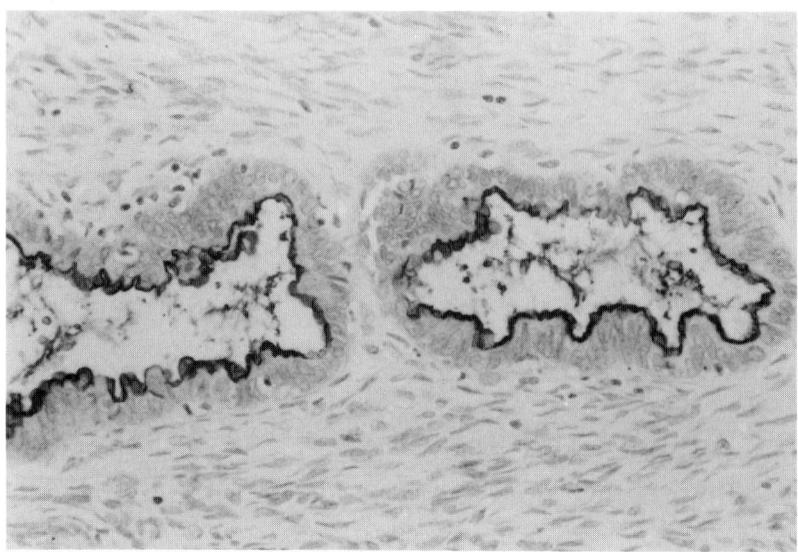

Fig. 3.1   Ovarian serous carcinoma stains with antibody to placental alkaline phosphatase (immunoperoxidase, × 350).

be regarded as tissue-specific (Lazarides 1980). Epithelial cells express cytokeratin; mesenchymal cells, vimetin; muscle cells, desmin; glial cells, glial fibrillary acidic protein; and neuronal cells, neurofilament antigens. There is more and more evidence that intermediate filaments are not as tissue-specific as originally thought: intermediate filament expression in different tissues may be similar, and expression of one or more classes of intermediate filaments by the same cell may occur (Gould 1985). The main intermediate filaments expressed by ovarian epithelial tumours are cyto-keratin and vimentin (Dabbs & Geisinger 1988). Low molecular weight cytokeratins are universally expressed in concordance with the biochemical analysis of simple epithelial type cytokeratin polypeptides (Moll et al 1983). High molecular weight cytokeratins may be expressed focally. Vimentin is expressed by some carcinomas. Distinct differences, however, are apparent in its expression by different types of ovarian carcinoma. In one study vimentin was present in 71% of endometrioid carcinomas, 42% of serous carcinomas and 7% of clear cell carcinomas, but was not detected in mucinous carcinomas (Dabbs & Geisinger 1988). It is of interest that the demonstration of vimentin in ovarian carcinoma parallels its expression in Müllerian tract epithelia. Fallopian tube epithelium and endometrium express vimentin, and endocervical mucinous epithelium does not. Ovarian surface epithelium, which is not of Müllerian derivation but has a similar embryological origin from coelomic epithelium, also expresses vimentin. Desmin, indicative of smooth muscle differentiation, may be detected in the stroma of ovarian carcinomas: smooth muscle actin is also expressed (Czernobilsky et al 1989).

Other markers

Epithelial markers such as epithelial membrane antigen, human milk fat globule antigens, and the epithelial cell surface antigen AuA1 are all expressed by ovarian carcinomas (Nouwen et al 1987, Benjamin 1987, Aguirre et al 1989) in common with carcinomas elsewhere. They may be of use in the differential diagnosis of ovarian carcinomas and sex cord–stromal tumours as described later. α_1-Antitrypsin and α_1-antichymotrypsin may be expressed by most carcinomas, whilst human chorionic gonadotrophin (hCG) and human placental lactogen are expressed in occasional cases (Ishikura & Scully 1987, Khalifa & Sesterhen 1990).

The rare hepatoid carcinomas of the ovary may express α-fetoprotein (Ishikura & Scully 1987). α-Fetoprotein expression has also been described rarely in mucinous adenocarcinomas (Konishi et al 1988). Neuroendocrine markers such as chromogranin A, neurone specific enolase, serotonin and peptide hormones have been detected in neuroendocrine cells of ovarian carcinoma, with the highest prevalence in mucinous tumours (Sasaki et al 1989).

The histogenesis of small cell carcinoma of ovary associated with hypercalcaemia (Dickersin et al 1982) is not known. The tumour cells express cytokeratin and often vimentin; neurone-specific enolase is expressed in most cases. The presence of immunoreactive parenchymal hormone has been reported in some cases and may be causally related to the hypercalcaemia (Abeler et al 1988).

Brenner tumours

Immunohistochemical studies of the epithelial component of Brenner tumours have confirmed that this is antigenically similar to transitional epithelium (Shevchuck et al 1980, Santini et al 1989), which supports the concept of urothelial differentiation. Brenner tumour epithelium expresses low and high molecular weight cytokeratins. Nests of transitional epithelium contain cytokeratin 18, whilst those with squamoid features contain cytokeratins 10 and 11; mixed nests with both keratin groups also occur (Lifschitz-Mercer et al 1988). Vimentin is not demonstrable (Santini et al 1989), a feature in common with mucinous ovarian neoplasms and urothelium. Vimentin is, however, demonstrable in the stromal cells of a Brenner tumour. Evidence of smooth muscle differentiation, characterized by desmin positivity may also be found in the stroma (Seldenrijk et al 1986). CEA has been detected in most benign, proliferating and malignant Brenner tumours (Shevchuck et al 1980, Charpin et al 1982). Positive staining for chromogranin, serotonin and neurone-specific enolase may be found in Brenner epithelium, consistent with the presence of argyrophilic cells in these tumours (Aguirre et al 1986, Santini et al 1989).

Mixed Müllerian tumours

These tumours are more common in the uterus than in the ovary and are discussed with uterine tumours (see p. 52).

Metastatic ovarian carcinomas

These are most commonly from the colon, stomach or breast. Of these, metastatic colonic carcinomas can be the most difficult to distinguish from primary ovarian tumour (Lash & Hart 1987). Immunostains for CA125 and placental alkaline phosphatase may be helpful as they are usually expressed by ovarian carcinomas, but are also occasionally present in colonic carcinomas. Immunostains for placental alkaline phosphatase are positive in metastatic gastric carcinomas. Conventional antibodies to CEA immuno-stain most metastatic colonic carcinomas (Lash & Hart 1987) and also mucinous and some non-mucinous ovarian carcinomas. Some of the monoclonal antibodies to specific epitopes of CEA may prove to be more useful in this respect. Three such markers (CD14, CEJ065 and SP-625) have been reported to show positive immunostaining with virtually all primary and metastatic colonic carcinoma, but to have little reactivity with ovarian carcinoma (Pavelic et al 1991). They were less useful, however, in differentiating between metastatic gastric and breast carcinomas. Another potentially useful marker is cytokeratin-7, which is expressed by ovarian carcinoma but not by colonic carcinoma (Raemekers et al 1990).

Sex cord–stromal tumours

Immunocytochemical studies on sex cord–stromal tumours are limited. The main markers studied have been hormones and intermediate filaments.

Hormonal markers

Studies that correlate hormone production with morphology have demon-strated that there is considerable overlap in hormone content of different types of sex cord–stromal tumours (Kurman & Nadji 1985). Furthermore, simply by immunohistochemical localization of a hormone one cannot distinguish between its synthesis, storage or receptor binding at the site. Hormone localization studies have several technical problems, including a high level of background staining and loss of antigenicity when using fixed tissues (Kurman & Nadji 1985).

Granulosa–theca cell tumours have been shown to have oestradiol and sometimes testosterone and progesterone in granulosa cells, whilst theca cells contain oestradiol and progesterone, and occasionally testosterone. In Sertoli–Leydig cell tumours, the Sertoli cells contain testosterone and oestradiol, and less commonly progesterone, or they may be devoid of hormones. The Leydig cells contain testosterone and oestradiol, and sometimes progesterone (Kurman & Nadji 1985). Confirmation of steroid hormone production by these tumours may be obtained by in vivo hormone measurements and in vitro incubation studies and steroid receptor assays.

A more recent immunohistochemical avenue of investigation of steroid hormone production has involved the demonstration of the steroidogenic enzymes aromatase, 17 α-hydroxylase and cholesterol side-chain cleavage cytochrome P-450, necessary for oestrogen, androgen and progesterone production respectively (Sasano et al 1989). Immunostaining for 3 β-hydroxysteroid dehydrogenase, which converts pregnenolone to progesterone, has also been investigated (Sasano et al 1990). These studies have revealed little evidence of steroid synthesis in granulosa cells, but the luteinized cells of thecomas show evidence of androgen and oestrogen production. In Sertoli–Leydig cell tumours, there is evidence of progesterone, androgen and oestrogen production.

Intermediate filaments

Early studies of intermediate filaments in sex cord–stromal tumours reported immunostaining for vimentin but not cytokeratins (Miettinen et al 1985). Granulosa and theca cells of normal ovaries were also reported to show this pattern of expression. Subsequent studies, however, have shown that granulosa cells and Sertoli cells can express both cytokeratin and vimentin (Benjamin et al 1987). In adult and fetal ovaries, granulosa cells express cytokeratin and vimentin, whilst theca cells and apparently undifferentiated stromal cells express vimentin only. This pattern of intermediate filament expression is also seen in fetal ovaries in the early stages of development.

Granulosa cell tumours

Adult and juvenile granulosa cell tumours may both express cytokeratin (Fig. 3.2A): it has been demonstrated in one-third to two-thirds of cases studied using antibodies to low molecular weight cytokeratins such as CAM 5.2 (Benjamin et al 1987), Aguirre et al 1989). The extent of positive staining varies and may be more prominent in tumours with insular, macrofollicular and microfollicular growth patterns. Biochemical analysis has confirmed the presence of cytokeratins 8 and 18 (Czernobilsky et al 1987). Vimentin filaments are universally present (Fig. 3.2B). Desmoplakins have also been demonstrated immunohistochemically and correspond to the presence of desmosomes. It has been shown by immunoelectronmicroscopy that vimentin filaments attach to desmoplakin in desmosomes. The unusual

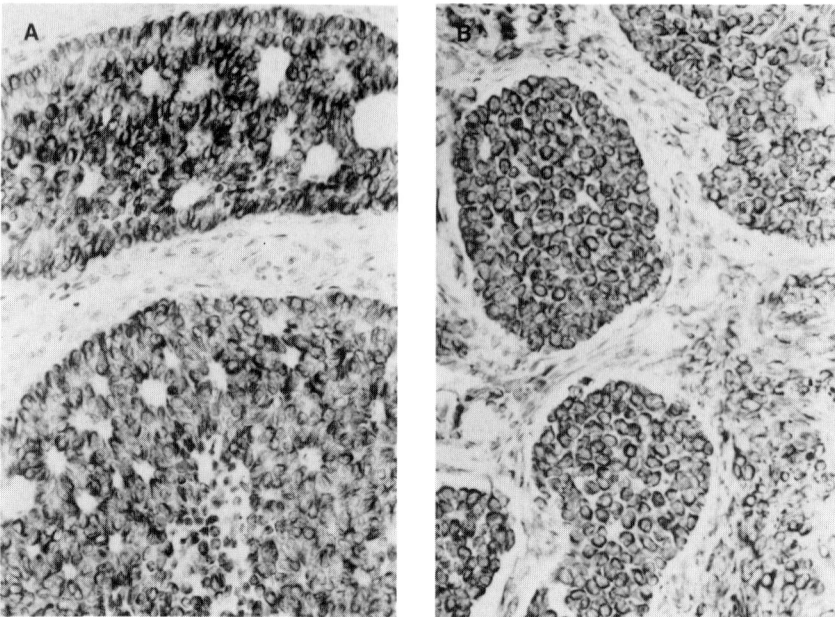

Fig. 3.2 Granulosa cell tumour showing: **A** cytoplasmic staining for cytokeratin antibody (CAM 5.2); **B** perinuclear staining with anti-vimentin which also stains stromal cells (immunoperoxidase, × 300).

combination of vimentin and desmoplakin may be a useful marker of granulosa cell tumours and an aid in distinguishing them from mesenchymal tumours (Czernobilsky et al 1987).

The histogenesis of granulosa cell tumours is not settled: whether the origin of normal granulosa cells is from coelomic mesothelium or gonadal mesenchyme is still disputed. The presence of desmosomes and the immunohistochemical demonstration of cytokeratin and desmoplakins indicates that granuloma cells have epithelial differentiation, but does not resolve the issue of histogenesis. A recently described marker of granulosa cell tumours is the peptide hormone inhibin, which is produced by granulosa and Sertoli cells. In the cases studied so far, increased serum concentrations of inhibin are correlated with the presence of tumour tissue (Lappohn et al 1989, Nishida et al 1991).

Pure thecomas and fibromas

These uniformly express vimentin but not cytokeratins, a similar pattern to normal theca and ovarian stromal cells (Benjamin et al 1987, Miettinen et al 1985).

Sertoli–Leydig cell tumours

The Sertoli cells in well-differentiated Sertoli–Leydig cell tumours express low molecular weight cytokeratins (Benjamin et al 1987). Poorly differentiated tumours may show focal expression, which sometimes corresponds with the presence of poorly formed tubular structures. Vimentin may also be expressed but tends to be focal. Leydig cells have been reported to express only vimentin, but cytokeratin has been demonstrated in testicular Leydig cell tumours (Duek et al 1989). Sertoli–Leydig cell tumours with heterologous elements may additionally express intermediate filaments corresponding to their component tissues, and also neuroendocrine peptide hormones corresponding to the presence of argyrophilic cells. α-Fetoprotein has been demonstrated in neoplastic Sertoli and Leydig cells, and in tumour cells resembling liver cells (Chada et al 1987, Young et al 1984, Tetu et al 1986).

DIFFERENTIAL DIAGNOSIS OF SEX CORD–STROMAL TUMOURS

Several neoplasms can mimic sex cord–stromal tumours. They include endometrioid carcinoma (which may resemble Sertoli–Leydig cell tumours and granulosa cell tumours), metastatic carcinoma (especially Krukenberg tumours of ovarian type) and ovarian carcinoid tumours (Young & Scully 1987). Conventional mucin stains are not always helpful in distinguishing these tumours: periodic acid–Schiff positive, diastase-resistant material resembling mucin may occur in granulosa cell and Sertoli–Leydig cell tumours. Similarly, expression of intermediate filaments (cytokeratin and vimentin) also does not differentiate these tumour groups.

The epithelial markers human milk fat globule antigen, epithelial membrane antigen and AuA1, however, do appear to be useful in distinguishing them (Fig. 3.3). Carcinomas consistently express these markers, and sex cord–stromal tumours do not (Benjamin 1987). Aguirre et al (1989) also failed to demonstrate staining with epithelial membrane antigen in 15 cases of adult granulosa cell tumours: all of their cases of endometrioid carcinoma expressed the antigen. They did, however, find positive staining for epithelial membrane antigen in one of their 14 cases of Sertoli–Leydig cell tumour. This highlights the value of these epithelial markers in differential diagnosis. Carcinoid tumours express human milk fat globule antigen and epithelial membrane antigen but not usually AuA1 (unpublished data), and they can be distinguished by reactivity with neuroendocrine markers.

Germ cell tumours

Germ cell tumours were among the earliest tumours to be studied immunohistochemically with the oncofetal markers β-hCG and α-feto-

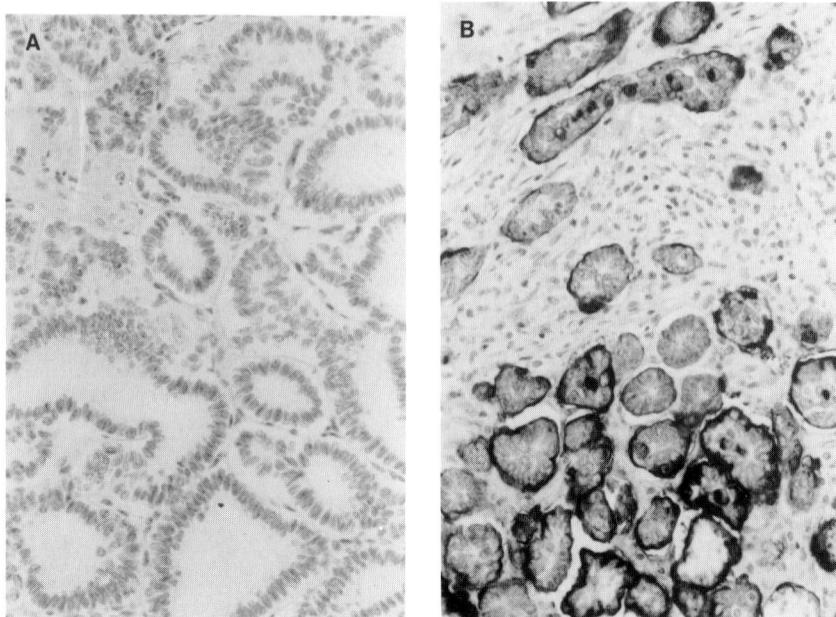

Fig. 3.3 Antibody to human milk fat globule antigen, **A** fails to stain an ovarian Sertoli–Leydig cell tumour, **B** shows strong reactivity in an ovarian carcinoma (immunoperoxidase, × 250).

protein. The main application of these markers is in clinical monitoring, as serum levels often closely reflect the histological composition and bulk of these tumours. The β subunit of hCG can be detected at a relatively low concentration and withstands routine fixation. Detection of α-fetoprotein in fixed tissue is more likely to be hampered by denaturing of the antigen during processing (Kurman & Nadji 1985). Serum concentrations of placental alkaline phosphatase and similar enzymes are most consistently raised in germ cell tumours (Hamilton-Dutoit et al 1990). These enzymes are, however, sensitive rather than specific markers of germ cells. Reactivity of germ cell tumours has been shown to be mainly with the placental alkaline phosphatase-like (Nagao) isoenzymes rather than the placental (Regan) isoenzymes.

Dysgerminoma

Among available markers the most consistent immunohistochemical marker of dysgerminoma, and of testicular seminoma, is placental alkaline phosphatase and placental alkaline phosphatase-like enzymes. In a study of gonadal dysgerminomas and seminomas, this enzyme was detected in 86%

of cases (Niehans et al 1988). Placental alkaline phosphatase immuno-reactivity in dysgerminomas is diffuse, whereas it is patchy in other germ cell tumours. In the 3–5% of tumours that have syncytiotrophoblast giant cells, hCG is demonstrable and is localized within these cells; such cases may be associated with raised serum concentrations of hCG. α-Fetoprotein is not usually detectable in pure seminomas.

Although cytokeratin expression was not found in early studies of dysgerminoma (Miettinen et al 1985), it has been described in 14–80% of seminomas (Raemekers et al 1985, Denk et al 1987) and has now also been detected in dysgerminomas. Vimentin reactivity is found in 30% of seminomas and dysgerminomas (Niehans et al 1988). Epithelial membrane antigen is generally not expressed by seminomas, nor by most germ cell neoplasms other than choriocarcinomas, syncytiotrophoblast giant cells and teratomas.

Yolk sac tumour

This is the second commonest malignant ovarian germ cell tumour. α-Fetoprotein is the most important immunohistochemical marker and often correlates with raised serum levels; its localization may be diffuse or focal within the tumour. Hyaline globules in yolk sac tumours rarely show reactivity for α-fetoprotein (Eglen & Ulbright 1987). Placental alkaline phosphatase is demonstrable in about half the cases (Niehans et al 1988), whilst epithelial membrane antigen is rarely expressed. Cytokeratin, CEA and α-antitrypsin may also be demonstrable in yolk sac tumours.

Embryonal carcinoma

Ovarian embryonal carcinomas usually form part of a mixed germ cell tumour. The cells of embryonal carcinoma may show focal expression of α-fetoprotein. Syncytiotrophoblast giant cells are often present and contain immunoreactive hCG (Kurman & Norris 1976). A high proportion of embryonal carcinomas express placental alkaline phosphatase but not epithelial membrane antigen; most contain cytokeratin and occasionally vimentin (Niehans et al 1988). The Ki-1 antigen (CD30), which is thought to be restricted to haemopoietic and lymphoid tissues, has recently been shown to be expressed by embryonal carcinomas of testis and embryonal elements of mixed germ cell tumours, but not by other germ cell neoplasms (Pallesen & Hamilton-Dutoit 1988). The significance of this finding is uncertain, but it may be of value as a marker of embryonal carcinoma. α_1-Antitrypsin, transferrin, ferritin and CEA have been demonstrated in embryonal carcinoma cells: in contrast, human placental lactogen and pregnancy specific glycoprotein have been found in syncytiotrophoblast giant cells (Krag-Jacobsen et al 1981, Kurman & Nadji 1985).

Choriocarcinoma

Non-gestational ovarian choriocarcinoma is usually part of a mixed germ cell tumour and rarely occurs as a pure tumour. As with gestational choriocarcinoma, β-hCG is the main immunohistochemical marker for this tumour. It is found in syncytiotrophoblastic cells. Human placental lactogen is also expressed and placental alkaline phosphatase is demonstrable in about half the cases (Niehans et al 1988). Epithelial membrane antigen is also found in syncytiotrophoblastic cells, though focal CEA expression can occur in cytotrophoblastic cells. Cytokeratins are expressed by both cell types.

Teratomas

Ovarian teratomas contain elements derived from the three germ cell layers. Intermediate filament expression occurs in line with tissue differentiation, and epithelial, mesenchymal and muscle components can be identified by immunostains for cytokeratin, vimentin and desmin, respectively. Mature glial tissue immunostains for glial fibrillary acidic protein, and antibodies to neurofilament mark neuronal cells and fibres. Primitive neural epithelium of immature teratomas does not stain for glial fibrillary acidic protein (Fig. 3.4).

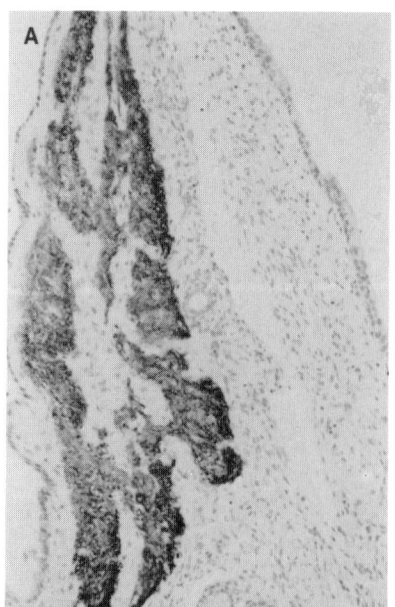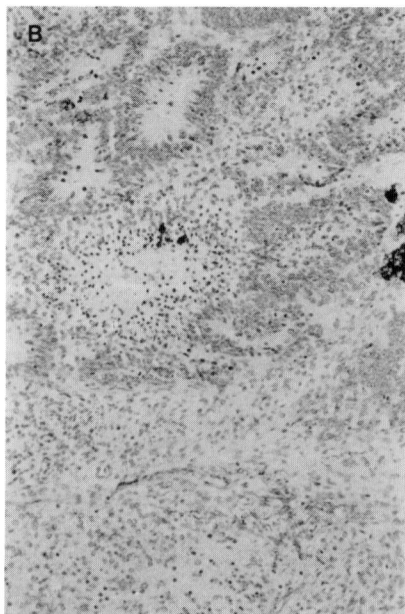

Fig. 3.4   Ovarian teratoma: **A** staining for glial fibrillary acidic protein in mature glial tissue. **B** primitive neuroepithelium with foci of melanin pigment fails to stain with glial fibrillary acidic protein. (Immunoperoxidase, × 250.)

Endoderm-derived epithelium may focally stain for α-fetoprotein and may occasionally be associated with a raised serum α-fetoprotein concentration (Ishiguro et al 1981). Staining for hCG has been found in syncytiotrophoblast giant cells in immature teratomas (Krag-Jacobsen et al 1981, Calame & Shaberg 1989). In a study of solid teratomas Calame & Shaberg (1989) found argyrophilic cells in all cases and immunoreactivity of these cells was reported to a range of peptides and proteins, including glucagon, insulin, gastrin, secretin, somatostatin and pancreatic polypeptide. All of the solid teratomas also showed CEA reactivity.

The differential diagnosis of solid teratoma and malignant mixed Müllerian tumour is usually not difficult, in part because of the different age groups affected. Where difficulty does arise, because of the range of tissues in the ovarian tumour, the presence of markers such as glial fibrillary acidic protein, neurofilament, α-fetoprotein, hCG and neuroendocrine markers are more in favour of a teratoma than a mixed Müllerian tumour (Calame & Shaberg 1989). There have, however, recently been reports of the presence of glial tissue (and therefore glial fibrillary acidic protein and neurofilament protein) in uterine and ovarian mixed Müllerian tumours (Gershell et al 1989, Erhmann et al 1990).

Struma ovarii and ovarian carcinoid tumours are monodermal or monophyletic teratomas. The presence of thyroglobulin and thyroid hormones can be demonstrated immunohistologically in struma ovarii (Hasleton & Whittaker 1978). Primary ovarian carcinoid tumours contain neuroendocrine markers such as chromogranin A (Wolpert et al 1989) and a variety of endocrine peptides, including pancreatic polypeptides, glucagon enkephalin and somatostatin. Immunoreactive cells to such peptides have been found in 53% of trabecular carcinoids, 42% of strumal carcinoids and 7% of insular carcinoids (Sporrong et al 1982). Strumal carcinoids may also contain thyroglobulin (Fig. 3.5) and calcitonin (Dayal et al 1979).

UTERUS

Endometrium

Tumour-associated antigens

Many tumour-associated antigens have been studied to determine their value in distinguishing between normal endometrium, atypical hyperplasia and endometrial carcinoma. CEA has been demonstrated in all cases of atypical hyperplasias and 60% of carcinomas (Hustin 1978). CA-1 antigen, a mucin-like glycoprotein, was found in some cases of atypical hyperplasia and endometrial carcinoma, but reactivity was also present in secretory phase endometrium (Ferguson & Fox 1984); a monoclonal antibody to the tumour-associated glycoprotein TAG-72 showed a similar pattern of reactivity (Thor et al 1987). Binding of antibody to human milk fat globule membrane showed a luminal pattern of distribution in normal endometrium

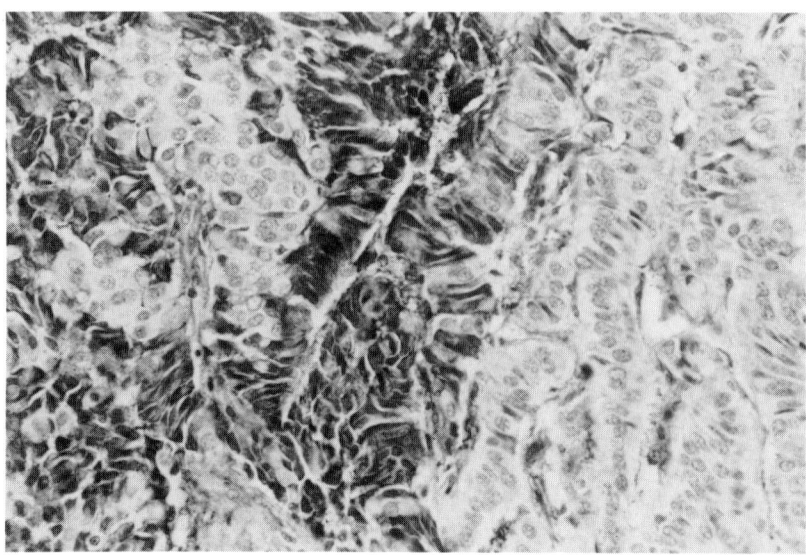

Fig. 3.5 Ovarian strumal carcinoid tumour showing cytoplasmic staining with antibody to thyroglobulin (immunoperoxidase, × 350).

and endometrial hyperplasia without atypia, whilst in atypical hyperplasia and endometrial carcinoma, cytoplasmic expression was also present (Morris et al 1989). None of these antibodies, however, has proved sufficiently discriminatory to be of value as a marker of neoplastic transformation. Some serum tumour markers that are raised in ovarian carcinomas may also be raised in endometrial carcinomas (Table 3.1), and have been used for clinical monitoring.

Intermediate filaments

Endometrial carcinomas, in common with normal endometrial glands, express cytokeratin polypeptides 7, 8, 18 and 19 (Moll et al 1983), which can be demonstrated by low molecular weight cytokeratin antibodies. Higher molecular weight cytokeratin antibodies show focal immunostaining of glands and areas of squamous differentiation. Vimentin positivity occurs in 70–80% of proliferative glands but drops to 20% or less in secretory glands (Dabbs et al 1986). Endometrial stromal cells express vimentin only. Vimentin immunoreactivity has been found in 65% of endometrial carcinoma; mucinous and clear cell carcinomas are negative. This contrasts with lack of immunoreactivity in endocervical adenocarcinomas and normal endocervical glands (Dabbs et al 1986). Demonstration of the presence of vimentin, therefore, may be a useful way of distinguishing between endometrial and endocervical adenocarcinomas (Fig. 3.6). It is likely,

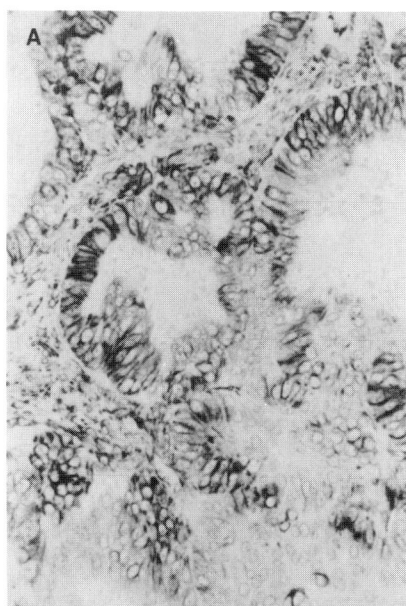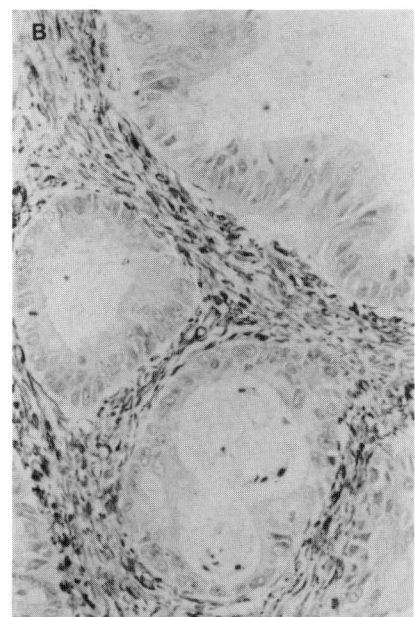

Fig. 3.6 Antibody to vimentin: **A** stains glands of endometrial adenocarcinoma; **B** fails to stain mucinous epithelium of endocervical adenocarcinoma (immunoperoxidase, × 250).

however, that in this context vimentin marks endometrioid differentiation rather than endometrial origin.

Mesenchymal tumours

Smooth muscle tumours

Leiomyomas and leiomyosarcomas express vimentin and desmin. An unexpected immunohistochemical finding has been the demonstration of low molecular weight cytokeratin positivity in uterine and extrauterine leiomyomas and leiomyosarcomas (Brown et al 1987, Norton et al 1987). It is unclear whether positive staining indicates the presence of cytokeratin, or cross-reactivity (Gusterson 1987). Immunoreactivity to epithelial membrane antigen has also been described in extrauterine leiomyosarcomas (Miettenen 1988), indicating that the presence of these epithelial markers cannot be taken, in isolation from their morphological features, as specific for carcinoma.

Endometrial stromal sarcoma

Vimentin is expressed by all stromal sarcomas, but the expression of cytokeratin is more controversial. Binder et al (1991) detected cytokeratin in three of five tumours in which no obvious epithelial differentiation was present, but other studies have not supported this finding (Lifschitz-Mercer et al 1987, Puts et al 1987). Tumour cells that immunostain for desmin may also be present (Del Poggetto et al 1983). In stromal sarcoma cells, β- and γ-actin have been detected biochemically, and they are also present in normal endometrial stromal cells (Lifschitz-Mercer et al 1987). One example of stromomyoma was positive for desmin and vimentin but not cytokeratin, and two uterine tumours that had sex cord–stromal features expressed cytokeratin and vimentin (Binder et al 1991). It is likely that the diverse immunostaining patterns of stromal tumours reflect their postulated histogenesis from a primitive stem cell that can differentiate along both epithelial and mesenchymal cell lines.

Mixed mesodermal tumours

These contain epithelial and mesenchymal elements and comprise adenofibroma, adenosarcoma, carcinofibroma and carcinosarcoma (mixed Müllerian tumour). Immunohistochemical studies have concentrated on mixed Müllerian tumours. The epithelial component stains for cytokeratin and epithelial membrane antigen, and also focally for vimentin (Geisinger et al 1987, Auerbach et al 1988, Bitterman et al 1990). CEA has also been demonstrated (Calame & Shaberg 1989). Epithelial differentiation may also be identified with these markers in spindle-shaped stromal cells and giant cells (Deligdisch et al 1988). Homologous stromal sarcoma cells are vimentin-positive and may focally express cytokeratin (Fig. 3.7). Desmin immunoreactivity has been found in 50% of cases (Auerbach et al 1988), and some of these also stain for myoglobin, indicative of striated muscle differentiation. Cross striations are usually identified only in differentiated rhabdomyoblasts, whereas myoglobin staining may help to identify skeletal muscle differentiation at an earlier stage (Sahin & Benda 1988). Other markers such as S100 may stain foci of chondrosarcoma, and α_1-antichymotrypsin stains stromal and giant cells (Auerbach et al 1988).

Recently, neuroectodermal differentiation in uterine and ovarian mixed Müllerian tumours has been reported (Gershell et al 1989, Erhmann et al 1990); they have positive staining for glial fibrillary acidic protein in mature glial tissue. This is contrary to the previously held view that neural tissues never occur in mixed Müllerian tumours (Dehner et al 1971). Clearly it is questionable whether these tumours are mixed Müllerian tumours or are in fact teratomas. Glial fibrillary acidic protein may be found in spindle cells of mixed Müllerian tumours in which no glial differentiation is present, and can be produced by cultured cells of mixed Müllerian tumours and normal endometrial stromal cells (Liao & Choi 1986, 1987). This indicates that mixed Müllerian tumours are capable of a wider range of differentiation than was hitherto thought. The histogenesis of mixed Müllerian tumours, whether from primitive stem cells giving rise to epithelial and mesenchymal

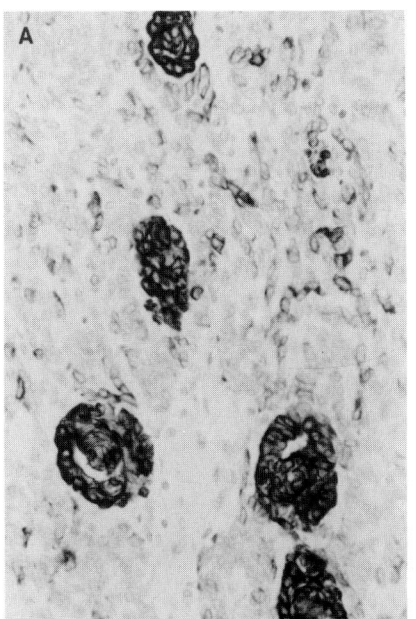 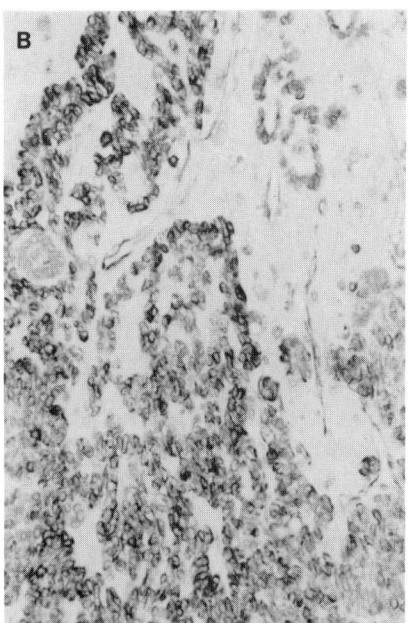

Fig. 3.7   Mixed Müllerian tumour.   **A** cytokeratin (CAM 5.2) staining of poorly formed epithelial structures and scattered stromal cells.   **B** perinuclear staining of homologous stromal sarcoma cells with anti-vimentin. (Immunoperoxidase, × 250.)

elements or from two independent stem cell lines developing in concert, is controversial. The immunocytochemical profile of these tumours almost certainly reflects their differentiation rather than their origin.

CERVIX

Immunohistochemical studies have been directed towards the demonstration of viral antigens and tumour markers of cervical neoplasms. Markers that may be of use in predicting malignant transformation of squamous and glandular epithelium, and in differentiating endocervical from endometrial adenocarcinoma, have also been investigated.

Viral antigens

Human papillomavirus and herpes simplex virus antigens have been demonstrated in cervical lesions. It is now clear that immunohistochemical methods are not sufficiently specific or sensitive for detection of viral antigens: they have largely been superseded by DNA hybridization techniques and the polymerase chain reaction (see p. 83).

Tumour-associated markers

Squamous cell carcinoma antigen/TA-4 antigen. The squamous cell carcinoma antigen is a subfraction of the glycoprotein TA-4 derived from a cervical squamous cell carcinoma. Both markers have been used in monitoring squamous and adenosquamous carcinomas of the cervix (Kato & Tongae 1977, Duk et al 1990). The antigen has been demonstrated immunohistochemically in keratinizing and large cell non-keratinizing tumours. Undifferentiated and small cell carcinomas do not immunostain.

Carcinoembryonic antigen. Elevated serum CEA levels may be found in both squamous cell carcinoma and adenocarcinomas of the cervix, and may be of value in predicting recurrence in patients who have tumours that contain CEA. It has been detected in 50–82% of cervical squamous cell carcinomas and 75–100% of adenocarcinomas (Van Nagell et al 1982, Bychkov et al 1983).

Squamous lesions

Intermediate filaments

Cytokeratin expression in the uterine cervix is complex. Endocervical epithelium contains simple epithelial type keratins 8, 18 and 19, and ectocervical epithelium has stratification type keratins 5 and 17 as well as several other cytokeratin polypeptides (Syrjanen et al 1988). Low molecular weight (simple epithelial) cytokeratins have been investigated for use as markers of potential invasion in cervical intraepithelial neoplasia, but results are conflicting. Some studies have shown that cases of cervical intraepithelial neoplasia (CIN) 1 and 2 do not express these cytokeratins, whereas some cases of CIN 3 and most invasive squamous carcinomas do express them (Bobrow et al 1986, Angus et al 1988). Others have disputed this, having found staining in only a small proportion of squamous cell carcinomas (Raju 1988) and lack of staining in microinvasive squamous carcinoma (Wells et al 1986). In HPV infected cervical epithelium and CIN, disturbances in the pattern of cytokeratin expression have also been described (Morris et al 1983, Syrjanen et al 1988).

Involucrin

This is a differentiation antigen of squamous epithelium, unrelated to keratin. It is expressed in normal squamous epithelium, squamous meta-plasia and viral condylomas. Its expression is less in CIN (Warhol et al 1982), but its value as a marker of CIN is reduced when there is significant inflammation, which itself results in decreased expression. It may be of some value in distinguishing CIN 1 from immature metaplasia and flat condylomas.

Glandular lesions

Carcinoembryonic antigen

As well as being a serum tumour marker in cervical adenocarcinoma, CEA has been reported to be of use in distinguishing benign glandular lesions from endocervical adenocarcinoma. Normal endocervix and 95% of cases of microglandular hyperplasia do not express CEA, whereas 64% of adeno-carcinomas do (Speers et al 1983). Other studies have confirmed this (Michael et al 1984, Steeper & Wick 1986) and, furthermore, have shown that cases of minimal deviation adenocarcinoma consistently expressed CEA. Reports of CEA expression in adenocarcinoma in situ are more conflicting. Hurliman & Gloor (1984) detected CEA in six of nine cases (67%), while Tobon & Dave (1988) detected it in only one of 11 cases. α-Amylase and human milk fat globule antigen have also been investigated as markers of endocervical glandular atypia; the pattern of human milk fat globule antigen staining is reported to be useful in distinguishing atypia from benign endocervical proliferations (Brown et al 1987). Results of staining for amylase are conflicting (Lee & Raju 1988, Griffin et al 1989).

The distinction between adenocarcinomas of endocervical and endo-metrial origin can sometimes be difficult in a cervical biopsy. The use of CEA to differentiate between these tumours was described by Wahlstrom et al (1979), who showed that 80% of endocervical tumours stained, in contrast to 8% of endometrial tumours. Other studies have shown no significant differences between the frequency and extent of expression of CEA in the two tumours, irrespective of whether monoclonal or polyclonal antibodies were used (Maes et al 1988).

Vimentin may be more useful than CEA in distinguishing endocervical from endometrial adenocarcinomas, as already described. Vimentin, how-ever, can be expressed by the rare mesonephric carcinoma of the cervix, and by mesonephric hyperplasia, in which vimentin positivity occurs in 10–30% of cells (Lang & Dallenbach-Hellweg 1990). These entities do not express CEA, and the combination of vimentin positivity and absence of CEA may help to distinguish them from typical endocervical adeno-carcinoma. Kudo et al (1990) have described a monoclonal antibody, IC5, that has a reactivity which they claim to be superior to that of CEA in invasive and in situ adenocarcinomas and adenosquamous carcinoma. Immunostains to the antibody were reported to be negative in intra-epithelial and invasive squamous cell carcinomas, and so could be used to distinguish between glandular and squamous neoplasms. The authors also claimed that it was useful in distinguishing endocervical from endometrial adenocarcinoma.

Small cell neuroendocrine cervical carcinoma

Hormone production by cervical carcinomas is well recognized. Serotonin, somatostatin and adrenocorticotrophin hormone may occasionally be detected. Small cell undifferentiated carcinomas express cytokeratin and sometimes epithelial membrane antigen and CEA. The most commonly demonstrated neuroendocrine markers include chromogranin A, Leu 7, neurone-specific enolase and synaptophysin (Gershell et al 1988, Ueda et al 1988).

Adenoid cystic carcinomas and adenoid basal carcinomas

These tumours have been studied immunohistochemically and express cytokeratin; CEA and epithelial membrane antigen are present focally. Adenoid cystic carcinomas differ from their salivary gland counterparts by failing to stain for S100 protein, which in salivary glands is expressed by the myoepithelial component. Ferry & Scully (1988) postulated that this tumour is a carcinoma resembling an adenoid cystic carcinoma rather than a true adenoid cystic carcinoma.

CONCLUSION

Immunocytochemical markers are useful for the clinical and pathological investigation of gynaecological disease. There are inherent limitations because of antigen heterogeneity in tumour cell populations and variation in the specificities of currently available antibodies. As newer antibodies are introduced and information on currently available ones grows, more selective immunotyping of tumours may be possible. This is already becoming the case with the introduction of antibodies to specific cytokeratin polypeptides and to specific CEA epitopes, and no doubt represents a growth area for the future.

REFERENCES

Abeler V, Kjorstad K E, Nesland J M 1988 Small cell carcinoma of the ovary: a report of six cases. International Journal of Gynecological Pathology 7: 315–329
Aguirre P, Scully R E, Wolfe H J et al 1986 Argyrophil cells in Brenner tumors: histochemical and immunohistochemical analysis. International Journal of Gynecological Pathology 5: 223–234
Aguirre P, Thor A D, Scully R E 1989 Ovarian endometrioid carcinomas resembling Sex-cord–stromal tumors. An immunohistochemical study. International Journal of Gynecological Pathology 8: 364–373
Angus B, Kiberu S, Purvis J, Wilkinson L, Horne C H W 1988 Cytokeratins in cervical dysplasia and neoplasia: a comparative study of immunohistochemical staining using monoclonal antibodies NCL-5D3, CAM 5.2, and PKK1. Journal of Pathology 155: 71–75
Atkinson B F, Ernst C S, Herlyn M, Steplewski Z, Sears H F, Koprowski H 1982 Gastrointestinal cancer associated antigen in immunoperoxidase assay. Cancer Research 42: 4820–4823
Auerbach H E, Livolsi V A, Merino M J 1988 Malignant mixed Mullerian tumours of uterus: an immunohistochemical study. International Journal of Gynecological Pathology 7: 123–130
Bast R C, Fenney M, Lazarus H, Nadler L M, Colvin R B, Knapp R C 1981 Reactivity of a

monoclonal antibody with human ovarian carcinoma. Journal of Clinical Investigation 68: 1331–1337

Benjamin E 1987 Sex cord-stromal tumour or ovarian carcinoma? Use of epithelial surface markers in differential diagnosis. Journal of Pathology 152: 192A

Benjamin E, Law S, Bobrow L G 1987 Intermediate filaments cytokeratin and vimentin in ovarian sex cord-stromal tumours with correlative studies in adult and fetal ovaries. Journal of Pathology 152: 253–266

Berkowitz R, Kabawat S, Lazarus H, Colvin R B, Knapp R, Bast R C 1983 Comparison of a rabbit heteroantiserum and a murine monoclonal antibody raised against a human epithelial ovarian carcinoma cell line. American Journal of Obstetrics and Gynecology 146: 607–612

Bhattacharya M, Chatterjee S K, Barlow J J, Fuji H 1982 Monoclonal antibodies recognising tumour associated antigen of human ovarian mucinous cystadenocarcinomas. Cancer Research 42: 1650–1654

Bhattacharya M, Chatterjee S K, Barlow J J 1985 Ovarian tumour antigens and other markers. In: Hudson C N (ed) Ovarian carcinoma. Oxford University Press, Oxford, p 169–189

Binder S W, Nieberg R K, Cheg L, Al-Jitawi S 1991 Histological and immunohistochemical analysis of nine endometrial stromal tumors: an unexpected high frequency of keratin protein positivity. International Journal of Gynecological Pathology 10: 191–197

Bitterman P, Chun B, Kurman R J 1990 The significance of epithelial differentiation in mixed mesodermal tumors of the uterus. American Journal of Surgical Pathology 14: 317–328

Bobrow L G, Makin C A, Law S et al 1986 Expression of low molecular weight cytokeratin proteins in cervical neoplasia. Journal of Pathology 148: 135–140

Breitenecker G, Neunteufel W, Bieglmayer C, Kolbl H, Schieder K 1989 Comparison between tissue and serum content of CA 125, CA 19-9 and carcinoembryonic antigen in ovarian tumors. International Journal of Gynecological Pathology 8: 97–102

Brown D G, Theaker J M, Banks P M, Gatter K C, Mason D Y 1987 Cytokeratin expression in smooth muscle and smooth muscle tumours. Histopathology 11: 477–486

Brown L J R, Griffin N R, Wells W 1987 Cytoplasmic reactivity with the monoclonal antibody HMFG1 as a marker of cervical glandular atypia. Journal of Pathology 15: 203–208

Bruns D E, Mills S E, Savary J 1982 Amylase in fallopian tube and serous ovarian neoplasms. Immunohistochemical localisation. Archives of Pathology and Laboratory Medicine 106: 17–20

Bychkov V, Rothman M, Bardawil W A 1983 Immunocytochemical localisation of carcino-embryonic antigen (CEA) alpha-fetoprotein (AFP) and human chorionic gonadotropin (HCG) in cervical neoplasia. American Journal of Clinical Pathology 79: 414–420

Calame J J, Schaberg A 1989 Solid teratomas and mixed Müllerian tumors of the ovary: a clinical, histological and immunocytochemical comparative study. Gynecologic Oncology 33: 212–221

Chada S, Honnebier W J, Schaberg A 1987 Raised serum alpha fetoprotein in Sertoli–Leydig cell tumor (androblastoma of ovary): report of two cases. International Journal of Gynecological Pathology 6: 82–88

Charpin C, Bhan A K, Zurawski V R, Scully R E 1982 Carcinoembryonic antigens (CEA) and carbohydrate determinant 19-9 (CA 19-9) localisation in 121 primary and metastatic ovarian tumors. An immunohistochemical study with use of monoclonal antibodies. International Journal of Gynecological Pathology 1: 231–245

Czernobilsky B, Moll R, Leppien G, Schweikhart G, Franke W W 1987 Desmosomal plaque-associated vimentin filaments in human ovarian granulosa cell tumors of various histologic patterns. American Journal of Pathology 126: 476–486

Czernobilsky B, Shezen E, Lifschitz-Mercer B et al 1989 Alpha smooth muscle actin in normal human ovaries, in ovarian stromal hyperplasia and in ovarian neoplasms. Virchow Archives B Cell Pathology 57: 55–61

Dabbs D J, Geisinger K R 1988 Common epithelial ovarian tumors. Immunohistochemical intermediate filament profiles. Cancer 62: 368–374

Dabbs D J, Geisinger K R, Norris H T 1986 Intermediate filaments in endometrial and endocervical carcinomas. American Journal of Surgical Pathology 10: 568–576

Daunter B 1990 Tumor markers in gynecologic oncology. Gynecological Oncology 39: 1–15

Dayal Y, Tashijan A H, Wolfe H J 1979 Immunocytochemical localisation of calcitonin producing cells in a strumal carcinoid with amyloid stroma. Cancer 43: 1331–1338

Dehner L P, Norris H J, Taylor H B 1971 Carcinosarcomas and mixed Müllerian tumors of the ovary. Cancer 27: 207–216

Deligdisch L, Plaxe S, Cohen C J 1988 Extra-uterine pelvic malignant mixed mesodermal tumors: A study of 10 cases with immunohistochemistry. International Journal of Gynecological Pathology 7: 361–372

Del Poggetto C B, Virtanen I, Lehto V-P, Walstrom T, Saksela E 1983 Expression of intermediate filaments in ovarian and uterine tumors. International Journal of Gynecological Pathology 1: 359–366

Denk H, Moll R, Weybora W et al 1987 Intermediate filaments and desmosomal plaque proteins in testicular seminomas and non-seminomatous germ cell tumours as revealed by immunohistochemistry. Virchows Archives A Pathological Anatomy 410: 295–307

Dickersin R G, Kline I W, Scully R E 1982 Small cell carcinoma of the ovary with hypercalcemia: a report of eleven cases. Cancer 49: 188–197

Duek W, Dieckmann K P, Loy V, Stein H 1989 Immunohistochemical determinations of oestrogen receptor, progesterone receptor and intermediate filaments in Leydig cell tumours, Leydig cell hyperplasia and normal Leydig cells of the human testis. Journal of Pathology 157: 225–234

Duk J M, De Bruijn W A, Groenier H K H 1990 Cancer of the uterine cervix. Sensitivity and specificity of serum squamous cell carcinoma antigen determinations. Gynecological Oncology 29: 186–194

Eglen D E, Ulbright T M 1987 The differential diagnosis of yolk sac tumor and seminomas. American Journal of Pathology 88: 328–332

Ehrmann R L, Weidner N, Welch W R, Gleiberman I 1990 Malignant mixed Müllerian tumor of ovary with prominent neuroectodermal differentiation (teratoid carcinosarcoma). International Journal of Gynecological Pathology 9: 272–282

Epenetos A A, Hooker G E, Krauz T, Snook D, Bodmer W F, Taylor-Papadimitriou J 1986 Antibody-guided irradiation of malignant ascites in ovarian cancer: a new therapeutic method possessing specificity against cancer cells. Obstetrics and Gynecology 68: 71s–74s

Ferguson A M, Fox H 1984 The expression of Ca antigen in normal, hyperplastic and neoplastic endometrium. British Journal of Obstetrics and Gynaecology 91: 1042–1045

Ferry J A, Scully R E 1988 Adenoid cystic carcinoma and adenoid basal carcinoma of the uterine cervix: a study of 28 cases. American Journal of Surgical Pathology 12: 134–144

Geisinger K R, Dabbs D J, Marshall R B 1987 Malignant mixed Müllerian tumors. An ultrastructural and immunohistochemical analysis with histogenetic considerations. Cancer 59: 1781–1790

Gershell D J, Mazoujian G, Mutch D G, Rudloff M A 1988 Small cell undifferentiated carcinoma of the cervix. A clinicopathological, ultrastructural and immunocytochemical study of 15 cases. American Journal of Surgical Pathology 12: 684–698

Gershell D J, Duncan D A, Fulling K 1989 Malignant mixed Mullerian tumor of the uterus with neuro-ectodermal differentiation. International Journal of Gynecological Pathology 8: 169–178

Gould V E 1985 The co-expression of distinct classes of intermediate filaments in human neoplasms. Archives of Pathology and Laboratory Medicine 109: 984–985

Griffin N R, Wells M 1990 Immunolocalisation of alpha amylase in ovarian mucinous tumors. International Journal of Gynecological Pathology 9: 41–46

Griffin N R, Wells M, Fox H 1989 Modulation of the antigenicity of amylase in cervical glandular atypia, adenocarcinoma in situ and invasive adenocarcinoma. Histopathology 15: 267–279

Gusterson B A 1987 Commentary: is cytokeratin present in smooth muscle. Histopathology 11: 549–551

Hamilton-Dutoit S J, Lou H, Pallerson G 1990 The expression of placental alkaline phosphatase (PLAP) and PLAP-like enzymes in normal and neoplastic human tissues. Acta Pathologica, Microbiologica et Immunologica Scandinavica 98: 797–811

Hasleton P S, Whittaker J L 1978 Benign and malignant struma ovarii. Archives of Pathology and Laboratory Medicine 102: 180–183

Hurliman J, Gloor E 1984 Adenocarcinoma in-situ and invasive adenocarcinoma of the uterine cervix: an immunohistological study with antibodies specific for several epithelial markers. Cancer 54: 103–109

Hustin J 1978 Immunohistochemical demonstration of several tumor markers in neoplastic and preneoplastic states of the uterine mucosa. Gynecologic Obstetric Investigation 9: 3

Ishiguro T, Oshida Y, Tenzaki T, Oshima M, Susuki H 1981 AFP in yolk sac tumor and solid teratoma of ovary: significance of post operative serum AFP. Cancer 48: 2480–2482

Ishikura H, Scully R E 1987 Hepatoid carcinoma of the ovary. Cancer 60: 2775–2784

Jobling T W, Granowska K E, Britton K E et al 1990 Radioimmunoscintigraphy of ovarian tumors using a new monoclonal antibody SM-3. Gynecologic Oncology 38: 468–472

Kabawat S E, Bast R C, Bhan A K, Welch W R, Knapp R C, Colvin R B 1983 Tissue distribution of a coelomic-epithelium related antigen recognised by the monoclonal antibody OC125. International Journal of Gynecological Pathology 2: 275–285

Kato H, Tongae T 1977 Radioimmunoassay for tumor antigen of human cervical squamous cell carcinoma. Cancer 40: 1621–1628

Khalifa M A, Sesterhen I A 1990 Tumor markers of epithelial ovarian neoplasms. International Journal of Gynecological Pathology 9: 217–230

Knauf S, Urbach G H 1980 Identification, purification and radioimmunoassay of NB/70K, a human tumour associated antigen. Cancer Research 41: 1351–1357

Konishi I, Fujii S, Kataoka N et al 1988 Ovarian mucinous cystadenocarcinoma producing alpha-fetoprotein. International Journal of Gynecological Pathology 7: 182–189

Krag-Jacobsen G K, Jacobsen M, Clausen P P 1981 Distribution of tumor associated antigens in the various histologic components of germ cell tumor of the testis. American Journal of Surgical Pathology 5: 257–266

Kudo R, Sasano H, Kolzumi M, Orenstein J, Silverberg S G 1990 Immunohistochemical comparison of new monoclonal antibody IC5 and carcino-embryonic antigen in the differential diagnosis of adenocarcinoma of the uterine cervix. International Journal of Gynecological Pathology 9: 325–336

Kurman R J, Nadji M 1985 Immunocytochemistry of ovarian neoplasms. In: Roth L M, Czernobilsky B (eds) Tumors and tumor-like conditions of the ovary. Churchill Livingstone, New York, p 207–232

Kurman R J, Norris H J 1976 Embryonal carcinoma of the ovary. A clinicopathological entity distinct from endodermal sinus tumor resembling embryonal carcinoma of adult testis. Cancer 38: 2420–2433

Lang G, Dallenbach-Hellweg G 1990 This histogenetic origin of cervical mesonephric hyperplasia and mesonephric adenocarcinoma of the uterine cervix studied with immunohistochemical methods. International Journal of Gynecological Pathology 9: 145–157

Lappohn R E, Burger H G, Bouma J, Bangah M, Krans M, de Bruijn H W A 1989 Inhibin as a marker for granulosa-cell tumors. New England Journal of Medicine 321: 790–793

Lash R H, Hart W R 1987 Intestinal adenocarcinomas metastatic to ovaries: a clinico-pathological evaluation of 22 cases. American Journal of Surgical Pathology 1: 114–121

Lazarides E 1980 Intermediate filaments as mechanical integrators of cellular space. Nature 283: 249–250

Lee Y, Raju G C 1988 The expression and localisation of amylase in normal and malignant glands of the endometrium and endocervix. Journal of Pathology 155: 201–205

Liao S Y, Choi B H 1986 Expression of glial fibrillary acidic protein by neoplastic cells of Müllerian origin. Virchows Archives (Cell Pathology) 52: 185–193

Liao S Y, Choi B H 1987 The cultured cells of malignant mixed Müllerian tumors and normal endometrium express glial fibrillary acidic protein: a light and EM immunocytochemical study. Laboratory Investigation 56: 43A

Lifschitz-Mercer B, Czernobilsky B, Dgani R, Dallenbach-Hellweg G, Moll R, Franke W W 1987 Immunocytochemical study of an endometrial diffuse clear cell stromal sarcoma and other endometrial stromal sarcomas. Cancer 59: 1494–1499

Lifschitz-Mercer B, Czernobilsky B, Shezen E, Dgoni R, Leitner O, Geiger B 1988 Selective expression of cytokeratin polypeptides in various epithelia of human Brenner tumor. Human Pathology 19: 640–650

Masuko Y, Zalutsk M, Knapp R C, Bast R C 1984 Interaction of monoclonal antibodies with cell surface antigens of human ovarian carcinomas. Cancer Research 44: 2813–2819

Maes G, Flueren G J, Bara J, Nap M 1988 The distribution of mucins, carcino-embryonic antigen and mucus-associated antigens in endocervical and endometrial adenocarcinoma. International Journal of Gynecological Pathology 7: 112–122

Michael H, Grawe L, Kraus F T 1984 Minimal deviation endocervical adenocarcinoma: clinical and histological features, immunohistochemical staining for carcino-embryonic antigen and differentiation from confusing benign lesions. International Journal of Gynecological Pathology 3: 261–276

Miettenen M 1988 Immunoreactivity for cytokeratin and epithelial membrane antigen in leiomyosarcoma. Archives of Pathology and Laboratory Medicine 112: 637–640

Miettenen M, Wahlstrom T, Virtanen I, Talerman A, Astengo-Osuna C 1985 Cellular differentiation in ovarian sex cord–stromal and germ cell tumors studied with antibodies to intermediate filament proteins. American Journal of Surgical Pathology 145: 127–148

Moll R, Levy R, Czernobilsky B, Hohlweg-Majert P, Dallenbach-Hellweg G, Franke W W 1983 Cytokeratins of normal epithelia and some neoplasms of the female genital tract. Laboratory Investigations 49: 599–610

Morris H B, Gatter K C, Pulford et al 1983 Cervical wart virus infection, intraepithelial neoplasia and carcinoma: an immunohistochemical study using a panel of monoclonal antibodies. British Journal of Obstetrics and Gynaecology 90: 1069–1081

Morris W P R, Griffin N R, Wells M 1989 Patterns of reactivity with the monoclonal antibodies HMFG 1, and HMFG 2 in normal endometrium, endometrial hyperplasia and adenocarcinoma. Histopathology 15: 179–186

Motoyama T, Watanabe H, Takeuchi S, Watanabe T, Gotoh S, Okazaki E 1990 Cancer antigen 125, carcinoembryonic antigen and carbohydrate determinant 19-9 in ovarian tumors. Cancer 66: 2628–2635

Niehans G A, Manivel C, Copland G T, Scheithauer B W, Wick M R 1988 Immunohistochemistry of germ cell and trophoblastic neoplasms. Cancer 62: 1113–1123

Nishida M, Jimi S, Haji M, Hayashi I, Kai T, Tasaka H 1991 Case report: juvenile granulosa cell tumor in association with a high serum inhibin level. Gynecologic Oncology 40: 90–94

Norton A J, Thomas J A, Isaacson P G 1987 Cytokeratin specific monoclonal antibodies are reactive with tumours of smooth muscle derivation. An immunohistochemical and biochemical study using antibodies to intermediate filament cytoskeletal proteins. Histopathology 11: 487–500

Nouwen E J, Hendrix P G, Dauwe S, Eerdekens M W, de Broe M E 1987 Tumor markers in the human ovary. American Journal of Pathology 126: 230–241

Ordonez N G, Manning J T, Brooks T E 1988 Effect of trypsinisation on the immunostaining of formalin fixed, paraffin-embedded tissues. American Journal of Surgical Pathology 12: 121–129

Pallesen G, Hamilton-Dutoit S J 1988 Ki-1(CD30) antigen is regularly expressed by tumor cells of embryonal carcinoma. American Journal of Pathology 133: 446–450

Pavelic Z P, Pavelic L, Pavelic K, Peacock J S 1991 Utility of carcinoembryonic antigen monoclonal antibodies for differentiating ovarian adenocarcinoma from gastrointestinal metastasis to ovary. Gynecologic Oncology 40: 112–117

Poels L G, Peters D, van Megen Y et al 1986 Monoclonal antibody against human ovarian tumor associated antigens. Journal of the National Cancer Institute 76: 781–791

Polak J M, van Noorden S 1988 An introduction to immunocytochemistry: current techniques and problems, revised edn. Microscopy Handbooks II. Oxford University Press, Oxford

Puts J J G, Moesker O, Aldeweireldt H, Vooijs G P, Raemaekers F C S 1987 Application of antibodies to intermediate filaments in simple and complex tumors of the female genital tract. International Journal of Gynecological Pathology 6: 257–274

Raju G C 1988 Expression of cytokeratin markers CAM 5.2 in cervical neoplasia. Histopathology 12: 437–438

Ramaekers F, Feitz W, Moesker O et al 1985 Antibodies to cytokeratin and vimentin in testicular tumour diagnosis. Virchows Archives A Pathological Anatomy 405: 127–142

Ramaekers F, van Niekerk C, Poels L et al 1990 Use of monoclonal antibodies to keratin in differential diagnosis of adenocarcinomas. American Journal of Pathology 136: 641–655

Sahin A, Benda J A 1988 An immunohistochemical study of primary ovarian sarcoma. International Journal of Gynecological Pathology 7: 268–279

Santini D, Gelli M C, Mazzoleni et al 1989 Brenner tumor of the ovary: a correlative, histologic, histochemical, immunohistological and ultrastructural investigation. Human Pathology 20: 787–795

Sasaki E, Sasano N, Kimura N, Andoh N, Yajima A 1989 Demonstrations of neuroendocrine cells in ovarian mucinous tumors. International Journal of Gynecological Pathology 8: 189–200

Sasano H, Oakamoto M, Mason J I et al 1989 Immunohistochemical studies of steroidogenic enzymes (aromatose, 17 alpha hydroxylase and cholesterol side-chain cleavage cytochromes P-450) in sex cord-stromal tumors of the ovary. Human Pathology 20: 452–457

Sasano H, Mason J I, Sasaki E et al 1990 Imumunohistochemical study of 3 beta hydroxy steroid dehydrogenase in sex cord-stromal tumors of the ovary. International Journal of Gynecological Pathology 9: 325–336

Seldenrijk C A, Willig A P, Baak J P A et al 1986 Malignant Brenner tumor. Cancer 58: 754–760

Shevchuck M M, Fenoglio C M, Richart R M 1980 Histogenesis of Brenner tumors. II Histochemistry and CEA. Cancer 46: 2617–2622

Smith L H, Teng N H 1987 Clinical applications of monoclonal antibodies in gynecologic oncology. Cancer 60: 2068–2074

Speers W C, Picaso L G, Silverberg S G 1983 Immunohistochemical localisation of carcino-embryonic antigen in microglandular hyperplasia and adenocinoma of the endocervix. American Journal of Clinical Pathology 79: 105–107

Sporrong B, Falkmer S, Robboy S J 1982 Neuro-hormonal peptides in ovarian carcinoids. Cancer 49: 68–74

Steeper T A, Wick M R 1986 Minimal deviation adenocarcinoma of the uterine cervix ("adenoma malignum"). An immunohistochemical comparison with microglandular endocervical hyperplasia and conventional adenocarcinoma. Cancer 58: 1131–1138

Syrjanen S, Cintorino M, Armellini D et al 1988 Expression of cytokeratin polypeptides in human papilloma virus (HPV) lesions of the uterine cervix. 1. Relationship to grade of CIN and HPV type. International Journal of Gynecological Pathology 7: 23–38

Tagliabue E, Menord S, Torre G D et al 1985 Generation of monoclonal antibodies reacting with human epithelial ovarian cancer. Cancer Research 45: 379–385

Tetu B, Ordonez N G, Silva E G 1986 Sertoli-Leydig cell tumor of the ovary with alpha fetoprotein production. Archives of Pathology and Laboratory Medicine 110: 65–68

Thor A, Ohuchi N, Szpak C A, Johnson W W, Schlom J 1986 Distribution of neofetal antigen tumour associated glycoprotein-72 defined by monoclonal antibody B72.3. Cancer Research 46: 3118–3124

Thor A, Viglione M J, Muraro R, Ohuchi N, Schlom J, Gorstein F 1987 Monoclonal antibody B72.3. reactivity with human endometrium: A study of normal and malignant tissues. International Journal of Gynecological Pathology 6: 235–247

Tobon H, Dave H 1988 Adenocarcinoma in situ of the cervix: clinicopathologic observations of 11 cases. International Journal of Gynecological Pathology 7: 139–151

Tsuji Y, Suzuki T, Nishiara H, Takemura T, Isojima S 1985 Identification of two different surface epitopes of human ovarian epithelial carcinomas by monoclonal antibodies. Cancer Research 45: 2358–2362

Ueda G, Shimizu C, Shimizu H et al 1988 An immunohistochemical study of small-cell and poorly differentiated carcinomas of the cervix using neuroendocrine markers. Gynecologic Oncology 34: 164–169

Van Nagell J R, Hudson S, Gay E C et al 1982 Carcinoembryonic antigen in carcinoma of the uterine cervix. Cancer 49: 379–383

Vergote I, Mathias O, Nustad K 1987 Placental alkaline phosphatase as a tumor marker in ovarian carcinoma. Obstetrics and Gynecology 69: 228–232

Wagener C, Petzold P, Kohler W, Totovic V 1984 Binding of five monoclonal anti-CEA antibodies with different epitope specificities to various carcinoma tissues. International Journal of Cancer 33: 469–475

Wahlstrom T, Lindgren J, Korhonen M, Segala M 1979 Distinction between endocervical and endometrial adenocarcinoma with immunoperoxidase staining of carcinoembryonic antigen in routine histological tissue specimens. Lancet 2: 1159–1160

Warhol M J, Antonioli D A, Pinkus G S, Burke L, Rice R H 1982 Immunoperoxidase staining for involucrin. A potential diagnostic aid in cervico-vaginal pathology. Human Pathology 13: 1095–1099

Wells M, Brown L J R, Jackson P 1986 Low molecular weight cytokeratin proteins in cervical neoplasia (letter). Journal of Pathology 150: 69–70

Wolpert H R, Fuller A F, Bell D A 1989 Primary mucinous carcinoid tumor of the ovary. International Journal of Gynecological Pathology 8: 156–162

Young R H, Scully R E 1987 Sex cord-stromal, steroid cell and other ovarian tumors with endocrine, paraendocrine and paraneoplastic manifestations. In Kurman R J (ed) Blaustein's pathology of the female genital tract. Springer-Verlag, New York, p 607–658

Young R H, Perez-Atayde A R, Scully R E 1984 Ovarian Sertoli–Leydig cell tumor with retiform and heterologous components. Report of a case with hepatocytic differentiation and elevated serum alpha-fetoprotein. American Journal of Surgical Pathology 8: 709–718

4. Oncogenes in gynaecological cancer

Marigold Curling   James V. Watson

INTRODUCTION

Abnormality of specific gene function has long been proposed as a contributory factor in malignant transformation (Huebner & Todaro 1967), and retroviral oncogenes have been described which are responsible for oncogenesis in animals (Cooper & Neiman 1980, Bishop 1984). Genes resembling the oncogenes of retroviruses have been found to be normal cellular constituents (Stehlin et al 1976, Bishop 1984, Cooper & Lane 1984, Varmus 1984). These are variously referred to as cellular oncogenes (c-*onc*) or proto-oncogenes, and derangement of their expression is associated with cancer (Krontiris 1983).

These genes can be divided into two major categories, those encoding cytoskeleton elements (Naharro et al 1984, Martin-Zanca et al 1986), about which little is known except that they may be involved with metastasis, and those encoding proteins involved in proliferation control. The latter may also be subdivided into two categories: those with positive- and those with negative-feedback control functions. Six subclasses of genes with positive growth regulatory control functions have now been defined: extracellular signal transmitters, membrane receptors, transmembrane transducers, cytoplasmic signal transmitters, nuclear signal receivers and nuclear transducers. A number of genes encode proteins that are responsible for growth suppression; the loss of normal function results in increased proliferation because of failure of part of a negative feedback mechanism.

VIRUSES AND CANCER

It is now accepted that cancer has a genetic basis; the original experiments that established this were performed by Peyton Rous, who observed that cell free filterable tumour extracts could transmit sarcomas in chickens (Rous 1911). However, the first suspicion that hereditary factors might be involved in cancer was voiced by Norris (1820), based on observations of what was probably malignant melanoma occurring in successive generations of the same family. Other than Rous' work, little of significance took place in the first half of this century. In 1951 it was reported that a virus induced murine leukaemia could be transmitted vertically from one generation to the next (Gross 1951). In 1958 it was shown that mouse parotid tumours grown in vitro resulted in propagation of an oncogenic virus (Stewart et al 1958). This virus was subsequently shown to induce tumours in rats, mice, hamsters, rabbits and guinea-pigs, and was called polyoma in recognition of its cross-species oncogenic potential. Furthermore, purified DNA from polyoma virus was found to be oncogenic, and Friend (1965) showed that this virus could transform cells in vitro.

Many of the oncogenic viruses, including the Rous sarcoma pathogen, are RNA viruses. The discovery of this had profound consequences not only for oncology but also for the whole of biology. The transcription of DNA to RNA and translation of RNA to protein are thermodynamically driven towards protein, but the reaction is also possible in the other direction. The very existence of RNA viruses containing no DNA signalled that there must be a mechanism for converting the message in the RNA sequence back into DNA. The enzyme responsible for this retroconversion, reverse transcriptase, was isolated from Rous sarcoma virus in 1970 by Baltimore and by Temin and Mizutani, and this work ushered in the era of recombinant DNA technology.

The genome of the non-oncogenic RNA viruses is small, with only three genes. These are *gag*, *pol* and *env*, encoding core protein, reverse transcriptase and envelope respectively. When infection with RNA virus takes place the cell accepts the injected RNA as its own messenger, which is then translated to protein. The protein product of the *pol* gene is reverse transcriptase. This constructs a DNA copy complementary to the RNA of the virus, which is spliced into the host cell's genome. The term retrovirus derives from this ability to perform the retroconversion of RNA into DNA and hence replication using the DNA synthesis mechanisms of the cell. Duesberg & Vogt (1970), using ribonuclease-induced partial deletions, showed that the Rous sarcoma virus contains an extra gene, *src* (an acronym derived from sarcoma). The genomes of most of the oncogenic retroviruses also contain an extra gene, which may be one of many; each is named after the tumour with which that particular oncogene is associated. The gene associated with chicken myelocytomatosis is called *myc*; *myb* derives from chicken myeloblastosis; and *ras* from rat sarcoma. There are two major *ras* gene families named after the discoverers of the transmitting agents, Harvey (Ha- or H-*ras*) and Kirsten (Ki- or K-*ras*).

The various non-human oncogenic viruses were regarded as interesting curiosities with little or no relevance to human cancer until Stehlin et al (1976) reported that the *src* gene has a homologue in perfectly normal cells. This was a seminal discovery and absolute confirmation of a genetic basis of cancer was obtained by transfection—incorporation of DNA foreign to the cell into its genome. Although the frequency of transfectants is generally low, it was shown that DNA from human bladder and lung cancers could give rise to transformation of 3T3 mouse fibroblasts (Weinberg 1981). The genes responsible for the malignant change were found to belong to the *ras* family (Der et al 1982).

By 1982 it had been shown that many oncogenes in RNA viruses have cellular homologues (Bishop and Varmus 1982). This gave rise to a nomenclature problem, which was resolved by adding a 'v-' prefix to the viral gene identifier and a 'c-' prefix to the cellular counterpart (Coffin et al 1981). It is now clear that oncogenes of RNA viruses were derived from cellular genes. The evidence for this comes firstly from a comparison of the genetic structure in RNA viruses and eukaryotes. A typical gene of, say, 1000 bases in eukaryotic cells may in fact span 20–30 kb in the genome and is divided into regions called introns and exons. The whole of the gene is transcribed to RNA. The introns are excised and the exons are spliced end-to-end to form the messenger RNA which is then translated to protein. The genetic code of RNA viruses does not contain introns. Furthermore, the RNA is constructed by a cell and must originally have been derived from the DNA of a cell. Initial confirmation of this was obtained by Hanafusa et al (1977). Rous sarcoma virus mutants deficient in segments of the v-*src* oncogene were used to infect chickens but the characteristic sarcomas did not develop. However, when virus was recovered and used to reinfect different animals, the tumours were induced. The partially deleted v-*src* gene had been reconstituted in the virus particles after one passage through animals, and could only have been reconstructed from the cellular homologue.

MOLECULAR PATHOLOGY IN ONCOGENES

It has been known for years that various chromosomal abnormalities are associated with cancer (see review by Gilbert 1983). Some of these are gross, with duplication of one, several or all chromosomes, and others are more subtle. A number of molecular mechanisms, including gene amplification, mutation, promoter insertion, translocation, deletion and rearrangements, are now known to be implicated in cancer. The 'Philadelphia' chromosome (Rowley 1973) is a not infrequent finding in chronic myeloid leukaemia and results from a 9:22 translocation. The c-*abl* oncogene is located at the breakpoint (de Klein et al 1982). The c-*mos* gene is associated with the 8:21 translocation in acute myeloid leukaemia (Neel et al 1982). The c-*myc* gene is translocated from chromosome 8 to 14 (most commonly) or to chromosomes 2 or 22 in Burkitt's lymphoma. The 8:14 translocation joins c-*myc* to the immunoglobulin γ_1 genes (Hamlyn & Rabbitts 1983), possibly removing c-*myc* from its normal control region and so giving rise to activation. c-Ki-*ras* is amplified, over-expressed and associated with karyotypic abnormalities in mouse adrenocortical tumour cells (Schwab et al 1983a).

Any chromosome abnormality which can be demonstrated by existing banding patterns represents massive genomic rearrangements in molecular terms. However, very subtle changes, not apparent by banding, may have profound consequences. The avian leukosis virus, unlike most retroviruses, does not contain an extra gene (Cooper & Neiman 1980). In cells infected with this virus, the new DNA complementary to the viral RNA was found to have been inserted close to the c-*myc* gene. This gave rise to a 50-fold increase in the number of c-*myc* mRNA copies with concomitant malignant transformation (Hayward et al 1981). Apart from the specific genes, the retroviruses contain flanking long terminal repeats. These genomic segments are thought to be involved in the insertion process and in 'promoting' activation of the genes after insertion. Complementary avian leukosis virus DNA close to the c-*myc* gene may, therefore, activate the gene by alteration of normal promoter function or by insertion of the viral promoter.

Gene amplification has been found in a myelocytic cell line and in the primary tumour from which the cell line was derived (Favera et al 1982). In one patient with chronic myelocytic leukaemia, the c-*myc* gene was amplified 16-fold and rearranged within the genome during episodes of transformation (McCarthy et al 1984). Amplification of the c-*myc* gene has also been reported in cell lines derived from a group of patients with small cell lung cancer who had a very poor prognosis (Little et al 1983). A gene which bears some homology with c-*myc* is amplified up to 100-fold in both neuroblastoma (Schwab et al 1983b) and retinoblastoma (Lee et al 1984), and is called N-*myc*. As yet, we have very little idea of how these tumours are produced in humans. However, a variety of carcinogens can each induce reliable mutation of specific cellular genes that are associated with oncogenic tumours in experimental animals. These include a methylbenzanthracine-induced mouse papilloma and c-Ha-*ras* (Balmain et al 1984), γ-radiation-induced thymic lymphoma and c-Ki-*ras* in the mouse (Guerrero et al 1984a), a number of nitrosourea compounds associated with mouse breast carcinoma and c-Ha-*ras* (Sukumar et al 1983), mouse thymic lymphoma and N-*ras* (Guerrero et al 1984b), and rat neuroblastoma and c-*neu* (Schechter et al 1984).

Cellular homologues of viral oncogenes were found to be often associated with translocation breakpoints, and this finding gave rise to searches for oncogenes at known chromosome breakpoints and deleted regions. Perhaps the best example is the heritable tumour, retinoblastoma (Knudson 1971, 1978), in which a visible deletion involving band 14 on the long arm of chromosome 13 (13q14) is found in a small proportion of cases (Knudson et al 1976, Yunis & Ramsey 1978). It is now established that genetic abnormalities in retinoblastoma are consistently present at 13q14 and are not random (Benedict et al 1983a). Patients who have one affected and one normal chromosome 13 have a predisposition to retinoblastoma (Benedict et al 1983b, Cavenee et al 1983). Development of the tumour is a consequence of somatic mutation at 13q14 in the single normal chromosome. The retinoblastoma gene (RB) has now been cloned (Friend et al 1986). Similar phenomena have been identified in a number of hereditary human tumours (Knudson 1985), including Wilms' tumour and familial adenomatous polyposis. The latter carries a well-defined risk of carcinoma which, at any given age, is about three times greater than that in the normal population (McKusic 1962, Ashley 1969). The molecular pathology in familial adenomatous polyplasia and associated tumours is more complex than in retinoblastoma: lesions at a number of chromosome sites have been implicated including 5q21–q22, 17p12–p13 and 18q21–qterminus and genes from the latter two regions have been cloned (Baker et al 1989, Fearon et al 1990).

ONCOPROTEIN FUNCTION

Although specific biochemical functions have been assigned to some of the oncoproteins (Bishop 1985) we do not, as yet, know how those functions, or the derangement of those functions, produce the neoplastic phenotype. Duesberg (1985), playing devil's advocate, has pointed out that the only 'true' oncogenes are those found in retroviruses. These genes have the capacity not only to induce but also to maintain malignant transformation, apparently in a single step by insertion of either a gene or a long terminal repeat, or both. Moreover, the oncogenes found in retroviruses are not identical to their cellular homologues (Hunter 1984); as a result of the molecular pathology induced by carcinogenesis, either the coding or control regions of the proto-oncogenes are modified (Krontiris 1983, Cooper & Lane 1984). These changes can alter the normal growth control processes by increased, or inappropriate, production of normal oncogene products, or by expression of aberrant proteins (Der & Cooper 1983, Stewart et al 1984). However, although our lack of physiological understanding is great, there are some very interesting observations which should eventually come together into a coherent principle.

The c-*sis* gene encodes a subunit of platelet-derived growth factor (Doolittle et al 1983, Waterfield et al 1983): the v-*sis* protein can transform appropriate cells but platelet derived growth factor cannot. However, *sis* encodes only the $\beta 2$ subunit of the growth factor, and the product of either v-*sis* or its cellular homologue may not have to be secreted from the cell to produce transformation (Betsholtz et al 1984). Hence, inappropriately increased production of the $\beta 2$ subunit may short-circuit one of the normal proliferation control mechanisms in the cell.

v-*erb* and c-*fms* respectively encode the intracellular domain of epidermal growth factor receptor (Downward et al 1984) and the transmembrane receptor for the macrophage colony stimulating factor, CSF-1, (Scherr et al 1984). The c-*erb*-B2 gene, also called *HER2* and *neu*, encodes a membrane protein that is serologically related to epidermal growth factor receptor (Schechter et al 1984, Gullick 1990).

A regulatory group of proteins called G-proteins have been shown to have homology with *ras* proteins (Dhar et al 1984, Hurley et al 1984, Papageorge et al 1984, Powers et al 1984). The product of the N-*ras* gene, $p21^{N\text{-}ras}$, seems to link the effects of growth-factor stimulation of receptors with inositol phospholipid metabolism (Wakelman et al 1986), which is increased in cells stimulated into the division cycle. Increased phosphoinositol turnover is mediated via a guanine nucleotide regulatory G-protein which may, therefore, be $p21^{N-ras}$ or a closely related protein.

A number of nuclear-associated DNA-binding proteins that are likely to be growth-regulatory receivers and transducers are encoded by oncogenes. These include oestrogen receptor (Green et al 1986), which has extensive homology with c-*erb*-A encoding thyroid-hormone receptor (Sap et al 1986, Weinberger et al 1986), and the protein products of the c-*myc* and c-*fos* genes, $p62^{c-myc}$ and $p55^{c-fos}$, respectively. The normal c-*fos* protein is a factor necessary for transcription (Distel et al 1987, Lech et al 1988) and does not induce transformation but modification of the carboxy terminus by manipulation of the gene can give rise to transformation (Miller et al 1984). The functions of c-*myc* and related proteins of the myc family (encoded by the N-*myc*, L-*myc* and v-*myc* genes) are not known, although the evidence suggests that the c-*myc* product is involved in regulation of cell proliferation (Kelly et al 1983, 1984, Greenberg & Ziff 1984, Makino 1984, Rabbitts et al 1985) and possibly in differentiation (Pfeiffer-Ohlsson et al 1984, Stewart et al 1984a). The protein products of the mouse c-*myc* and human c-*myc*, and of N-*myc* and L-*myc* genes, share a common amino acid sequence, the 'leucine zipper', in conserved regions (Landschultz et al 1988). This is also found in $p55^{c-fos}$, the yeast DNA regulatory protein GCN4, and the protein encoded by the *jun* oncogene which also has transcriptional activity (Vogt et al 1987, Landschultz et al 1988). $p62^{c-myc}$ is one of a discrete set of non-histone and non-nuclear matrix proteins which elute from the nucleus at salt the concentrations below 200 mmol/l (Evan & Hancock 1985). This evidence, taken with the structure of the conserved region, suggests that these proteins have a DNA binding function that can be modulated rapidly by ionic changes within physiological concentrations. The turnover of both the protein and its mRNA is rapid, with half-lives in the order of 20–30 min in exponentially growing cells (Hann et al 1985, Rabbitts et al 1985). c-*myc* mRNA increases within 2 h of serum stimulation in serum-deprived cells but does not, thereafter, show a cyclical variation correlating with cell-cycle phase; it does not decrease in density-arrested cells cultured in the presence of growth factors (Thompson et al 1985). There is some evidence that $p62^{c-myc}$ is intimately involved in the replicon complex of proteins responsible for initiation and maintenance of DNA synthesis (Studzinski et al 1986). More recently, it has been shown that this protein induces a shortening of the cell cycle by shortening the G_1 phase, with no significant alteration of the S, G_2 or M phases (Karn et al 1989).

Many of these proteins, including those encoded by *erb*-B, *fms*, *yes*, *src*, *ras*, *mos* and *fes*, to mention but a few, have protein kinase activity (Hunter & Cooper 1985). $p60^{v-src}$ phosphorylates tyrosine (Hunter & Sefton 1980) is found in adhesion plaques of infected cells (Rohrschneider 1980); as with $p55^{c-fos}$, there is also a difference between the carboxy termini of $p60^{v-src}$ and $p60^{c-src}$ that may be related to the transforming capacity of the former

(Takeya & Hanafusa 1983). These findings aroused interest as tyrosine is one of the more unusual amino acids to undergo phosphorylation, and the cytoskeleton protein vinculin is abundant in adhesion plaques. It anchors actin microfilaments to the plasma membrane, as part of the mechanism responsible for adherence of cells to the substratum. The tyrosine residues of vinculin are specifically hyperphosphorylated by a factor of about eight in Rous sarcoma virus-infected cells compared with those that are not infected (Sefton et al 1981). This modifies the protein's normal function. In one study, cells infected with heat sensitive Rous sarcoma virus mutants (Martin 1970) exhibit dramatic cytoskeleton changes at $p60^{v-src}$-permissive temperatures. Within 15–20 min of a temperature decrease 'flowers', observed by fluorescence microscopy, appeared on the upper surface of infected cells. These 'flowers' were composed of myosin, tropomyocin, α-actin and actin (Boschek et al 1981). These observations may link growth regulatory signalling with cytoskeleton derangements and with metastatic potential.

The discovery of allelic loss at the RB 13q14 deletion site, and hence complete loss of normal function, led Knudson (1983) to use the term 'anti-oncogene' to describe the type of gene function that normally suppresses tumour formation. The abnormality results from failure of a negative feedback mechanism (Comings 1973) which has now been identified in a number of hereditary human tumours (Knudson 1985). The chromosome 17 deletions in colorectal carcinoma are associated with p53 gene mutations (Baker et al 1989); increasing evidence suggests that normal p53, discovered a decade ago in cells infected with the SV40 DNA virus (Lane & Crawford 1979, Linzer & Levine 1979), has tumour-suppressor function (Wolf & Rotter 1985, Masuda et al 1987, Munroe et al 1988, Finlay et al 1988). It is thought that p53 is involved not only in transformation (Eliyahu et al 1984) but also in cell proliferation (Milner & McCormick 1980, Milner & Milner 1981, Sarnow et al 1981, Mercer et al 1982). Raised concentrations are found in cells transformed by radiation and chemicals as well as by viral agents (Deleo et al 1979, Lane & Crawford 1979, Linzer & Levine 1979, Rotter et al 1981, Rotter 1983). It may play a part in regulation of DNA synthesis, as microinjection of an anti-p53 monoclonal antibody inhibits growth factor-induced DNA synthesis (Mercer et al 1982). However, p53 is a normal nuclear protein that has a part in the control of proliferation (Milner & McCormick 1980, Mercer et al 1982, Reich & Levine 1984).

We can surmise that expression of p53 must be under extremely strict regulation in normal cells in order to contain its oncogenic potential. This control could operate at several levels including regulation of transcription (Milner & Milner 1981), mRNA transcript copy number (Reich et al 1983) and protein turnover (Oren et al 1981, Reich et al 1983). It also appears to exist in at least two distinct forms. A number of antibodies have been raised to this protein; it has been shown that one antibody recognizes a p53 epitope in quiescent cells that is occluded after stimulation and becomes inaccessible to the antibody. A second antibody attaches to an epitope after stimulation that is not exposed before stimulation (Milner 1984, Milner & Watson 1990). Both antibodies immunoprecipitate at 53 kD. These results suggest that, after stimulation, there may be a conformational change in the protein related to the different functional states of quiescent and stimulated cells.

RELEVANCE OF ONCOGENES TO GYNAECOLOGICAL CANCER

Various aspects of oncogene expression have been studied in a number of gynaecological cancers. Over-expression of epidermal growth factor receptor has been found in carcinomas of the ovary (Bauknecht et al 1988, 1989, Battaglia et al 1989), vulva (Gullick et al 1986), endometrium (Berchuck et al 1989) and cervix (Bauknecht et al 1989, Battaglia et al 1989). About 40% of ovarian cancers and 60% of cervical tumours expressed moderate to high receptor levels. However, as Gullick (1990) has pointed out, these results are not easy to interpret as, in one study, 19 of 20 normal uteri expressed epidermal growth factor receptor but, in contrast, 13 of 40 endometrial adenocarcinomas did not.

Slamon et al (1989) studied *HER-2/neu* gene expression in breast and ovarian cancers and found a good correlation between immunocytochemical staining, Western blotting, and DNA and mRNA hybridization signals. These investigators stressed that it was important to identify which antibodies could be used for immunocytochemistry in formalin-fixed biopsies. Frozen sections had to be used for their studies, as completely negative staining was observed after formalin fixation. Patient survival correlated inversely with *HER-2/neu* gene amplification and its protein expression in ovarian cancer.

Riou et al (1984) studied c-*myc* and c-Ha-*ras* expression in patients with cervical carcinoma in whom there was papilloma virus, and detected both c-*myc* and *ras* gene amplification in over half of patients with FIGO Stage III and IV disease.

Leake & Owens (1990) studied the expression of oestrogen and progesterone receptors in ovarian tissue and found an unusual distribution in normal ovary. In most target tissues, synthesis of progesterone receptor is induced by oestrogens mediated via the oestrogen receptor. However, progesterone receptor are much more common than oestrogen receptor in normal ovary: 84% have significant amounts of soluble progesterone receptor, but only 35% had soluble oestrogen receptor, all of which also contained progesterone receptor (Soutter & Leake 1987). Leake & Owens (1990) stressed the need to quantitate functional receptors; they found significantly better survival in 35 patients who had advanced ovarian cancer that was progesterone receptor positive compared with 54 patients whose cancers were negative.

The various results reported above were obtained with bulk techniques or immunocytochemistry. The latter technique has the advantage that the architecture is preserved but suffers from the disadvantage of poor quantitation. Slamon et al (1989) were able to identify tumours that had 'low', 'medium' and 'high' *HER-2/neu* protein expression, and this had a meaningful clinical correlation. Bulk techniques have the disadvantage that the result is a 'grand average' from the whole sampled population, which may mask the values from minority subsets in heterogeneous populations. Our approach has been to use flow cytometric systems (Watson 1987) with fluorescence quantitation of antibody-probed oncogene-encoded proteins and DNA simultaneously, to try to overcome some of these problems (Watson et al 1985). However, as a single-cell suspension is mandatory with this method, we lose the morphological information that is obtained with immunocytochemistry. The technique was adapted from that of Hedley et al (1983); nuclei are released by cytoplasmic digestion after dewaxing and rehydration of tissue sections, and are subsequently probed for nuclear associated antigens.

In one study, 127 biopsies of cervical neoplasms were assayed for $p62^{c\text{-}myc}$ content (Hendy-Ibbs et al 1987). Biopsies of normal cervix had higher protein levels than carcinomas and there was a progressive decrease in level with progression from CIN 1 to CIN 3. Furthermore, the maximum fluorescence signal in the normal tissues occurred at a lower antibody concentration than in tumour tissue. There was no correlation with histological grade, stage, age or prognosis in patients with invasion. These results were totally unexpected, particularly in view of the findings of Riou et al (1984), who used Northern blotting for mRNA. An increase in either the gene or mRNA copy number (or both), which should give rise to an increased protein production rate, need not necessarily be reflected in a marked increase in the total protein content. There are two reasons for this. Firstly, inappropriately increased message may result in rate limitation at the protein synthesis level. Secondly, there may be an increase in protein degradation. The latter is most likely to occur with a protein that has a short half-life and, clearly, this is a distinct possibility for $p62^{c\text{-}myc}$, which has a half-life of 20–30 minutes in rapidly cycling and stimulated cells (Greenberg & Ziff 1984, Rabbitts et al 1985). The lower absolute levels in carcinoma of the cervix than in normal mucosa may therefore reflect increased protein turnover and an increased cell production rate in the former. A further possibility is that post-translational protein modification in cervical carcinoma gives rise to an alteration or partial occlusion of the epitope recognized by the antibody, and to an increase in the susceptibility of the protein to proteolysis in neoplastic cells during the preparation for the assay. There was some evidence that post-translational protein modification may occur in cervical carcinoma. The antibody used for these experiments was raised to a synthetic peptide corresponding to sequences of the normal protein; maximum binding was observed at different antibody concentrations in the normal and malignant cells. This may indicate a change in binding constant and hence a difference in protein structure.

This technique was also used to study serous papillary ovarian carcinoma, which expressed significantly higher $p62^{c-myc}$ levels compared with normal ovary (Watson et al 1987). Biopsies classified as 'borderline' or 'low potential malignancy' had levels between normal ovary and invasive carcinoma. The difference between normal tissue and borderline tumours was significant, but no difference between levels in borderline and invasive tumours was found. No difference was found in $p62^{c-myc}$ in the different histological grades of carcinomas. All normal ovaries had a diploid DNA content as did 5 of 6 cases of 'borderline' tumour. Twenty-eight of the 36 cases of carcinoma were aneuploid. There was a statistically significant difference in the distribution of aneuploidy between invasive carcinomas and borderline tumours. It would seem that elevation of $p62^{c-myc}$ preceded the development of aneuploidy in the evolution of the malignant phenotype in ovarian cancer, but there is no evidence to suggest that these are causally related.

CONCLUSIONS

The fundamental pathological diad of cancer is disordered proliferation and metastasis. We are entering a very exciting phase in oncology which has important implications in diagnosis, prognosis, monitoring and therapy, as oncogenes are intimately involved in proliferation regulation and possibly metastasis.

At present, a diagnosis of cancer is confirmed by classical histological methods, predominantly using haemotoxylin and eosin stained sections, which have been with us for over 100 years. These can now be augmented with immunocytochemistry, blotting techniques for DNA, RNA and protein, hybridization and polymerase chain reaction methods, and flow cytometry directed towards specific oncogenes and their products, for identification, localization and quantitation purposes. This will enable biochemical classifications of disease states to be made that are based on the fundamental pathology at the molecular level and not just on the morphological appearances.

As a consequence of this 'neo-pathology', we will obtain better prognostic factors. There is already evidence of this in ovarian cancer with the work of Slamon et al (1989). It is not sufficient, however, simply to produce better prognostic stratification. If that is all we do, we will have fewer and fewer patients in the good prognostic groups and more and more in the bad, with no change in the overall results. Better prognostic factors will enable us to identify those patients who require more aggressive therapy.

Furthermore, when all the intricate growth-regulation pathways have been unravelled and understood, which will take a long time, we may be able specifically to interrupt pathological regulation mechanisms. This possibility already exists: epidermal growth factor receptor encoded by c-*erb*-B and expressed in many tumours is truncated, and if this does not occur in *any* normal tissues there is a basis for specific therapy. This would be affected by specific antibodies to the truncated extracellular domain coupled with complement or ricin α-chain-mediated cell lysis. This type of specific therapy, directed towards the individual biochemical 'oncogenic' phenotype of a particular tumour in an individual patient, irrespective of its classical histological appearances, is the 'holy grail' of cancer therapy. It is unlikely to be realized within the first few decades of the next millenium, but it will take place.

REFERENCES

Ashley D J B 1969 Colonic cancer arising in polyposis coli. J Med Genet 6: 376–378

Baker S J, Fearon E R, Nigro J M et al 1989 Chromosome 17 deletions and p53 gene mutations in colorectal carcinoma. Science 244: 217–221

Balmain A, Ramsden M, Bowden G T, Smith J 1984 Activation of the mouse Harvey-*ras* gene in chemically induced benign skin papillomas. Nature 307: 658–660

Baltimore D 1970 RNA-dependent DNA polymerase in virons of RNA tumour viruses. Nature 226: 1209–1211

Battaglia F, Scambia G, Benedetti Panici P et al 1989 Epidermal growth factor receptor expression in gynaecological malignancies. Gynaecol Obstet Invest 27: 42–44

Bauknecht T, Runge M, Schwall M, Pfleiderer A 1988 Occurrence of epidermal growth factor receptors in human adnexal tumours and their prognostic value in advanced ovarian carcinomas. Gynecol Oncol 29: 147–157

Bauknecht T, Kohler M, Janz I, Pfleiderer A 1989 The occurrence of epidermal growth factor receptors and the characterisation of EGF-like factors in human ovarian, endometrial, cervical and breast cancer. J Cancer Res Clin Oncol 115: 193–199

Benedict W F, Banerjee A, Mark C, Murphee A L 1983a Non-random chromosomal changes in untreated retinoblastoma. Cancer Genet Cytogenet 10: 311–333

Benedict W F, Murphee A L, Banerjee A et al 1983b Patient with 13 chromosome deletion: evidence that the retinoblastoma gene is a recessive cancer gene. Science 219: 973–975

Berchuck A, Soisson A P, Olt G J et al 1989 Epidermal growth factor receptor expression in normal and malignant endometrium. Am J Obstet Gynecol 161: 1247–1252

Betsholtz C, Wetermark B, Ek B, Heidin C H 1984 Coexpression of a PDGF-like growth factor and PDGF receptors in a human osteosarcoma cell line: implications for autocrine receptor activation. Cell 39: 447–457

Bishop J M 1984 Trends in oncogenes. Trends Genet 1: 245–249

Bishop J M 1985 Viral oncogenes. Cell 32: 23–36

Bishop J M, Varmus H 1982 Functions and origins of retroviral transforming genes. In: Weiss R, Teich N, Varmus H, Coffin J, (eds) Molecular biology of tumor viruses, Part III, RNA tumor viruses. Cold Spring Harbor Press, New York, p 999–1108

Boschek C B, Jockusch B M, Friis R R, Back R, Grundmann E, Bauer H 1981 Early changes in the distribution and organization of microfilament proteins during cell transformation. Cell 24: 175–184

Cavenee W K, Dryja T P, Phillips R A et al 1983 Expression of recessive alleles by chromosomal mechanisms in retinoblastoma. Nature 305: 779–784

Coffin J H, Varmus H E, Bishop J M et al 1981 Proposal for naming host cell derived inserts in retrovirus genomes. J Virol 40: 953–957

Comings D E 1973 A general theory of carcinogenesis. Proc Natl Acad Sci USA 70: 3324–3328

Cooper G M, Lane M A 1984 Cellular transforming genes and oncogenes. Biochem Biophys Acta 738: 9–20

Cooper G M, Neiman E 1980 Transforming genes of neoplasms induced by avian leukosis virus. Nature 287: 656–659

Deleo A B, Jay G, Appella E, Dubois G C, Law L W, Old J 1979 Detection of a transformation-related antigen in chemically induced sarcomas and other transformed cells in the mouse. Proc Natl Acad Sci USA 76: 2420–2424

Der C J, Cooper G M 1983 Altered gene products are associated with activation of cellular ras^K genes in human lung and colon carcinomas. Cell 32: 201–208

Der C J, Krontiris T G, Cooper G M 1982 Transforming genes of human bladder and lung carcinoma cell lines are homologous to the ras gene of Harvey and Kirsten sarcoma viruses. Proc Natl Acad Sci USA 79: 3637–3640

Dhar R, Nieto A, Koller R, DeFeo-Jones D, Scolnick E M 1984 Nucleotide sequence of two ras^H related-genes isolated from the yeast *Saccharomyces cerevisiae*. Nucleic Acid Res 12: 3611–3619

Distel R J, Ro H-S, Rosen B S, Groves D L, Spiegelman B M 1987 Nucleoprotein complexes that regulate gene expression in adipocyte differentiation: direct participation of *fos*. Cell 49: 835

Doolittle R F, Hunkerpiller M W, Hood L E et al 1983 Simian sarcoma virus *onc* gene, v-*sis*, is derived from the gene (or genes) encoding a platelet derived growth factor. Science 211: 275–276

Downward J, Yardem Y, Mayes E et al 1984 Close similarities of epidermal growth factor receptor and v-*erb* B oncogene protein sequences. Nature 307: 521–527

Duesberg P H 1985 Activated proto-oncogenes: Sufficient or necessary for cancer? Science 228: 660–677

Duesberg P H, Vogt P K 1970 Differences between the ribonucleic acids of transforming and non-transforming avian tumor viruses. Proc Natl Acad Sci USA 67: 1673–1680

Eliyahu D, Raz A, Gruss P, Gival D, Oren M 1984 Participation of p53 cellular tumour antigen in transformation of normal embryonal cells. Nature 312: 646–649

Evan G I, Hancock D C 1985 Studies on the interaction of the human c-*myc* protein with cell nuclei: $p62^{c-myc}$ as a member of a discrete subset of nuclear proteins. Cell 43: 253–261

Favera D R, Wong-Staal F, Gallo R. 1982 Oncogene amplification in promyelocytic leukaemia cell line (HL-60) and in the primary from the same patient. Nature 299: 61–63

Fearon E R, Cho K R, Nigro J M et al 1990 Identification of a chromosome 18q gene that is altered in colorectal cancer. Science 247: 1083–1093

Finlay C A, Hinds P W, Levine A J 1988 The p53 proto-oncogene can act as a suppressor of transformation. Cell 57: 1083–1093

Friend M 1965 Cell transformation ability of a temperature sensitive mutant of polyoma virus. Proc Natl Acad Sci USA 53: 486–491

Friend S H, Bernards R, Rogelj S et al 1986 A human DNA segment with properties of the gene that predisposes to retinoblastoma and osteosarcoma. Nature 323: 643–646

Gilbert F 1983 Chromosome aberrations and oncogenes. Nature 303: 475

Green S, Walter P, Kurman V et al 1986 Human oestrogen receptor cDNA: sequence, expression and homology to v-*erb*-A. Nature 320: 134–139

Greenberg M E, Ziff E B 1984 Stimulation of 3T3 cells induces transcription of the c-*fos* proto-oncogene. Nature 311: 433–438

Gross L 1951 Spontaneous leukaemia developing in C3H mice following innoculation, in infancy, with AK-leukaemia extracts, or AK-embryos. Proc Soc Exp Biol Med 76: 27–32

Guerrero I, Villasante A, Corces V, Pellicer A 1984a Activation of a c-K-*ras* oncogene by somatic mutation in mouse lymphomas induced by γ-radiation. Science 225: 1159–1162

Guerrero I, Villasante A, D'Eustachio P, Pellicer A 1984b Isolation, characterization, and chromosome assignment of mouse N-*ras* gene from carcinogen-induced thymic lymphoma. Science 225: 1041–1043

Gullick W J 1990 The role of oncogenes in ovarian cancer. In: Sharp F, Mason W P, Leake R E (eds) Ovarian cancer: Biological and therapeutic challenges. Chapman and Hall, London, p 63–68

Gullick W J, Marsden J J, Whittle N et al 1986 Expression of epidermal growth factor receptors on human cervical, ovarian and vulval carcinomas. Cancer Res 46: 285–292

Hamlyn P H, Rabbitts, T H 1983 Translocation joins the c-*myc* and the immunoglobulin $\gamma\pm$ genes in Burkitt's lymphoma revealing a third exon in the c-*myc* oncogene. Nature 304: 135–139

Hanafusa H, Haplern C C, Buckhagen D L, Kawai S 1977 Recovery of avian sarcoma viruses from tumours induced by transformation-defective mutants. J Exp Med 146: 1735–1747

Hann S R, Thompson C B, Eisenman R N 1985 c-*myc* oncogene protein is independent of the cell cycle in human and avian cells. Nature 314: 366–369

Hayward W S, Neel B G, Ashin S M 1981 Activation of a cellular oncogene by promoter insertion in ALV-induced lymphoid leukaemias. Nature 290: 475–479

Hedley D W, Friedlander M I, Taylor I W, Rugg C A, Musgrove E A 1983 Method for analysis of cellular DNA content of paraffin-embedded pathological material using flow cytometry. J Histochem Cytochem 31: 1333–1335

Hendy-Ibbs P, Cox H, Evan G I, Watson J V 1987 Flow cytometric quantitation of DNA and c-*myc* oncoprotein in archival biopsies of uterine cervix neoplasia. Brit J Cancer 55: 275–282

Huebner R J, Todaro G J 1967 Oncogenes of RNA viruses as determinants of cancer. Proc Natl Acad Sci USA 64: 1087–1094

Hunter T 1984 Oncogenes and proto-oncogenes: How do they differ? J Natl Cancer Inst 73: 773–785

Hunter T, Cooper J A 1985 Protein-tyrosine kinases. Ann Rev Biochem 54: 897–930

Hunter T, Sefton B M 1980 Transforming gene product of Rous sarcoma virus phosphorylates tyrosine. Proc Natl Acad Sci USA 77: 1311–1315

Hurley J B, Simon M I, Teplow D B, Robinshaw J D, Gilman A G 1984 Homologies between signal transducing G proteins and *ras* gene products. Science 226: 860–863

Karn J, Watson J V, Lowe A D, Green S M, Vedeckis W 1989 Regulation of cell cycle duration by c-*myc* levels. Oncogene 4: 773–787

Kelly K, Cochran B H, Stiles C D, Leder P 1983 Cell specific regulation of the c-*myc* gene by lymphocyte mitogens and platelet derived growth factor. Cell 35: 603–610

Kelly K, Cochran B H, Stiles C D, Leder P 1984 The regulation of c-*myc* by growth signals. Curr Topics Microbiol Immunol 113: 117–126

de Klein A, Kessel A G, Grosveld G et al 1982 A cellular oncogene is translocated to the Philadelphia chromosome in chronic myelocytic leukaemia. Nature 300: 765–707

Knudson A G 1971 Mutation and cancer: statistical study of retinoblastoma. Proc Natl Acad Sci USA 68: 820–823

Knudson A G 1978 Retinoblastoma: a prototypic hereditary neoplasm. Semin Oncol 5: 57–60

Knudson A G 1983 Hereditary cancers of man. Cancer Invest 1: 187–193

Knudson A G 1985 Hereditary cancer, oncogenes and antioncogenes. Cancer Res 45: 1437–1443

Knudson A G, Meadows A T, Nichols W W, Hill R 1976 Chromosomal deletion and retinoblastoma. N Engl J Med 295: 1120–1123

Krontiris T G 1983 The emerging genetics of human cancer. N Engl J Med 309: 404–409

Landschultz W H, Johnson P F, McKnight S L 1988 The Leucine Zipper: A hypothetical structure common to a new class of DNA binding proteins. Science 240: 1759

Lane D P, Crawford L V 1979 T-antigen is bound to a host protein in SV40-transformed cells. Nature 278: 261–263

Leake R E, Owens O 1990 The prognostic value of steroid receptors, growth factors and growth factor receptors in ovarian cancer. In: Sharp F, Mason W P, Leake R E (eds) Ovarian cancer: Biological and therapeutic challenges. Chapman and Hall, London, p 65–75

Lech K, Anderson K, Brent R 1988 DNA bound *fos* proteins active transcription in yeast. Cell 52: 179

Lee W W, Murphee A L, Benedict W F 1984 Expression and amplification of the N-*myc* gene in primary retinoblastoma. Nature 309: 458–460

Linzer D I H, Levine A J 1979 Characterization of a 54K dalton cellular SV40 tumour antigen present in SV40-transformed cells and uninfected embryonal carcinoma cells. Cell 17: 43–52

Little C D, Nau M M, Carney D N, Gazdar A F, Minna J D 1983 Amplification and expression of the c-*myc* oncogene in human lung cancer cell lines. Nature 306: 194–196

McCarthy D M, Rassool F V, Goldman J M, Graham S V, Binnie G D 1984 Genomic alterations involving the c-*myc* proto-oncogene locus during the evolution of a case of chronic granulocytic leukaemia. Lancet 2: 1362–1365

McKusic V A 1962 Genetic factors in intestinal polyposis. J Am Med Ass 182: 271–277

Makino R, Hayashi K A, Sugimura T 1984 c-*myc* is induced in rat liver at a very early stage of regeneration or by cycloheximide treatment. Nature 310: 697–698

Martin G S 1970 Rous sarcoma virus; a function required for the maintenance of the transformed state. Nature 227: 1021–1023

Martin-Zanca D, Hughes S H, Barbacid M 1986 A human oncogene formed by the fusion of truncated tropomyosin and protein tyrosine kinase sequences. Nature 319: 743–748

Masuda H, Miller C, Koeffler H P, Battifora H, Cline M J 1987 Rearrangement of the p53 gene in human osteogenic sarcoma. Proc Natl Acad Sci USA 84: 7716–7719

Mercer W E, Nelson D, Deleo A B, Old L J, Baserga R 1982 Microinjection of monoclonal antibody to protein p53 inhibits serum-induced DNA synthesis in 3T3 cells. Proc Natl Acad Sci USA 79: 6309–6312

Miller A D, Curran T, Verma I M 1984 c-*fos* protein can induce cellular transformation: A novel mechanism for activation of a cellular oncogene. Cell 36: 51–60

Milner J 1984 Different forms of p53 detected by monoclonal antibodies in non-dividing and dividing lymphocytes. Nature 310: 143–145

Milner J, McCormick F 1980 Lymphocyte stimulation: concanavalin A induces the expression of a 53K protein. Cell Biol (Int Rep) 4: 663–667

Milner J, Milner S 1981 SV40–53K antigen: A possible role for 53K in normal cells. Virology 112: 785–788

Milner J, Watson J V 1990 Addition of fresh medium induces cell cycle and conformation changes in p53, a tumour suppressor protein. Oncogene 5: 1683–1690

Munroe D G, Rovinski R, Bernstein A, Benchimol S 1988 Loss of highly conserved domain on p53 as a result of gene deletion during Friend virus-induced erythroleukaemia. Oncogene 2: 621–624

Naharro G, Robins K, Reddy E P 1984 Gene product of v-*fgr* onc: hybrid protein contains a portion of actin and a tyrosine-specific protein kinase. Science 223: 63–66

Neel B G, Jhan War S C, Chaganti R S K, Hayward W S 1982 Two human c-*onc* genes are located on the long arm of chromosome 8. Proc Natl Acad Sci USA 79: 7842–7846

Norris W 1820 Case of fungoidal disease. Edinburgh Med Surg J 16: 562–565

Oren M, Malzman W, Levine A J 1981 Post-translational regulation of the 54K cellular tumour antigen in normal and transformed cells. Mol Cell Biol 1: 101–110

Papageorge A G, DeFeo-Jones D, Robinson P, Temeies G, Scolnick E M 1984 *Saccharomyces cerevisiae* synthesizes proteins related to the p21 *ras* found in mammals. Mol Cell Biol 4: 23–29

Pfeiffer-Ohlsson S, Goustin A S, Rydnert J et al 1984 Spatial and temporal pattern of cellular *myc* oncogene expression in developing human placenta; Implications for embryonic cell proliferation. Cell 38: 585–596

Powers S, Kataoka T, Fasano O et al 1984 Genes in S. cerevisiae encoding proteins with domains homologous to the mammalian *ras* proteins. Cell 36: 607–612

Rabbitts P H, Watson J V, Lamond A et al 1985 Metabolism of c-*myc* gene products: c-*myc* mRNA and protein expression in the cell cycle. EMBO J 4: 2009–2015

Reich N C, Levine A J 1984 Growth regulation of a cellular tumour antigen, p53, in non-transformed cells. Nature 308: 199–201

Reich N C, Oren M, Levine A J 1983 Two distinct mechanisms regulate the level of a cellular tumour antigen, p53. Mol Cell Biol 3: 2143–2150

Riou G, Barrois M, Tordjman I, Dutronquay V, Orth G 1984 Presence de genomes de papillonavirus et amplification des oncogenes c-*myc* et c-Ha-*ras* dans des cancers envahissants du col de l'uterus. C R Acad Sci Paris 299: 575–580

Rohrschneider L R 1980 Adhesion plaques of Rous sarcoma virus transformed cells contain the *src* gene product. Proc Natl Acad Sci USA 77: 3514–3518

Rotter V 1983 p53, a transformation-related cellular-encoded protein, can be used as a biochemical marker for the detection of primary mouse tumour cells. Proc Natl Acad Sci USA 80: 2613–2617

Rotter V, Boss M A, Baltimore D J 1981 Increased concentration of an apparently identical cellular protein in cells transformed by either Ableson murine leukaemia or other transforming agents. J Virol 38: 336–346

Rous P 1911 Transmission of a malignant new growth by means of a cell-free filtrate. J Am Med Assoc (Chic) 6: 198–202

Rowley J D 1973 A new consistent chromosomal abnormality in chronic myelogenous leukaemia identified by quinacrine fluorescence and Giemsa staining. Nature 243: 290–293

Sap J, Munoz A, Damm K et al 1986 The c-*erb*-A protein is a high-affinity receptor for thyroid hormone. Nature 324: 635

Sarnow P, Ho Y S, Williams J, Levine A J 1981 Adenovirus Elb-58K tumour antigen and SV40 large tumour antigen are physically associated with the same 54kd cellular protein in transformed cells. Cell 28: 387–394

Schechter A L, Stern D F, Vaidyanathan L et al 1984 The *neu* oncogene: an *erb*-B-related gene encoding a 185,000-M^r tumour antigen. Nature 312: 513–517

Scherr C J, Rettenmier C W, Sacca R et al 1985 The c-*fms* proto-oncogene product is related to the receptor for the mononuclear phagocytic growth factor, CSF 1. Cell 41: 665–676

Schwab M, Alitalo K, Varmus H E, Bishop J M, George D 1983a A cellular oncogene c-Ki-*ras* is amplified, overexpressed and located with karyotypic abnormalities in mouse adrenocortical tumour cells. Nature 303: 497–501

Schwab M, Alitalo K, Klempenauer K H et al 1983b Amplified N-*myc* with limited homology to *myc* cellular oncogene is shared by human neuroblastoma cell lines and a neuroblastoma tumour. Nature 305: 245–248

Sefton B M, Hunter T, Ball E H, Singer S J 1981 Vinculin: a cytoskeletal target for the transforming protein of Rous sarcoma virus. Cell 24: 165–174

Slamon D J, Godolphin W, Jones L A et al 1989 Studies of the HER-2/*neu* proto-oncogene in human breast and ovarian cancer. Science 244: 707–712

Soutter W P, Leake R E 1987 Steroid hormone receptors in gynaecological cancers. In: Bonnar J (ed) Recent advances in obstetrics and gynaecology. Churchill Livingstone, London, p 175–194

Stehlin D, Varmus H E, Bishop J M, Vogt P K 1976 DNA related to transforming genes of avian sarcoma virus is present in normal avian DNA. Nature 260: 170–173

Stewart S E, Eddy B E, Borgese N G 1958 Neoplasms in mice inoculated with a tumour agent carried in tissue culture. J Natl Cancer Inst 20: 1223–1243

Stewart T A, Bellve A R, Leder P 1984a Transcription and promoter usage of the c-*myc* gene in normal somatic and spermatogenic cells. Science 226: 707–710

Stewart T A, Pattengale P K, Leder P 1984 Spontaneous mammary adenocarcinomas in transgenic mice carry and express *MTV*/*myc* fusion genes. Cell 38: 627–637

Studzinski G P, Brelvi Z S, Feldman S C, Watt R A 1986 Participation of c-*myc* in DNA synthesis of human cells. Science 234: 467–470

Sukumar S, Notorio V, Martin-Zanca D, Barbacid M 1983 Induction of mammary carcinomas in rats by nitros-methylurea involves malignant activation of H-*ras*-1 locus by single point mutation. Nature 306: 658–661

Takeya T, Hanafusa H 1983 Structure and sequence of the cellular gene homologous to the RSV *src* gene and the mechanism for generating the transforming virus. Cell 32: 881–890

Temin H, Mizutani S 1970 RNA-dependent DNA polymerase in virons of Rous sarcoma virus. Nature 226: 1211–1213

Thompson C B, Challoner P B, Neiman P E, Groudine M 1985 Levels of c-*myc* oncogene mRNA are invariate throughout the cell cycle. Nature 314: 363–366

Varmus H E 1984 The molecular genetics of cellular oncogenes. Ann Rev Genet 18: 553–612

Vogt P K, Bos T J, Doolittle R F 1987 Homology between the DNA-binding domain of the GCN4 regulatory protein of yeast and the carboxyl-terminal region of a protein coded for by the oncogene *jun*. Proc Natl Acad Sci USA 84: 3316–3319

Wakelman M J O, Davies S A, Houslay M D, McKay I, Marshall C J, Hall A 1986 Normal p21^{N-ras} couples bombesin and other growth factors to inositole phosphate production. Nature 323: 173–176

Waterfield M D, Scrace G T, Whittle N et al 1983 Platelet derived growth factor is structurally related to the putative transforming protein p28^{sis} of simian sarcoma virus. Nature 304: 35–39

Watson J V 1987 Flow cytometry in biomedical science. Nature 325: 741–742

Watson J V, Sikora K E, Evan G I 1985 A simultaneous flow cytometric assay for c-*myc* oncoprotein and cellular DNA in nuclei from paraffin embedded material. J Immunol Methods 83: 179–192

Watson J V, Curling O M, Munn C F, Hudson C H 1987 Oncogene expression in ovarian cancer. A pilot study of the c-*myc* oncoprotein in serous papillary ovarian cancer. Gynecol Oncol 28: 137

Weinberg R A 1981 Use of transfection to analyse genetic information and malignant
    transformation. Biochem Biophys Acta 651: 25–35
Weinberger C, Thompson C C, Ong E S, Lebo R, Gruol D J, Evans R M 1986 The c-*erb*-A
    gene encodes a thyroid hormone receptor. Nature 324: 641
Wolf D, Rotter V 1985 Major deletions in the gene encoding the p53 tumor antigen cause lack
    of p53 expression in HL-60 cells. Proc Natl Acad Sci USA 82: 790–794
Yunis J J, Ramsay N 1978 Retinoblastoma and sub-band deletion of chromosome 13. Am J
    Dis Child 132: 161–163

5. Human papillomavirus associated lesions of the lower female genital tract

Michael Wells

INTRODUCTION

The occurrence of sexually transmitted anogenital warts or condylomata acuminata has been recognized since classical times, but a viral aetiology was suggested only in the 1920s. In the late 1950s, it was first suggested that 'koilocytosis', characterized by cytoplasmic cavitation and nuclear pyknosis in squamous epithelium, was a manifestation of viral infection (Koss & Durfee 1956). In the late 1960s, electron microscopy first showed viral particles in anogenital condylomata (see Schneider 1987), but it was not until 1976 that viruses were demonstrated in condylomas of the cervix (Meisels & Fortin 1976). Around this time, there was also a gradual realization that these condylomata could rarely undergo malignant trans-formation. In the early 1980s it was realized that human papillomavirus (HPV) could also cause so-called noncondylomatous infection of the cervix or flat warts (Reid et al 1980). In the 1980s an increasing association between HPV infection and squamous cell neoplasia of the lower female genital tract emerged (Pfister 1987) and, with the application of a variety of molecular biological techniques, certain 'high risk' viral types have been identified (Anderson & Tidy 1991).

The morphological expression of human papillomavirus infection with or without accompanying intraepithelial neoplasia has led to considerable terminological confusion in the histopathological assessment of biopsy material (Fox & Buckley 1990). Recently, use of the more sensitive technique of the polymerase chain reaction has suggested that the distri-bution of 'high risk' types of virus may be widespread even in histologically normal epithelium (Griffin et al 1990). The relation between the presence of HPV and neoplastic transformation, therefore, is far from clear-cut and it seems likely that other co-factors such as the constituents of tobacco smoke also play a role (Barton et al 1988). It also remains questionable whether the knowledge that tissue is infected by HPV (and, if so, by what particular type) should influence the clinical management of an individual patient.

The general properties of human papillomaviruses have recently been well reviewed (Arends et al 1990, Chang 1990). They are small double-stranded DNA viruses; the virions consist of a central core of DNA enclosed in an outer capsid of viral protein. The viral genome contains a series of protein coding sequences or open reading frames that can be classified as early (E) or late (L), depending on when genes are 'turned on' in the course of a productive infection. The biological function of most open reading frames is established; E6 and E7 open reading frames, for example, code for the major transforming proteins, and the L region largely comprises open reading frames that code for the structural proteins of the viral capsid.

Sixty HPV types have been described so far; new types are identified on the basis of less than 50% homology of their nucleic acids with known types rather than by serology. In future, comparisons of HPV sequences may provide a more logical rationale on which a classification can be based.

METHODS OF DEMONSTRATION

Electron microscopy

Human papillomavirus particles can be demonstrated in only about 50% of condylomata of the external female genital tract, mainly in the nuclei of koilocytic cells (Schneider 1987) (Fig. 5.1). Cervical intraepithelial neoplasia (CIN) grade 3 and invasive cervical carcinoma have been found to be negative for virus particles in all studies. The reason for these disappointing ultrastructural results is that complete viral assembly is required for a positive result and such a manifestation of late gene expression is not always present, particularly in neoplastic lesions.

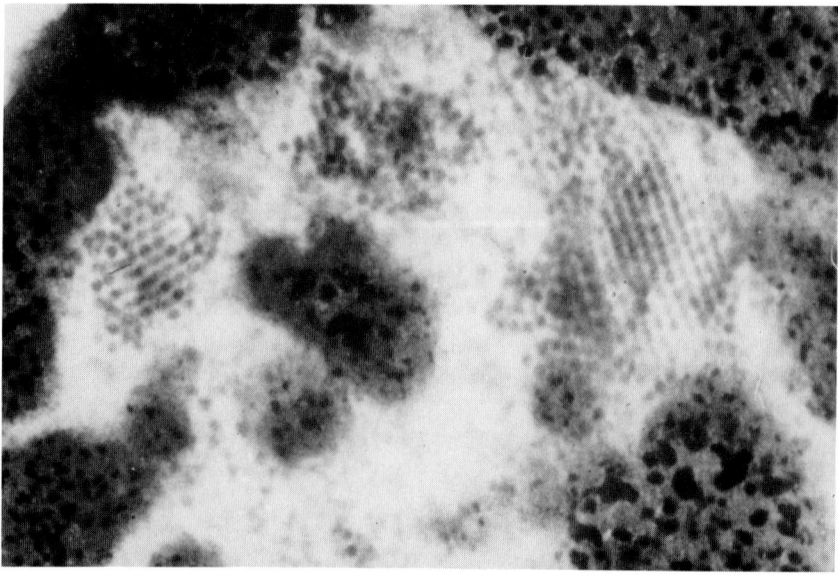

Fig. 5.1   Intranuclear crystalline array of papillomavirus particles demonstrated electron microscopically. (Courtesy of Dr C M Stanbridge.)

Immunohistochemistry

Antibodies against papillomavirus capsid antigen prepared by detergent disruption of bovine papillomavirus type 1 have been available for a number of years and detect a group-common epitope that has been mapped in HPV 16 to a 15-amino-acid region on the L1 capsid protein (Cason et al 1989, Patel et al 1989). The presence of viral capsid protein, however, is a manifestation of late gene expression and viral DNA may be present in host cells without the capsid protein being demonstrable. Positive immunocytochemical reactions with these antibodies are usually seen in the upper epithelial layers and correlate with the presence of koilocytes, though even these cells are often negative.

Until very recently it was not possible to produce type-specific antibodies because human papillomaviruses do not replicate in tissue culture and because the amount of viral DNA present in genital lesions was low. These difficulties have now been overcome by cloning in bacterial vectors of sequences of individual open reading frames of different HPV types and the production of fusion proteins (Banks et al 1987). The availability of a series of monoclonal antibodies against the major capsid protein L1 of HPV 16 prompted an immunohistochemical study of L1 protein in the diagnosis of HPV 16 infection of the cervix (Lacey et al 1991). Only one of 10 known HPV 16 positive cases showed L1 protein expression, which apparently occurred shortly after the onset of clinical infection (Fig. 5.2). It is uncertain

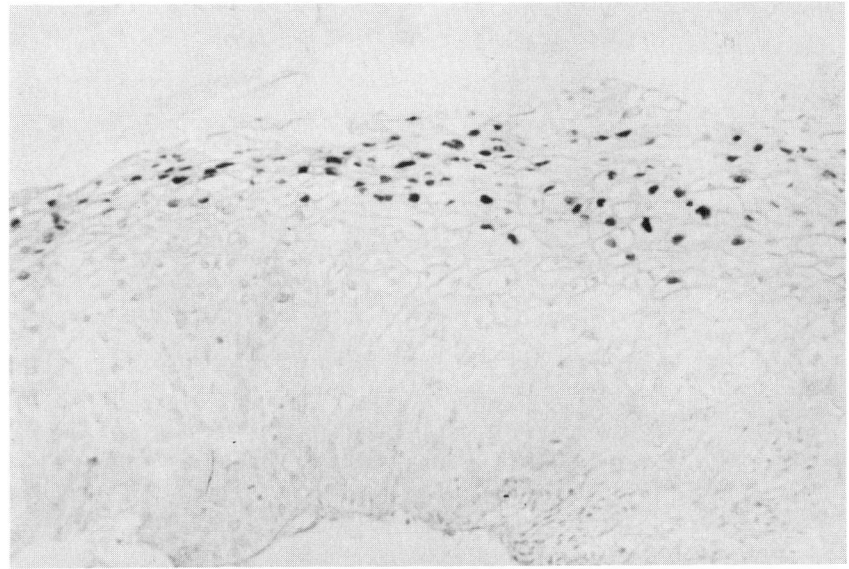

Fig. 5.2   Immunoreactivity of superficial cervical squamous cell nuclei for human papillomavirus with a monoclonal antibody to the L1 protein of HPV-16.

whether major capsid protein expression reflects episodes of viral replication. The serious limitations of immunohistochemistry for the demonstration of human papillomaviruses should be borne in mind when the value
of commercially available diagnostic kits is assessed.

Hybridization

Five different hybridization techniques are available for the molecular
biological diagnosis of HPV infection: Southern blot hybridization, dot–
blot hybridization, sandwich hybridization, filter in situ hybridization and
in situ hybridization. Discussion here will concentrate on the latter
methods.

The extraction of single-stranded human DNA, separation by gel
electrophoresis, transfer to a nitrocellulose filter (Southern blotting) and
subsequent hybridization with a radioactively labelled viral probe consisting of a complementary DNA sequence, form the fundamental basis of
the now well-established technique of DNA hybridization. Dot–blot
hybridization is a more rapid variation of this basic technique.

Since 1985 there has been an increasing number of publications on the
subject of in situ hybridization to demonstrate HPV DNA (Wells 1990).
Only this technique allows direct localization of the virus (Fig. 5.3).
Numerous detection systems have been developed to visualize labelled gene
probes. Autoradiography has been used to detect radiolabelled probes in

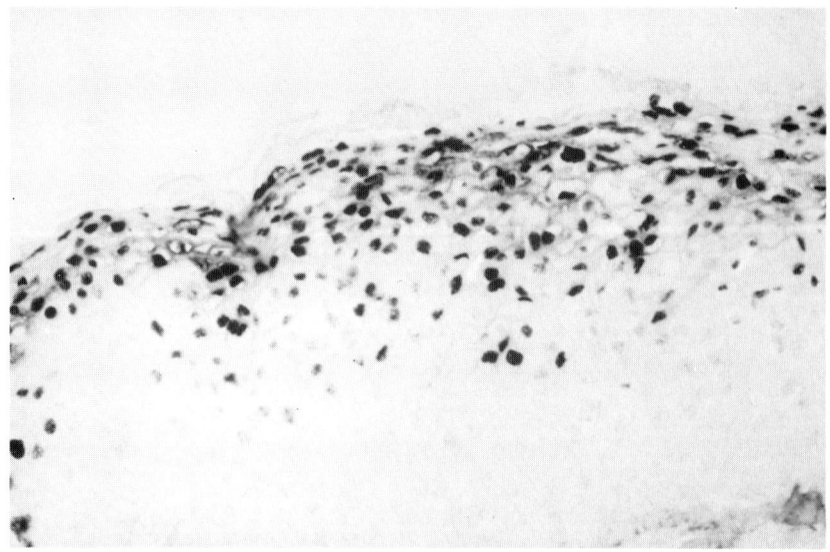

Fig. 5.3 In situ DNA hybridization of HPV 16 in a cervical biopsy specimen using a biotin/
polyalkaline phosphatase complex. (Reproduced with permission of the Editor, J Clin
Pathol.)

cell smears and paraffin-wax sections; whilst this method is very sensitive, it is unsuitable for most routine applications (Gupta et al 1985). The introduction of biotinylated DNA probes and the development of methods applicable to formalin-fixed material have enabled these techniques to become almost routine (Crum et al 1988, Amortegui et al 1990). Lewis et al (1987) developed a method for the detection of in situ hybridized DNA probes using a streptavidin/polyalkaline phosphatase complex.

Whereas dot–blot hybridization can detect one viral genome copy per cell provided sufficient cellular DNA is analysed, successful visualization by in situ hybridization using biotinylated probes on tissue requires that some cells contain 200–800 copies of the viral genome.

Polymerase chain reaction

The polymerase chain reaction is a method of amplifying a desired segment of DNA by attaching a piece of complementary DNA (primer) to the template strand to prepare or 'prime' it for the action of DNA polymerase, which extends the primer by adding further nucleotides complementary to the template. As the newly synthesized DNA is also complementary to and capable of binding to the primers, each replication cycle doubles the amount of DNA synthesized in the previous cycle. The result is a logarithmic increase in the desired DNA segment (Goudie 1989).

The use of the polymerase chain reaction improved sensitivity by many orders of magnitude so that, in theory, a single copy of HPV can be detected in a background of 10 cells (Taylor & Quirke 1989). Its application to cytological and histological preparations (including paraffin-wax embedded material) should allow the absolute prevalence of HPV infection to be determined (Shibata et al 1988a,b, Griffin et al 1990).

After amplification, samples can be taken for electrophoresis on poly-acrylamide gels and the reaction products visualized by ethidium bromide staining. The specificity of the amplified product can be confirmed by Southern blotting and standard hybridization to appropriate ^{32}P-labelled oligonucleotide probes (Fig. 5.4).

HISTOLOGICAL FEATURES OF HUMAN PAPILLOMAVIRUS INFECTION

The histological feature that has been linked most frequently with HPV infection is koilocytosis, but it is important that koilocytosis is not over diagnosed. To warrant recognition as a koilocyte the nucleus of the cell should be enlarged and hyperchromatic and have a wrinkled outline, and there should be cavitation of the cytoplasm. Koilocytes are rarely present in the basal layers of the cytoplasm and then only when they are present more superficially. The changes are often quite focal. It is particularly important

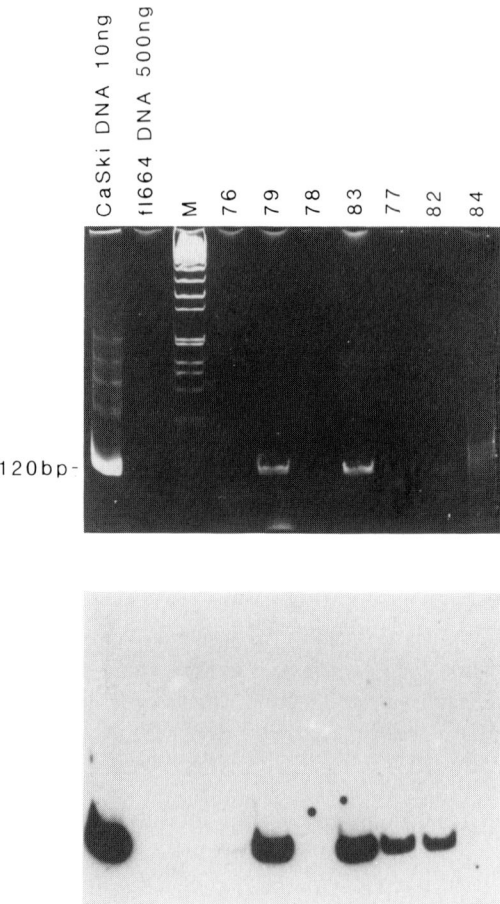

Fig. 5.4 Amplification of DNA isolated from paraffin-wax embedded cervical tissue with HPV 16-specific oligonucleotide primers. Upper: polyacrylamide gel electrophoresis and ethidium bromide staining of products of the polymerase chain reaction on DNA isolated from CaSki cells (HPV 16 positive cervical carcinoma line), fetal liver (f1664-negative control) and paraffin-wax embedded cervical carcinomas (samples 76, 79, 78, 83, 77, 82, 84). M = DNA size markers. Lower: Southern blot of amplified polymerase chain reaction products from the gel, confirming specificity for HPV 16 DNA. Amplified products from gel were electroblotted on to Hybond-N + membrane (Amersham) and hybridized with an oligonucleotide probe of 40 nucleotides end-labelled with ^{32}P and taken from the region between the two HPV 16 E6 region primers. (Reproduced with permission of the Editor, J Clin Pathol.)

that koilocytosis is not confused with the 'basket-weave' appearance of the normal, mature squamous epithelium.

The two other main histological features of HPV infection are individual cell keratinization (dyskeratosis) and multinucleation. The other features of HPV infection are acanthosis, parakeratosis and papillomatosis.

Vulva

Vulval condylomata associated with HPV types 6 and 11 are the best characterized examples of HPV infection. Bowenoid papulosis refers to a clinical appearance of the vulva and should not be regarded as a distinct pathological entity. Histologically, it is a high-grade vulval intraepithelial neoplasia which is usually associated with HPV 16 (Bergeron et al 1987).

Interestingly, in a recent study HPV 16 was found to be no more likely to be associated with vulval intraepithelial neoplasia than HPV 6/11 (Cone et al 1991). This finding contrasted strongly with previous reports, suggesting that HPV 16 was the major subtype associated with vulval intraepithelial neoplasia (Bergeron et al 1987, Buscema et al 1988, Twiggs et al 1988). The overall prevalence of HPV DNA in colposcopically defined lesions was relatively low (14%), there was no strong correlation between 'subclinical' vulval lesions and HPV DNA positivity by in situ hybridization (Cone et al 1991).

Thirty cases of vulval intraepithelial neoplasia were recently studied by in situ hybridization and the polymerase chain reaction (Park et al in press). HPV type 16 was found in half of the cases. Women with HPV-positive vulval intraepithelial neoplasia were significantly younger than those with HPV-negative vulval intraepithelial neoplasia, suggesting that there may be at least two different types of vulval intraepithelial neoplasia, with different clinical, pathological and virological features. The invasive potential of vulval intraepithelial neoplasia is generally thought to be low (see p. 152), and HPV is infrequently associated with the usual type of squamous cell carcinoma of the vulva.

Younger women are more likely to have tumours containing HPV, and these tumours are typically associated with vulval intraepithelial neoplasia (Toki et al 1991). There are two types of tumours that occur in younger women and that are frequently associated with HPV. One type is termed basaloid carcinoma and the other has been designated warty carcinoma and has condylomatous features (Toki et al 1991).

Squamous cell papillae of the vulva are controversial lesions: a number of different pathological processes may present with the same clinical appearances. Some investigators believe they are variations of normal anatomy, whilst others have found that the changes were associated with severe local symptoms and human papillomavirus infection. In a recent study of vulval squamous cell papillae, vulval biopsies from 46 women with colposcopic evidence of squamous cell papillae but no evidence of vaginal or cervical disease showed koilocytosis, and HPV DNA was detected in 76% of these cases. Thus, if koilocytosis is present the lesions are likely to be positive for viral DNA (Wang et al 1991).

Vagina

Invasive carcinoma of the vagina is relatively rare. Ostrow et al (1988) showed HPV DNA in only 21% of samples from 14 cases of vaginal carcinoma. This low figure, however, may reflect the inability of in situ hybridization to give a true picture of viral status when the virus is present in low copy number.

Cervix

Human papillomavirus infection of the cervix may be divided into two groups. First, HPV 6, 11, 31 and 35 are predominantly associated with condylomata acuminata (Fig. 5.5), non-condylomatous wart virus infection, low-grade cervical intraepithelial neoplasia (CIN 1) and only rarely with invasive tumours. This is regarded as the low-risk or 'benign' HPV group. Second, HPV types 16, 18 and 33 are associated with low-grade CIN

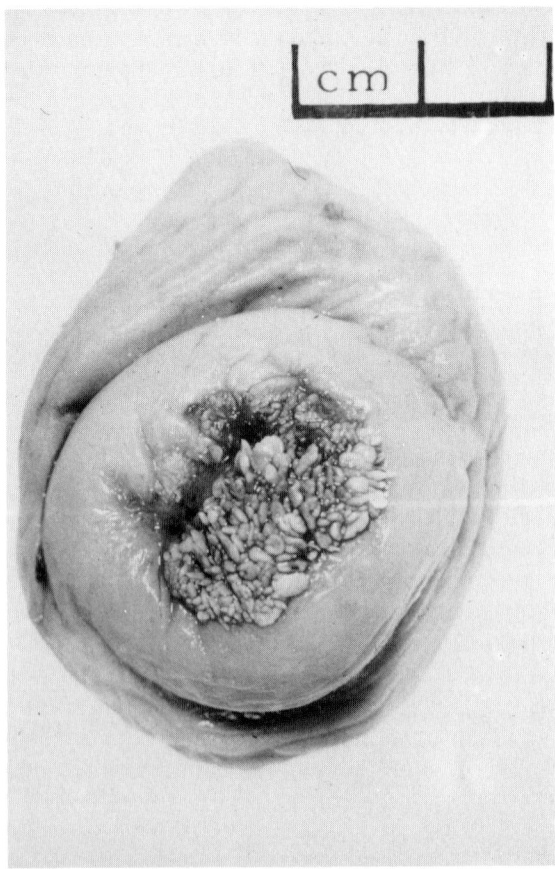

Fig. 5.5   A large cervical condyloma protruding through the external os.

that progresses, high-grade CIN (grades 2 and 3), and invasive carcinomas, and form the high-risk or 'malignant' HPV group (Willett et al 1989).

Cervical intraepithelial neoplasia

Human papillomaviruses 6 and 11 have been detected by some workers in only a small number of CIN lesions (Pfister 1987, Koutsky et al 1988), but Syrjanen et al (1986) detected HPV 6 or 11 in most of the cases of CIN examined: CIN 1 = 73%, CIN 2 = 67% and CIN 3 = 75%. Gupta et al (1987a) reported the presence of HPV 6/11 in 20% of CIN cases. In another study of the same group, HPV 6/11 was found in 8% of cases of CIN 1, in 40% of CIN 2, but in no cases of CIN 3 (Gupta et al 1987b). Recently, Pao et al (1989) found HPV 6/11 in 13% of cases of CIN. Schneider et al (1991) did not find a single positive case of CIN containing HPV 6/11.

By morphometry, cervical epithelium infected with HPV 6/11 and 16/18/33 can be distinguished on the basis of cellularity, standard deviation of nuclear perimeter in the intermediate and superficial epithelial cell layers, and the standard deviation of the nuclear area in the intermediate layers. The HPV 16/18/33 group show high total and abnormal mitotic counts (Fu et al 1988).

Squamous cell carcinoma

Many studies have confirmed that a high proportion of cervical squamous cell cancers contain HPV DNA and in particular HPV 16, 18 and 33. Most cervical tumours and cell lines derived from cervical tumours contain a proportion of HPV DNA that, instead of being episomal or extra-chromosomal, is integrated into the host genome. Integration disrupts the viral genome in the E1–E2 region, resulting in failure of transcription of the late genes and possibly in uncontrolled transcription of the E6 and E7 genes. As a result, the viral life cycle is aborted and infectious virus is not produced. Integration with transcription of the E6 and E7 genes is associated with malignant transformation (Ambros & Kurman 1990).

Human papillomaviruses and adenocarcinoma of the cervix

Human papillomavirus types 16 and 18 have been demonstrated in cervical adenocarcinoma and adenosquamous carcinoma by Southern blotting and DNA hybridization (Smotkin et al 1986, Wilczynski et al 1988a,b). These findings have been supported by other workers using in situ hybridization of formalin-fixed, paraffin-wax embedded tissues and radiolabelled probes (Tase et al 1988, 1989, Farnsworth et al 1989). Human papillomavirus DNA was detected in 17 cases (42.5%) of adenocarcinoma and 16 cases (36.4%) of adenosquamous carcinoma using mixed probes (Tase et al 1988). This latter study and other studies have suggested that HPV 18 may be particularly implicated in the aetiology of adenocarcinoma.

To investigate further the possibility that human papillomaviruses play a role in the aetiology of cervical glandular neoplasia, Griffin et al (1991) examined 16 cases of invasive cervical adenocarcinoma and eight cases of in situ adenocarcinoma by in situ DNA hybridization using biotinylated probes to HPV 6, 11, 16, 18 and 31 and by the polymerase chain reaction with sequences to HPV types 11, 16 and 18. Of the invasive adeno-carcinomas, 4 of 16 contained HPV 16 sequences demonstrable by the polymerase chain reaction. Only one invasive adenocarcinoma and one case of adenocarcinoma in situ showed a positive in situ hybridization signal, suggesting that there was a low copy number in the PCR positive cases. This low rate of HPV carriage suggested to Griffin et al that these viruses do not play a major role in the aetiology of cervical glandular neoplasia in a British population, and that there may be population differences in the carriage of HPV in cervical glandular lesions.

DIFFICULTIES AND CONFUSION IN HISTOPATHOLOGICAL REPORTING

The difficulties in interpreting biopsies from epithelia infected with HPV have been well described by Fox & Buckley (1990). The issues were also constructively discussed in an editorial board symposium published in the *International Journal of Gynecological Pathology* (Crum et al 1989). Many confusing terms have been used to describe human papillomavirus in-fection, including flat condyloma, koilocytic atypia, HPV-associated atypia and subclinical papillomavirus infection.

Subclinical HPV infection presents only mild histological abnormalities, such as elongated rete pegs, acanthosis, 'mild' koilocytosis, lack of glyco-genization, and para- or hyperkeratosis (Anderson & Tidy 1991). Sensi-tivity and specificity of these criteria are controversial and low. These facts are reflected in the low reproducibility and high inter-observer variability in the histological diagnosis of subclinical HPV infection. When 12 consultant histopathologists examined cervical specimens that were thought to show signs of HPV infection in the absence of CIN, there was practically no histological agreement (κ value 0.08) (Ismail et al 1989).

The most important questions are:

- Can non-condylomatous wart virus infection (so-called flat condyloma) be distinguished from CIN 1 with or without superimposed features of papillomavirus infection?
- Can histopathologists predict the HPV type from the histopathological appearances alone?
- Is knowledge of HPV type important in the management of an individual patient with an intraepithelial vulval or cervical lesion?

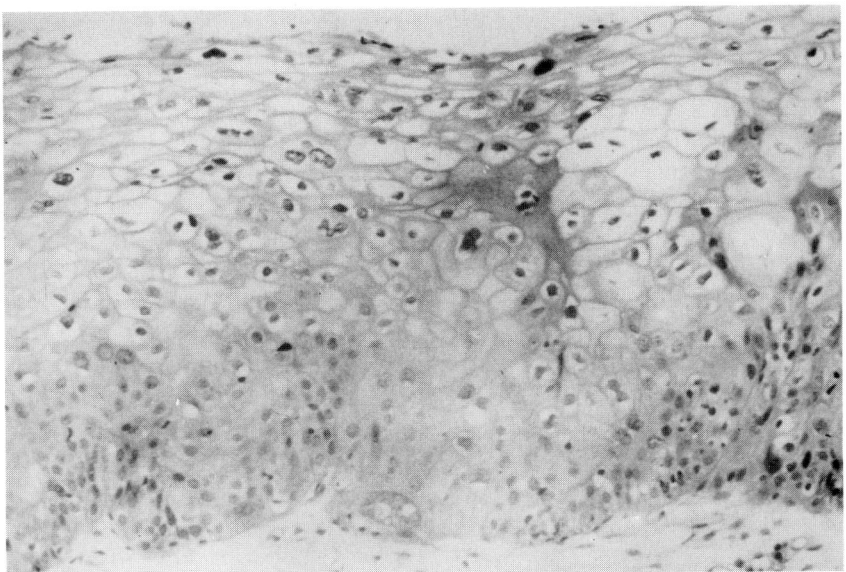

Fig. 5.6 Florid koilocytosis of cervical squamous cell epithelium indicating non-condylomatous wart virus infection in the absence of cervical intraepithelial neoplasia.

In my opinion, the answers are *yes* (Fig. 5.6), *no* and *no*, respectively. At a meeting convened in 1989 by the National Cancer Institute to develop a suitable classification to replace the Papanicolau Class system, the 'Bethesda System for Reporting Cervical and Vaginal Cytological Diagnoses' was developed. In this classification, squamous cell lesions are divided into three groups: squamous cell atypia, squamous cell intraepithelial lesions and invasive squamous cell carcinoma. Squamous intraepithelial lesions are further divided into two sub-groups: low grade and high grade. The low grade group comprises condylomatous atypia (koilocytotic atypia) and mild dysplasia. Kurman has advocated that this classification should be adopted by histopathologists as well as by cytopathologists (Ambros & Kurman 1990).

Other workers have suggested that cases now categorized as either flat condyloma or CIN 1 should be classed as 'borderline CIN' (Ismail et al 1989). Fox and Buckley (1990) reject this suggestion, arguing that the term 'borderline CIN' should be reserved for cases in which it is uncertain whether CIN 1 is superimposed on a flat wart. The accuracy with which morphological characteristics predict the presence and type of HPV infection is controversial.

It is now clear that high-risk types of HPV are detectable in up to a quarter of flat condylomas and in a similar proportion of cases of CIN 1 (Franquemont et al 1989). The study by Willett et al (1989) showed that there is a heterogeneous but broadly similar distribution of HPV types, including 6/11, 16, 18, 31 and as yet uncharacterized types, in lesions classified as flat condyloma and CIN 1. CIN 2 lesions also showed a mixture of HPV types, but had a proportionately greater percentage of lesions that contained HPV 16. In contrast, a more homogeneous distribution of HPV types was observed in typical exophytic condylomas (the majority of which contained HPV 6/11) and CIN 3 lesions which mostly contained HPV 16. Abnormal mitotic figures are predominantly seen in CIN 3 but only rarely in CIN 1 and flat condylomata (Franquemont et al 1989).

If the changes of CIN and HPV infection coexist, the changes of CIN are superimposed on those of HPV infection, resulting in nuclear pleo-morphism of the basal layers with koilocytosis in the superficial layers, the nuclear changes of which often appear exaggerated. The tendency to attribute too high a grade of CIN should be resisted. In addition, it should be borne in mind that the features of HPV infection may be seen in all grades of CIN.

In the opinion of a recent working party (Anderson et al 1991), not all examples of CIN 1 are an expression of HPV infection. They maintained that it was possible and indeed desirable to distinguish between CIN 1 with HPV infection and CIN 1 without HPV infection. For this reason, and also because of the therapeutic implications, the working party rejected systems of terminology that grouped epithelia that had only HPV-associated changes with epithelia showing CIN 1.

EVIDENCE FOR THE ONCOGENIC ROLE OF HUMAN PAPILLOMAVIRUSES

The viral genes *E6* and *E7* from the HPV types associated with squamous cell carcinomas can convert normal cells to an unrestricted life span, but the cells most probably require further interacting factors for the development of full neoplastic transformation (McDougall 1990). The *E7* gene alone can induce immortalization of various cell types but the efficiency of this in human cells is enhanced by *E6*. The expression of these open reading frames is found consistently in transformed cells in vitro, in cell lines derived from cervical carcinomas and in cervical carcinomas. It seems clear, therefore, that *E6* and *E7* gene expression play a role in the development of malignancy, possibly by extending the proliferative capacity of HPV-infected cells and enabling them to become resistant to normal differ-entiation signals. As occurs with other small DNA viruses, the binding of putative tumour suppressor genes to viral oncogenes may be an important step in the multistep progression from normal to malignant cells. The observation that DNA integration is quite a common event in the progression of cervical lesions has fuelled much speculation, although its precise significance remains obscure.

A recent study has shown that the E6 protein of HPV 16 is capable of binding to cellular p53 protein (Werness et al 1990). It has been shown that E7 forms a complex with the protein product, RB, of the retinoblastoma gene, *Rb1* (Dyson et al 1989). Both these proteins are thought to play an important role in the regulation of the cell cycle. The E6 proteins from different HPV types form complexes with p53; this activity was assayed and found to correlate with the in vivo transforming activity of these different papillomaviruses. Protein p53 is thought to be important in the suppression of cell growth, and so viral proteins might act simply by binding to and effectively neutralizing the normal function of p53. Interestingly, E6 protein from the 'benign' HPV types 6 and 11 does not appear to form a complex with p53 (Werness et al 1990). Similarly, E7 proteins from the oncogenic HPV types 16 and 18 bind RB more strongly than E7 expressed by the benign types HPV 6 and 11 (Munger et al 1989). Human papillomaviruses encode proteins that bind to both RB and p53, which implies that the two proteins function in independent but complementary pathways. This has been supported by a recent report which shows that transformation by E7 (presumably by interfering with the RB pathway) can be greatly potentiated by cotransfection with mutant p53 (Vousden et al 1991).

EPIDEMIOLOGICAL CONSIDERATIONS

Enthusiasm for the view that HPVs have a central role in cervical oncogenesis has been tempered by reports of widely different prevalences of different HPV types in normal, dysplastic and neoplastic cervices. In a review of studies of prevalence of HPV in the UK, USA, FRG, Central and South America, and Japan, the incidence rates for HPV 16 or 18, or both, in invasive squamous cell carcinoma ranged from 15.4 to 94.0% (Munoz et al 1988). Similarly, ranges of 13.8–83.3% incidence of these HPV types in CIN, and 0–45% in healthy cervix, were recorded. Whilst this may reflect a true global variation in prevalence, it is likely that variation in study design and sensitivity of detection techniques have introduced some error into the studies.

The existence of HPV DNA in histologically normal squamous epithelium has recently been questioned and re-evaluated by Syrjänen & Syrjänen (1989). They consistently failed to demonstrate even weak signals of HPV DNA (6, 11, 16, 18, 31 or 33) in histologically normal epithelium adjacent to a range of virus-associated lesions. The authors concluded that HPV DNA rarely if ever appeared in histologically normal squamous or columnar epithelium in the female genital tract when sought using in situ hybridization. Results from the more sensitive polymerase chain technique do, however, seem to contradict these findings (Griffin et al 1990).

ROLE OF CO-FACTORS IN ONCOGENESIS

The evidence linking HPVs with cervical cancer remains incomplete and other co-factors may be involved, such as seminal plasma or spermatozoal DNA (Anderson & Tidy 1991, Singer & Jenkins 1991). Epidemiological evidence strongly implicates cigarette smoking as a co-factor in cervical carcinogenesis; some effects of materials in cigarette smoke on local immunocompetent cells in the cervix have been shown, with a reduction in the numbers of Langerhans' cells in cervical squamous cell epithelium (Barton et al 1988). This immunosuppression may play an important part in the outcome of HPV infection. Smoking may also act through chemical carcinogenesis and additional smoking-related products of DNA have been demonstrated in the cervix (Cuzick et al 1990).

It has also been suggested that herpes simplex virus may act as a co-factor in the development of malignancy (Anderson & Tidy 1991, Singer & Jenkins 1991). Herpes simplex virus and HPV can cooperate to transform cells into a tumorigenic phenotype (Iwasaka et al 1988) and herpes simplex virus-VMW65 protein can transactivate HPV 18 gene expression (Gius & Laimins 1989).

HUMAN PAPILLOMAVIRUSES AND PROGNOSIS

Cervical intraepithelial lesions induced by HPV 16 seem to run a more aggressive course than those caused by any of the other HPV types analyzed (Campion et al 1986). However, as pointed out by Willett et al (1989), the association of specific HPV types with particular morphological abnormalities is complex. The notion of low- and high-risk HPV types should be considered to be one of relative risk and not an all-or-none phenomenon. Infection with HPV 6/11 may lead to a lesion that progresses to CIN 2 but rarely goes further, whereas infection with HPV 16 has a greater risk of progression to CIN 3. Probably not all infections with HPV 16 progress; progression is likely to be determined by other environmental, genetic and immunological factors.

Recent reports on small series of patients have suggested that HPV 18 is associated with aggressiveness of cervical cancer (Kurman et al 1988, Barnes et al 1989). In a study of patients with HPV 18 containing tumours, they were more likely to give a history of recent normal Papanicolau smears than were those whose tumours contained HPV 16. The authors suggest that tumours containing HPV 18 can progress to invasion without a prolonged preinvasive period (Walker et al 1989). Another study showed no significant relationship between the risk of overall relapse and individual HPV types, though patients with no detectable HPV DNA sequences in their tumour had a 2.6 times higher risk of overall relapse and a 4.5 times higher risk of distant metastatic tumour than did HPV-positive patients (Riou et al 1990).

At present there is no clinical or diagnostic indication for HPV typing on a routine basis. Treatment is based on the extent and grade of CIN or VIN. A knowledge of the HPV type does not alter the fundamental approach to diagnosis and therapy of a vulval or cervical lesion.

THE FUTURE

A major restraint on research into HPV has been the inability to grow the virus in tissue culture. Recently, however, Sterling et al (1990) have developed an in vivo culture system to graft HPV-containing cervical squamous cells onto athymic mice. These cells were established in culture from a biopsy of CIN 1 and contained about 100 copies per cell of episomal HPV 16 DNA. In this system the virus seemed able to undergo its full replicative cycle. The demonstration that HPV 16 particles can be produced by a cell line that has episomal HPV 16 DNA revives hope that a system will be developed in which the factors involved in the regulation of the life cycle of the virus can be studied. It is important to discover what risk factors predispose established HPV lesions to undergo rapid progression.

Of considerable interest is the nature of the immune response to HPV. Antibodies specifically directed against proteins of HPV 6 and HPV 16 have recently been detected at high frequency both in patients attending sexually transmitted disease clinics and in young children (Galloway 1990). There appeared to be a higher level of antibodies against the HPV 16 E7 and E4 proteins in patients with cervical lesions than in controls. There is clear evidence of widespread exposure to HPV at an early age; it is not yet known whether the presence of antibodies is of any prognostic significance, though there are implications for the development of a prophylactic vaccine to HPV.

HIV-induced immunosuppression exacerbates HPV-mediated cervical abnormalities (Maiman et al 1990), and the increased incidence of cervical abnormalities in immunosuppressed women following renal transplantation is well recognized (Blessing et al 1990). Such findings again highlight the importance, in clarifying the natural history of HPV infection, of investigating the immunological response.

REFERENCES

Ambros R A, Kurman R J 1990 Current concepts in the relationship of human papillomavirus infection to the pathogenesis and classification of precancerous squamous lesions of the uterine cervix. Seminars in Diagnostic Pathology 7: 158–172

Amortegui A J, Meyer M P, McIntyre-Seltman K, Locker J 1990 Detection of human papillomavirus DNA in cervical lesions by in situ hybridization using biotinylated probes. International Journal of Gynecological Pathology 9: 306–315

Anderson M C, Tidy J A 1991 The aetiology of cervical cancer. In: Symmers W St (general ed) Systemic pathology, 3rd ed, vol 6; Anderson M C (ed) Female reproductive system. Churchill Livingstone, Edinburgh, p 73–89

Anderson M C, Brown C, Buckley C H, Fox H, Jenkins D, Lowe D G, Manners B T B, Melcher D H, Robertson A J, Wells M 1991 Current views on cervical intraepithelial neoplasia. Journal of Clinical Pathology 44: 969–978

Arends M J, Wyllie A H, Bird C C 1990 Papillomaviruses and human cancer. Human Pathology 21: 686–698

Banks L, Matlashewski G, Pim D, Churcher M, Roberts C, Crawford L 1987 Expression of human papillomavirus type 6 and type 16 capsid proteins in bacteria and their antigenic characterization. Journal of General Virology 68: 3081–3089

Barnes W, Delgado G, Kurman R J et al 1988 Possible prognostic significance of human papillomavirus type in cervical cancer. Gynecologic Oncology 29: 267–273

Barton S E, Maddox P H, Jenkins D, Edwards R, Cuzick J, Singer A 1988 Effects of cigarette smoking on cervical epithelial immunity: a mechanism for neoplastic change? Lancet ii: 652–654

Bergeron C, Naghashfar Z, Canaan C, Shah K, Fu Y, Ferenczy A 1987 Human papillomavirus type 16 in intraepithelial neoplasia (Bowenoid papulosis) and coexistent invasive carcinoma of the vulva. International Journal of Gynecological Pathology 6: 1–11

Blessing K, McLaren K M, Morris R et al 1990 Detection of human papillomavirus in skin and genital lesions of renal allograft recipients by in situ hybridization. Histopathology 16: 181–185

Buscema J, Nagashfar Z, Sawada E, Daniel R, Woodruff J D, Shah K 1988 The predominance of human papillomavirus type 16 in vulvar neoplasia. Obstetrics and Gynecology 71: 601–606

Campion M J, Singer A, Malcolm A D, Coleman D V 1986 Progressive potential of mild cervical atypia: prospective cytological, colposcopic and virological study. Lancet 2: 237–240

Cason J, Patel D, Naylor J et al 1989 Identification of immunogenic regions of the major coat protein of human papillomavirus type 16 that contain type-restricted epitopes. Journal of General Virology 70: 2973–2987

Chang F 1990 Role of papillomaviruses. Journal of Clinical Pathology 43: 269–276

Collins J E, Jenkins D, McCance D J 1988 Detection of human papillomavirus DNA sequences by in situ DNA–DNA hybridisation in cervical intraepithelial neoplasia and invasive carcinoma: a retrospective study. Journal of Clinical Pathology 41: 289–295

Cone R, Beckmann A, Aho M, Wahlstrom T, Ek M, Corey L, Paavonen J 1991 Subclinical manifestations of vulvar human papillomavirus infection. International Journal of Gynecological Pathology 10: 26–35

Crum C P, Nuova G, Friedman D, Silverstein S J 1988 A comparison of biotin and isotope-labelled ribonucleic acid in genital precancers. Laboratory Investigation 58: 354–359

Crum C, Fu Y-S, Kurman R J, Okagaki T, Twiggs L B, Silverberg S G 1989 Editorial board symposium. Practical approach to cervical human papillomavirus-related intraepithelial lesions. International Journal of Gynecological Pathology 8: 388–389

Cuzick J, Routledge M N, Jenkins D, Garner R C 1990 DNA adducts in different tissues of smokers and non-smokers. International Journal of Cancer 45: 673–678

Dyson N, Howley P M, Munger K, Harlow E 1989 The human papillomavirus-16 E7 oncoprotein is able to bind to the retinoblastoma gene product. Science 243: 934–937

Farnsworth A, Laverty C, Stoler M H 1989 Human papillomavirus messenger RNA expression in adenocarcinoma in situ of the uterine cervix. International Journal of Gynecological Pathology 8: 321–330

Fox H, Buckley C H 1990 Current problems in the pathology of intra-epithelial lesions of the uterine cervix. Histopathology 17: 1–6

Franquemont D W, Ward B E, Anderson W A, Crum C P 1989 Prediction of "high-risk" cervical papillomavirus infection by biopsy morphology. American Journal of Clinical Pathology 92: 577–592

Fu Y S, Huang I, Beaudenon S, Ionesco M, Barrasso R, de Brux J, Orth G 1988 Correlative study of human papillomavirus DNA, histopathology, and morphometry in cervical condyloma and intraepithelial neoplasia. International Journal of Gynecological Pathology 7: 297–307

Galloway D A 1990 HPV serology: an update. Papillomavirus Report 1(2): 1–3

Gius D, Laimins L A 1989 Activation of human papillomavirus type 18 gene expression by herpes simplex virus type 1 viral transactivators and a phorbol ester. Journal of Virology 63: 555–563

Goudie R B 1989 The polymerase chain reaction and histopathology. Journal of Pathology 158: 183–184

Griffin N R, Bevan I S, Lewis F A, Wells M, Young L S 1990 Demonstration of multiple HPV types in normal cervix and in cervical squamous cell carcinoma using the polymerase chain reaction on paraffin wax embedded material. Journal of Clinical Pathology 43: 52–56

Griffin N R, Dockey D, Lewis F A, Wells M 1991 Demonstration of low frequency of human papillomavirus DNA in cervical adenocarcinoma and adenocarcinoma in situ by the polymerase chain reaction and in situ hybridization. International Journal of Gynecological Pathology 10: 36–43

Gupta J, Gendelman H E, Nagashfar Z et al 1985 Specific identification of human papillomavirus type in cervical smears and paraffin sections by *in situ* hybridization with radioactive probes: a preliminary communication. International Journal of Gynecological Pathology 4: 211–218

Gupta J W, Gupta P K, Rosenshein N, Shah K V 1987a Detection of human papillomaviruses in cervical smears. Acta Cytologica 31: 387–396

Gupta J, Pilotti S, Rilke F, Shah K 1987b Association of human papillomavirus type 16 with neoplastic lesions of the vulva and other genital sites by in situ hybridization. American Journal of Pathology 127: 206–215

Ismail S M, Colclough A, Dinnen J S et al 1989 Observer variation in histopathological grading of cervical intraepithelial neoplasia (CIN)—is there a need for change? Journal of Pathology 159: 273–275

Iwasaka T, Yokoyama M, Hayashi Y, Sugimori H 1988 Combined herpes simplex type 2 and human papillomavirus type 16 or 18 deoxyribonucleic acid leads to oncogenic transformation. American Journal of Obstetrics and Gynaecology 159: 1251–1255

Koss L G, Durfee G R 1956 Unusual patterns of squamous epithelium of the uterine cervix. Cytologic and pathology study of koilocytic atypia. Annals of the New York Academy of Sciences 63: 1245–1261

Koutsky L A, Galloway D A, Holmes K K 1988 Epidemiology of genital human papillomavirus infection. Epidemiology Reviews 10: 122–163

Kurman R J, Schiffman M H, Lancaster W D et al 1988 Analysis of individual human papillomavirus types in cervical neoplasia: A possible role for type 18 in rapid progression. American Journal of Obstetrics and Gynaecology 159: 293–296

Lacey C J N, Wells M, Macdermott R I J, Gibson P E 1991 Human papillomavirus type 16 infection of the cervix—a comparison of differing DNA detection modes and the use of monoclonal antibodies against the major capsid protein. Genitourinary Medicine 67: 87–91

Lewis F A, Griffiths S, Dunnicliffe R, Wells M, Dudding N, Bird C C 1987 Sensitive *in situ* hybridisation technique using biotin–streptavidin–polyalkaline phosphatase complex. Journal of Clinical Pathology 40: 163–166

McDougall J K 1990 HPV immortalization and transformation. Papillomavirus Report 1(3): 1–4

Maiman M, Fruchter R G, Serur E et al 1990 Human immunodeficiency virus infection and cervical neoplasia. Gynecologic Oncology 38: 377–382

Meisels A, Fortin R 1976 Condylomatous lesions of the cervix and vagina. Cytlogic patterns. Acta Cytologica 20: 505–509

Munger K, Werness B A, Dyson N, Phelps W C, Harlow E, Howley P M 1989 Complex formation of human papillomavirus E7 proteins with the retinoblastoma tumour suppressor gene product. EMBO Journal 8: 4099–4105

Munoz N, Bosch X, Kaldor J W 1988 Does human papillomavirus cause cervical cancer? The state of the epidemiological evidence. British Journal of Cancer 57: 1–5

Ostrow R S, Manias D A, Clark B A et al 1988 The analysis of carcinomas of the vagina for human papillomavirus DNA. International Journal of Gynecological Pathology 7: 308–314

Pao C C, Lai C H, Wu S Y, Young K C, Chang P L, Soong Y K 1989 Detection of human papillomaviruses in exfoliated cervicovaginal cells by in situ DNA hybridization analysis. Journal of Clinical Microbiology 27: 168–173

Park J S, Jones R W, McLean M R et al 1991 Possible etiologic heterogeneity of vulvar intraepithelial neoplasia: a correlation of pathologic characteristics with human papillomavirus detection by in situ hybridization and polymerase chain reaction. Cancer 67: 1599–1607

Patel D, Shepherd P S, Naylor J A, McCance D J 1989 Reactivities of polyclonal and monoclonal antibodies raised to the major capsid protein of human papillomavirus type 16. Journal of General Virology 70: 69–77

Pfister H 1987 Human papillomaviruses and genital cancer. Advances in Cancer Research 48: 113–147

Reid R, Laverty C R, Coppleson M, Wiwatwong I, Hills E 1980 Noncondylomatous cervical wart virus infection. Obstetrics and Gynecology 55: 476–483

Riou G, Favre M, Jeannel D, Bourhis J, Le Doussal V, Orth G 1990 Association between poor prognosis in early stage invasive cervical carcinomas and non-detection of HPV DNA. Lancet 335: 1171–1174

Schneider A 1987 Methods of identification of human papillomaviruses. In: Syrjanen K, Gissmann L, Koss L G (eds) Papillomaviruses and human disease. Springer Verlag, Berlin, p 19–39

Schneider A, Meinhardt G, Kirchmayr R, Schneider V 1991 Prevalence of human papillomavirus genomes in tissues from the lower genital tract as detected by molecular in situ hybridization. International Journal of Gynecological Pathology 10: 1–14

Shibata D K, Araheim N, Martin W J 1988a Detection of human papilloma virus in paraffin embedded tissue using the polymerase chain reaction. Journal of Experimental Medicine 167: 225–230

Shibata D, Fu Y S, Gupta J W, Shah K V, Araheim N, Martin W J 1988b Detection of human papillomavirus in normal and dysplastic tissue by the polymerase chain reaction. Laboratory Investigation 59: 555–559

Singer A, Jenkins D 1991 Viruses and cervical cancers (Leading Article). British Medical Journal 302: 251–252

Smotkin D, Berek J S, Fu Y S, Hacker N F, Major F J, Weltstein F O 1986 Human papillomavirus deoxyribonucleic acid in adenocarcinoma and adenosquamous carcinoma of the uterine cervix. Obstetrics and Gynecology 68: 241–244

Sterling J, Stanley M, Gatward G, Minson T 1990 Production of human papillomavirus type 16 virions in a keratinocyte cell line. Journal of Virology 64: 6305–6307

Syrjänen K, Syrjänen S 1989 Concept of the existence of human papillomavirus (HPV) in histologically normal squamous epithelium of the genital tract should be evaluated. Acta Obstetrica Gynecologica Scandinavica 68: 613–617

Syrjänen S, Syrjänen K, Mantyjavi R et al 1986 Human papillomavirus (HPV) DNA sequences demonstrated by in situ DNA hybridization in serial paraffin-embedded cervical biopsies. Archives of Gynecology 239: 39–48

Tase T, Okagaki T, Clark B A 1988 Human papillomavirus types and localisation in adenocarcinoma and adenosquamous carcinoma of the uterine cervix: a study by *in situ* DNA hybridisation. Cancer Research 48: 993–998

Tase T, Okagaki T, Clark B A, Twiggs L B, Ostrow R S, Faras A J 1989a Human papillomavirus DNA in adenocarcinoma in situ, microinvasive adenocarcinoma of the uterine cervix, and coexisting cervical squamous intraepithelial neoplasia. International Journal of Gynecological Pathology 8: 8–17

Tase T, Okagaki T, Clark B A, Twiggs L B, Ostrow R S, Faras A J 1989b Human papillomavirus DNA in glandular dysplasia and microglandular hyperplasia: presumed precursors of adenocarcinoma of the uterine cervix. Obstetrics and Gynecology 73: 1005–1008

Taylor G, Quirke P 1989 Further applications of the polymerase chain reaction. Journal of Pathology 159: 277–279

The 1988 Bethesda system for reporting cervical/vaginal cytological diagnoses. Journal of the American Medical Association 262: 931–934

Toki T, Kurman R J, Park J S, Kessis T, Daniel R W, Shah K V 1991 Probable nonpapillomavirus etiology of squamous cell carcinoma of the vulva in older women: a clinicopathologic study using in situ hybridization and polymerase chain reaction. International Journal of Gynecological Pathology 10: 107–125

Twiggs L B, Okagaki T, Clark B, Fukushima M, Ostrow R, Faras A 1988 A clinical, histopathologic and molecular biologic investigation of vulvar intraepithelial neoplasia. International Journal of Gynecological Pathology 7: 48–55

Vousden K H, Wrede D, Crook T 1991 HPV oncoprotein function: releasing the brakes on cell growth control. Papillomavirus Report 2(1): 1–3

Walker J, Bloss J D, Liao S Y et al 1989 Human papillomavirus genotype as a prognostic indicator in carcinoma of the uterine cervix. Obstetrics and Gynecology 74: 781–785

Wang A C, Hsu J J, Hsueh S, Sun C F, Tsao K C 1991 Evidence of human papillomavirus deoxyribonucleic acid in vulvar squamous papillomatosis. International Journal of Gynecological Pathology 10: 44–50

Wells M 1990 The demonstration of viral DNA in human tissues by in-situ DNA hybridisation. In: Harris N, Williams D G, (eds) In-situ hybridisation: application to developmental biology and medicine, Society for Experimental Biology Seminar Series. Cambridge University Press, Cambridge, p 271–284

Werness B A, Levine A J, Howley P M 1990 Association of human papillomavirus types 16 and 18 E6 proteins with p53. Science 248: 76–79

Wilczynski S P, Walker J, Liao S-Y, Bergen S, Berman M 1988a Adenocarcinoma of cervix associated with human papillomavirus. Cancer 62: 1331–1336

Wilczynski S P, Bergen S, Walker J, Liao S-Y, Pearlman L F 1988b Human papillomaviruses and cervical cancer: analysis of histopathologic features associated with different viral types. Human Pathology 19: 697–704

Willett G D, Kurman R J, Reid R, Greenberg M, Jenson A B, Lorincz A T 1989 Correlation of the histologic appearance of intraepithelial neoplasia of the cervix with human papillomavirus types. Emphasis on low grade lesions including so-called flat condyloma. International Journal of Gynecological Pathology 8: 18–25

6. Vulval dermatoses and intraepithelial neoplasia

C. H. Buckley

INTRODUCTION

The study of vulval dermatoses and intraepithelial neoplasias has been made unnecessarily complicated by the confusion of terms used to describe the disease processes. In some instances the same disease has been classified differently by clinicians and pathologists, and sometimes more than one name has been given to the same disorder: terms from different classification systems have coexisted and have been used indiscriminately. Clinical descriptive terms, such as leucoplakia, have been used as pathological diagnoses, but such terms are imprecise and subject to misinterpretation, and have no place in modern terminology.

Our understanding of vulval skin disorders has been hindered by the difficulty in establishing precise histopathological criteria for the recognition and classification of the disease processes, particularly the intraepithelial neoplasias. We are also hampered by our inadequate knowledge of the natural history even of those conditions recognized as intraepithelial neoplasms, and by the fact that dermatological conditions in the vulva may, perhaps fortuitously, be complicated by carcinoma, particularly in the elderly.

This review of the current status of vulval dermatoses and intraepithelial neoplasia concentrates deliberately on those aspects which the author believes cause the most problems: these are the classification of vulval epithelial lesions, their correct identification and the pathological factors relating to their management.

CLASSIFICATION OF VULVAL DERMATOSES AND INTRAEPITHELIAL NEOPLASIAS

We commonly refer to the vulval dermatoses and intraepithelial neoplasms as if they were a single group of disorders because they are frequently confused both clinically and pathologically and may coexist, and because their clinical presentation may be remarkably similar. The term chronic vulval dystrophy was introduced in 1961 (Jeffcoate & Woodcock) to describe 'intractable skin changes for which a specific cause is not clear';

with the exception of lichen sclerosus, this definition excluded recognizable dermatological disorders (Jeffcoate & Woodcock 1961). It is still frequently used in a general way to describe any vulval dermatological abnormality until histopathological examination of the tissue provides a definite diagnosis. This practice is to be discouraged, however, because the clinician may act in the belief that a valid diagnosis has been made.

The early classifications were essentially clinical and, even when histopathological examination was introduced, clinical descriptive terms continued to be applied to histological appearances. A major problem was that diseases with a malignant potential were not distinguished from benign conditions.

The first attempt to apply some order to vulval skin abnormalities, and to understand their behaviour, began with Jeffcoate & Woodcock's introduction of the term chronic epithelial dystrophy. The term dystrophy encompassed benign conditions, premalignant conditions and intraepithelial neoplasms of varying invasive potential, and was a useful way of referring to a group of disorders of uncertain aetiology and prognosis. Nevertheless, apart from allowing analysis of the behaviour of certain of the cutaneous disorders, it did little to enhance our understanding of the nature of these enigmatic vulval skin disorders.

In 1969, Gardner & Kaufmann expanded the concept of vulval dystrophies to include hyperplastic dystrophy, atrophic dystrophy (lichen sclerosus) and mixed dystrophy (lichen sclerosus with squamous epithelial hyperplasia) (Gardner & Kaufmann 1969). This classification formed the basis of the recommendations of the International Society for the Study of Vulvar Diseases (ISSVD) (Friedrich 1976), which have been in use until the last few years (Table 6.1).

Even this classification was not entirely satisfactory, however. Several of the groups within it encompassed benign, premalignant conditions and intraepithelial neoplasms, and it drew an artificial distinction between squamous epithelium in which there were cytologically atypical cells with some cytoplasmic differentiation (hyperplastic dystrophy with atypia) and carcinoma in situ in which cells with little or no differentiation occupied more or less the full thickness of the epithelium. There were also problems associated with the fact that the diagnosis was entirely histopathological and

Table 6.1 Classification of vulval dystrophies (after Friedrich 1976)

Description
Hyperplastic dystrophy
a. Without atypia
b. With atypia
Lichen sclerosis
Mixed dystrophy
Carcinoma in situ

Table 6.2   Classification of vulval dermatoses and intraepithelial neoplasia (after Wilkinson et al 1986)

Description
Non-neoplastic epithelial disorders
a. Squamous (cell) epithelial hyperplasia
b. Lichen sclerosus
c. Other dermatoses
Mixed non-neoplastic and neoplastic epithelial disorders
Vulvar intraepithelial neoplasia (VIN)
Non-squamous epithelial intraepithelial neoplasia

clinical findings were not evaluated. As a consequence, inappropriately aggressive therapy might follow the detection of cytological atypia because it was taken to imply a neoplastic process (Ridley 1988).

More recently the International Society of Gynecological Pathologists and the ISSVD have made recommendations which seek to remedy these drawbacks (Wilkinson et al 1986) (Table 6.2). The classification draws a distinction between conditions that are believed to be non-neoplastic and those that are intraepithelial neoplasms. The former include lichen sclerosus, other dermatoses and squamous epithelial hyperplasia (hyperplastic dystrophy without cytological atypia) on the one hand, and vulval intraepithelial neoplasia (VIN—hyperplastic dystrophy with cytological atypia, and carcinoma in situ) on the other. It is also recommended, in order that management of the conditions can be properly planned, that when two or more conditions are present, each should be separately identified and that the term mixed dystrophy should be abandoned—indeed, the term dystrophy should no longer be applied. Intraepithelial neoplasms that are not squamous are separately identified.

Even this classification, which is an improvement on previous attempts to assign lesions correctly to specific categories, is not without its problems. Between 10 and 15% of patients will be found to have both a non-neoplastic and a neoplastic disorder and between 2 and 4% of women with lichen sclerosus, a non-neoplastic dermatological condition, will develop vulval carcinoma (though not necessarily in the area of the vulva affected by the disease). There are, however, no clinical features that will allow certain recognition of these mixed lesions prior to histological examination, nor is there any reason to believe that the various components of a mixed lesion behave differently when they are in combination.

NON-NEOPLASTIC DERMATOSES

Squamous epithelial hyperplasia (hyperplastic dystrophy without cytological atypia)

This is recognizable by some degree of epithelial acanthosis, elongation of the rete ridges, and hyperkeratosis or parakeratosis. It may occur in previously normal skin, in which case, if there is a chronic dermal inflammatory cell infiltrate, it is known as lichen simplex, or it may be superimposed upon a dermatosis, particularly lichen sclerosus (termed lichenification by the dermatologists and previously known as mixed dystrophy. The role of the pathologist is to determine whether there is an underlying causative disorder, and to check for the presence of an intraepithelial neoplasm. In all these conditions there may be a chronic inflammatory cell infiltrate in the underlying dermis and, on occasions, the epithelium may be diagnostically difficult to evaluate.

Lichen sclerosus

Lichen sclerosus is recognized histologically by the presence of a hyper-keratotic, shallow squamous epithelium with variable loss of rete ridges. Follicle plugging by keratin is not uncommon and 'liquefaction' de-generation of the basal layer of the epidermis is frequently present. The underlying papillary and reticular dermis is hyalinized or may be oedematous. A non-specific, chronic inflammatory cell infiltrate forms a band at the deep margin of the abnormal dermis (Fig. 6.1).

Involucrin, synthesized by maturing cells of stratified squamous epithelium, in which it is a marker for late keratinocyte differentiation and is thus limited

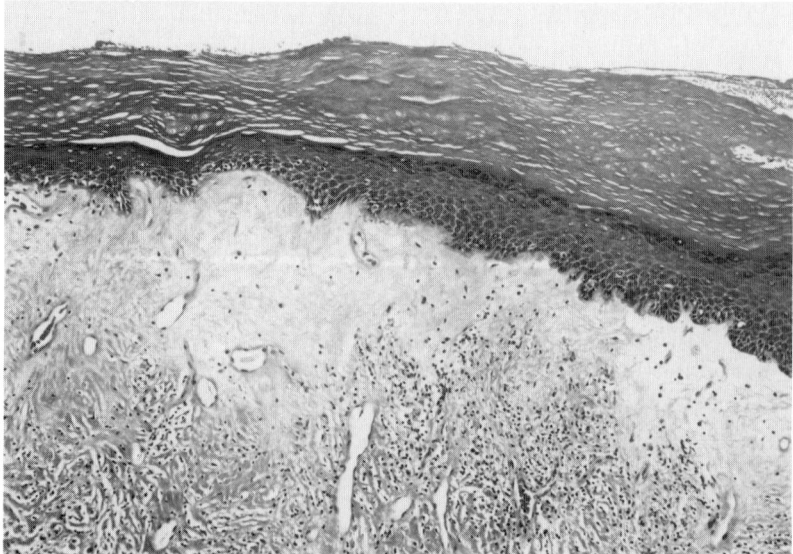

Fig. 6.1   Lichen sclerosus. The shallow epidermis with loss of rete ridges, dermal oedema and hyalinization and the deep, band-like chronic inflammatory cell infiltrate are typical of chronic lichen sclerosus. In this case there is also marked hyperkeratosis and mild secondary squamous epithelial hyperplasia to the right. H & E, × 95.

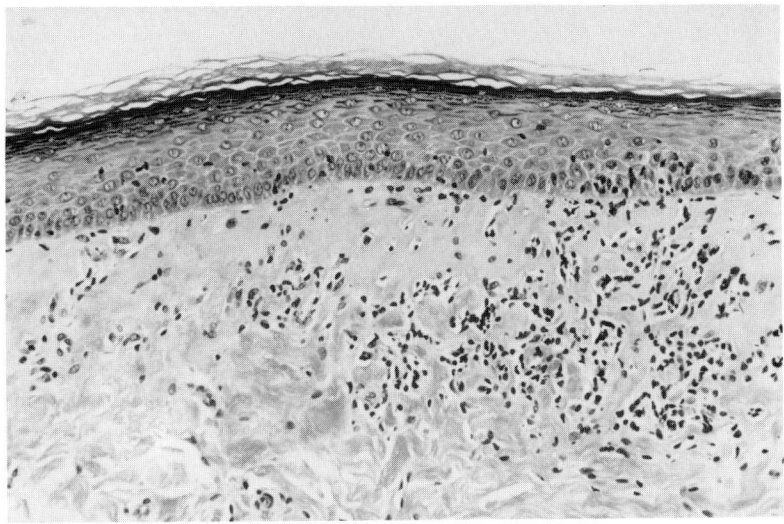

Fig. 6.2   Chronic lichen sclerosus. The epithelium is shallow with loss of rete ridges, but dermal hyalinization is limited to a narrow band and the chronic inflammatory cell infiltrate is sparse and partly overlies the dermoepidermal junction. H & E, × 185.

to the superficial cells in normal epithelium, is found in all but the basal layers of the epidermis in lichen sclerosus. This suggests that premature epithelial differentiation may be a feature of this disorder (de Oliviera & Saleiro 1986).

In chronic lichen sclerosus the dermal hyalinization and oedema, which is regarded as typical, may be minimal and limited to linear hyalinization and thickening of the basement membrane, or may even be absent at the site of a biopsy. In other cases, the chronic inflammatory cell infiltrate may be concentrated at the dermoepidermal junction, rather than lying deep in the dermis, producing a picture similar to that seen in lichen planus (Hewitt 1986). There are also cases of lichen sclerosus in which the chronic inflammatory cell infiltrate is minimal (Fig. 6.2). In these cases, however, loss of rete ridges is usual and may give a clue to the diagnosis, although this is less consistent in the vulva than elsewhere in the body. Curiously, when skin grafts have been used to replace tissue affected by vulval lichen sclerosus, the disease has developed in the grafted skin, and skin with the features of lichen sclerosus transferred to the thigh may become normal (Ridley 1988).

Patients with lichen sclerosus complicated by epithelial hyperplasia, even without cytological atypia, have been found by some authors to be at particular risk of developing carcinoma (Rodke et al 1988) and these patients should therefore be identified to the clinician who can institute adequate follow-up. In rare cases, the hyperplastic epithelium may develop the features of vulval intraepithelial neoplasia (see below).

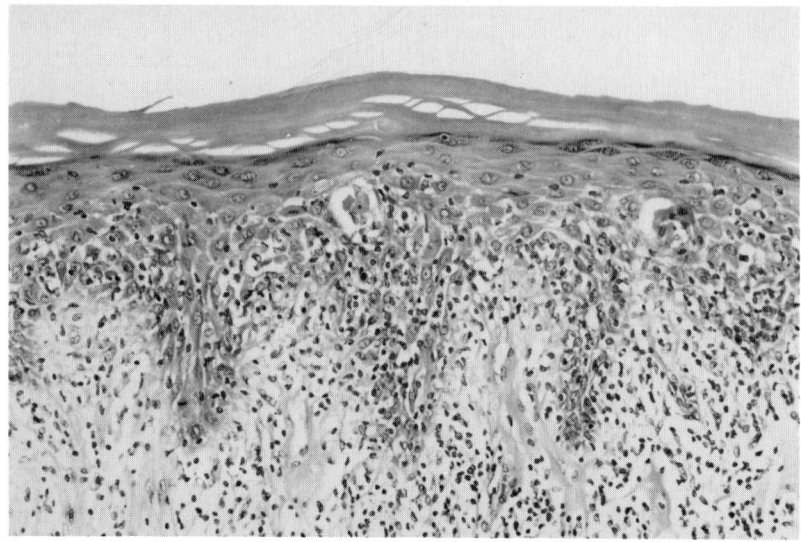

Fig. 6.3   Lichen planus. The epidermis is mildly acanthotic and hyperkeratotic with a prominent granular layer. A chronic inflammatory cell infiltrate overlies the dermoepidermal junction, where there is 'liquefaction' degeneration of the basal layer, with the formation of colloid bodies; the rete ridges are long and pointed or 'saw-toothed'. H & E, × 185.

Lichen planus

Lichen planus may also be difficult to recognize on a non-keratinizing skin surface, and clinicopathological collaboration is essential if these difficult cases are to be correctly diagnosed. Clinically, lichen planus may present diagnostic problems, as there may be little or no systemic disease and, on the vulva, the appearance of the lesions may be very variable. In mild disease the changes may be subtle, and in more severe disease there may be extensive erosions and scarring with, in the chronic phase, loss of the normal vulval contours due to resorption of the labia minora and atrophy similar to that seen in lichen sclerosus (Soper et al 1988, Edwards 1989, Bermejo et al 1990). The lesions (Fig. 6.3) are characterized by hyperkeratosis, acanthosis, an increased granular cell layer and a dense subepidermal band-like infiltrate, mainly composed of T-cells, which extends up to the basal layer where there may be 'liquefaction' degeneration and the formation of colloid bodies; the rete ridges become long and pointed (Ridley 1988).

Other dermatoses

A wide spectrum of other dermatoses, including psoriasis, eczema and bullous disorders, are also encountered on the vulva. Whilst their clinical appearance is often modified by the local conditions, the histological picture is similar to that seen elsewhere on the body. The management of these conditions is mainly the concern of the dermatologist and dermato-pathologist.

VULVAL INTRAEPITHELIAL NEOPLASIA

The adoption of the vulval intraepithelial neoplasia (VIN) terminology to encompass all forms of dystrophy with squamous epithelial cytological atypia, Bowen's disease and squamous carcinoma in situ is based partly on an analogy with cervical intraepithelial neoplasia (Buckley et al 1982, 1984, Crum 1982a, Reid et al 1984). The single most important factor responsible for the introduction of the terminology was, however, the finding, on Feulgen deoxyribonucleic acid microspectrophotometry, that the cells in most cases of mild or moderate atypia were aneuploid (Fu et al 1981, Crum et al 1982b). Most cases of vulval carcinoma in situ are also aneuploid (Friedrich et al 1980, Fu et al 1981), and there is no evidence that aneuploid

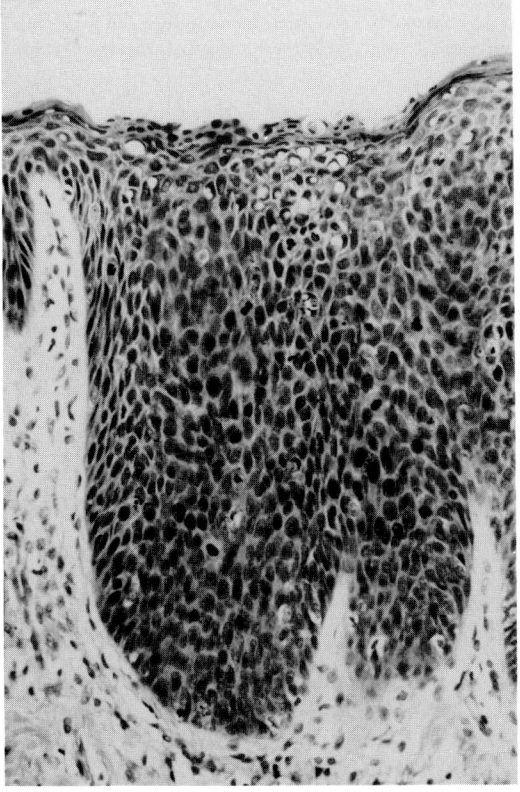

Fig. 6.4 Vulval intraepithelial neoplasia. Large cell basaloid VIN 3 has epithelium occupied by a population of cells resembling parabasal cells, with high nucleocytoplasmic ratios and hyperchromatic nuclei. There is overlying parakeratosis. H & E, × 230.

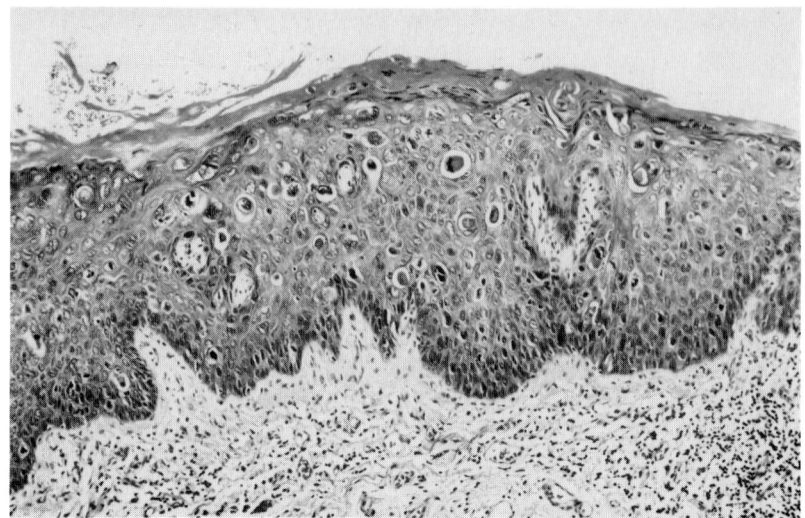

Fig. 6.5   Vulval intraepithelial neoplasia. Bowenoid or 'warty' VIN with preservation of cellular stratification (contrast with Fig. 6.4) but with cellular atypia characterized by premature cytoplasmic maturation, koilocytes and mitoses above the basal layer. H & E, × 120.

atypia and carcinoma in situ differ biologically from each other except in the degree of cytoplasmic maturation or differentiation.

VIN is characterized by disturbances of cellular stratification and maturation. Two basic patterns are seen (Buscema et al 1980): basaloid VIN, in which cells of basal or parabasal type (small cell or large cell VIN, respectively) extend into the upper layers of the epithelium (Fig. 6.4) (Abell 1965); and Bowenoid or 'warty' VIN, in which premature cytoplasmic maturation occurs often in association with epithelial multinucleation, corps ronds and koilocytosis, the latter being the hallmark of human papilloma virus infection (Abell & Gosling 1961) (Fig. 6.5). Common to both forms of VIN are:

● the presence of mitotic figures (often of atypical form) above the basal layer of the epithelium,
● cellular and nuclear pleomorphism (though this is more marked in the Bowenoid form),
● high nucleocytoplasmic ratios,
● irregular nuclear chromatin, and
● either parakeratosis or hyperkeratosis.

These two types of VIN are not mutually exclusive and commonly coexist. It is not unusual in both these forms of VIN for the underlying dermis to contain large numbers of melanin-laden macrophages, as pigmentary incontinence is common and in some cases sufficient to allow the VIN to appear heavily pigmented.

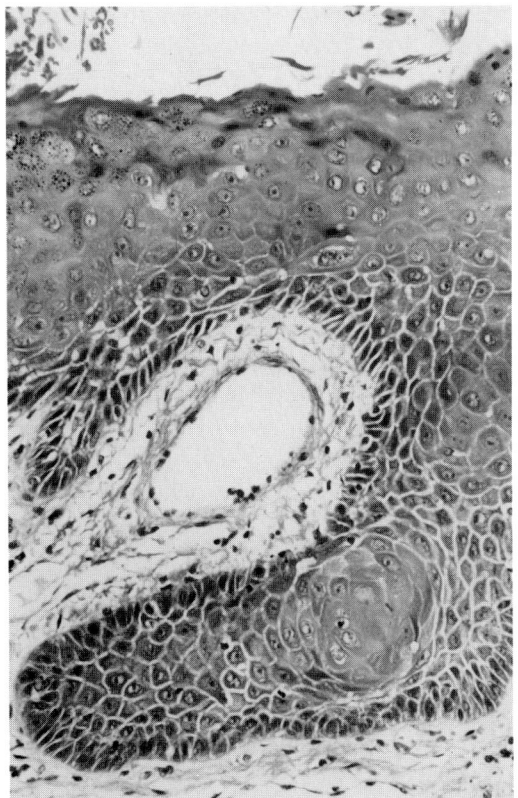

Fig. 6.6   Vulval intraepithelial neoplasia. 'Differentiated' VIN with an epithelial 'pearl' in the rete ridge. Note the prominent nucleoli but the marked cytoplasmic maturation. H & E, × 230.

A further lesion, which is sometimes regarded as a variant of VIN 3 (Friedrich 1976, Buscema & Woodruff 1980, Wilkinson et al 1986) is one in which the epidermis shows little evidence of cytological atypia but instead the principle abnormality is that squamous cells have prominent eosinophilic cytoplasm and there are intraepithelial 'pearls' in the rete ridges. The nuclei in these areas may have coarse chromatin and prominent nucleoli. The term 'differentiated intraepithelial neoplasia' has been suggested for such foci (Wilkinson et al 1986). Whether such an abnormality is really VIN is a matter of debate and further study, but such pearls are not uncommon in the minimally atypical epithelium adjacent to invasive squamous carcinoma (Fig. 6.6), which lends support to the argument for this to be recognized as a form of VIN.

Aetiology

There is a clear association between VIN, sexually transmitted diseases and neoplasms elsewhere, particularly in the lower genital tract. Thus 20–25% of patients with VIN 3 have concurrent, or metachronous, CIN (Buscema et al 1980, Friedrich et al 1980, Benedet & Murphy 1982, Caglar et al 1982, DiPaola et al 1982, Andreasson & Bock 1985, Spitzer et al 1989) whilst between 8 and 40% have concurrent or subsequent invasive neoplasms, most commonly in the genital tract but also elsewhere in the body. Sexually transmitted disease occurs in 22–60% of women who develop VIN (Collins et al 1970, Friedrich et al 1980). A history of herpetic vulvitis can be elicited in 10–12% patients, and 15–30% have condylomata acuminata (Abell 1965, Kovi et al 1974, Forney et al 1977, Buscema et al 1980, Friedrich et al 1980, Caglar et al 1982, Bernstein et al 1983, Daling et al 1984).

A clear association between Bowenoid VIN, Bowenoid papulosis and human papillomavirus (HPV) type 16 has been demonstrated (Pelisse et al 1985, Obalek et al 1986, Bergeron et al 1987, Gupta et al 1987, Reid et al 1987, Bender et al 1988, Nuovo et al 1990), although the virus is often identified only in those areas of VIN showing evidence of koilocytosis and surface maturation (Beckmann et al 1988) and is absent from those areas showing little or no cytoplasmic differentiation. It has been suggested that, in some cases, herpes simplex virus type 2 (HSV 2) may act synergistically with HPV in the development of VIN (Zur Hausen 1982).

Clinical aspects

A major problem when describing the clinical features of VIN is that most reports refer only to VIN 3 (see below) and not to lesser grades of the condition; this should be remembered when interpreting data.

In general, Bowenoid VIN occurs in younger women and is more likely to be multifocal than is the basaloid type (Jones & McClean 1986, Powell et al 1986, Beckman et al 1988, Husseinzadeh et al 1989). The most common presenting complaint of women with VIN is pruritus but a substantial proportion are asymptomatic (Buscema et al 1980, Friedrich et al 1980, Caglar et al 1982, DiPaola et al 1982, Bernstein et al 1983, Andreasson & Bock 1985, Powell et al 1986, Ragnarsson et al 1987, Fiorica et al 1988).

The appearance of the skin is very variable, non-specific and may resemble a variety of non-neoplastic conditions. A diagnosis of VIN can be made only by histological examination, and the multifocal nature of the disorder makes multiple sampling mandatory (Buckley et al 1984). Lesions may be discrete and sharply localized to the labia and/or perineum, or may affect the whole vulva. Between 70 and 75% of lesions are multifocal, especially the HPV-associated lesions (Powell et al 1986, Twiggs et al 1988, Husseinzadeh et al 1989). The lesions may be dull red and granular (Abell & Gosling 1961) or may present a variegated red and white, patchily pigmented appearance, with warty areas in 20% of cases (Buscema et al 1980). In many cases, intraepithelial and intradermal pigment is increased and the lesions are darkly pigmented. Some of these dark-brown or black, warty lesions are regarded as clinically distinct entities and described variably as multicentric pigmented Bowen's disease (Kimura et al 1978, Bhawan 1980) or Bowenoid papulosis (Wade et al 1979). The histological features and the behaviour of the disease appear to differ in no way from the non-pigmented forms of the disease (Obalek et al 1986, Bergeron et al 1987), being complicated in some instances by invasive carcinoma and having nuclear aneuploidy (Planner et al 1987). Such separate designation is, therefore, not recommended, especially as a pathological diagnosis.

Microscopic appearance

VIN may be found in an epithelium of normal thickness, in a hyperplastic epithelium, with or without the histological features of lichen sclerosus (Fig. 6.7), and in a condyloma. It is usual to grade VIN in a manner similar

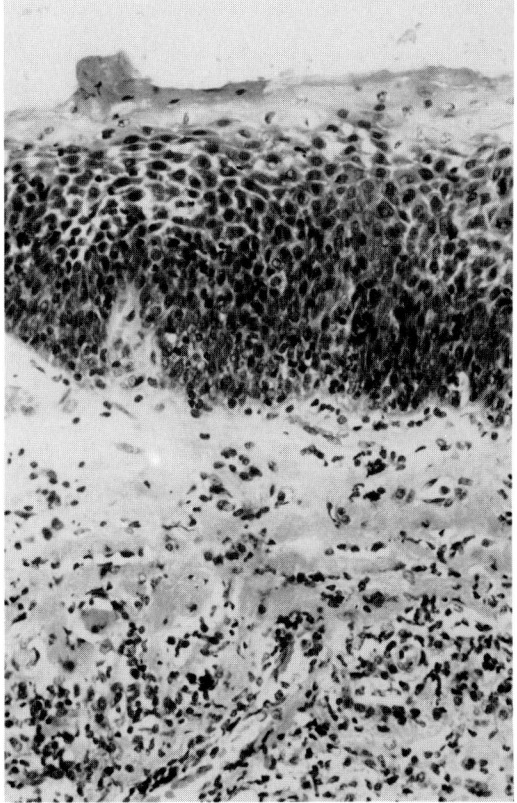

Fig. 6.7   Lichen sclerosus with vulval intraepithelial neoplasia. The epithelium has the features of basaloid VIN 3 and the underlying dermis is hyalinized and infiltrated by chronic inflammatory cells. These are the appearances previously classified as mixed dystrophy. H & E, × 230.

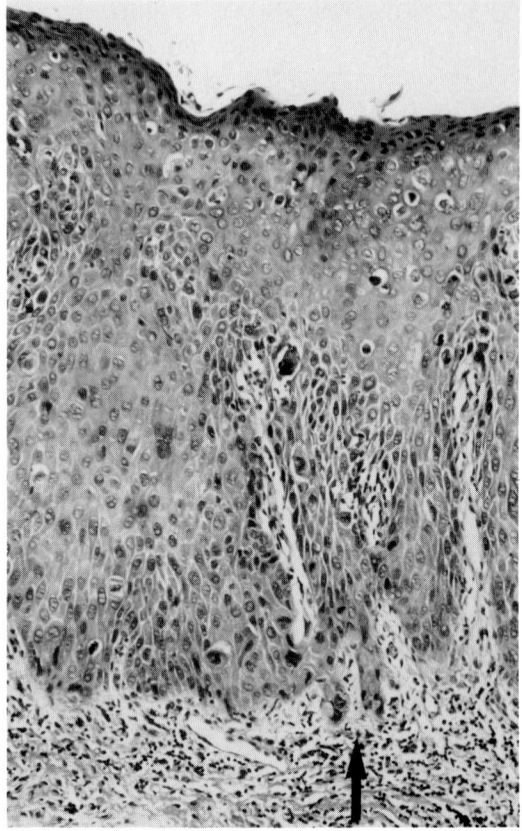

Fig. 6.8   Vulval intraepithelial neoplasia with superficial invasion of the stroma (arrow). The epithelium has the features of 'warty' VIN which is difficult to grade but, in view of the degree of cytoplasmic maturation, probably represents VIN 2. H & E, × 150.

to that used for cervical intraepithelial neoplasia: VIN 1, a well-differentiated intraepithelial neoplasm, VIN 2, a moderately differentiated intraepithelial neoplasm, and VIN 3, a poorly differentiated intraepithelial neoplasm (Buckley et al 1984, Buckley & Fox 1988). The validity of such grading is, however, open to debate. Histological examination rarely reveals the presence of lesions less than VIN 3, and the epithelium from which carcinomas arise is often so well differentiated that one questions whether it represents VIN at all (Fig. 6.6). It may be that some of the intraepithelial neoplasms of the vulva are as well differentiated as the carcinomas to which they give rise and may not fulfil the usual histological criteria for the recognition of an intraepithelial neoplasm. Be that as it may, it is usual to grade the lesions, when possible.

When cellular abnormalities and lack of both stratification and cyto-plasmic differentiation are limited to the lower third of the epithelium the lesion is classed as VIN 1. Extension of the abnormal cells into the middle third of the epithelium puts the lesion into the category of VIN 2 (Fig. 6.8). Involvement of the outer third of the epithelium warrants a diagnosis of VIN 3 (Figs. 6.4 and 6.5). Whilst it is, technically, relatively easy to grade large or small cell basaloid intraepithelial neoplasia of the vulva, it is more difficult to grade Bowenoid VIN with its superimposed HPV changes. A useful feature in distinguishing HPV changes from VIN with 'warty' features is to note that, in an uncomplicated condylomatous lesion, nuclear enlargement, hyperchromasia and atypia tend to become apparent only in the intermediate and superficial cell layers of the epithelium and frequently become progressively more marked in the more superficial layers. When VIN alone is present, nuclear enlargement and pleomorphism is present in the basal and parabasal cell layers and may diminish in the Malpighian and superficial cell layers. Typical HPV-associated VIN tends to be grade 1 or 2 because, as the VIN becomes less well differentiated, it tends to lose the 'warty' features and comes to resemble more closely large or small cell VIN with few or no HPV-associated features.

Pathological factors in prognosis

The behaviour of VIN appears to be very variable and the prognosis, in individual cases, is not predictable. That VIN 3 may lead to invasive carcinoma is not questioned, but spontaneous regression of histologically proven aneuploid VIN 3 has also been reported (Buckley & Fox 1988).

The invasive potential of VIN, particularly the Bowenoid type in the younger patient, appears to be low and is usually estimated to be no more than 3 or 4% (Fiorica et al 1988). The risk of invasion is not consistently low, however, and is reported to be greater in women with multifocal 'warty' VIN if they are older than the average patient with this form of the disease (Jones & McClean 1986). There also generally appears to be a greater risk of invasive carcinoma developing if the patient is old, immunocompromised for whatever reason (Penn 1986), and has a basaloid lesion with a low ploidy value (Fu et al 1981). Lesions with ploidy values in excess of three times normal tend, on the other hand, to recur or persist (Fu et al 1981) and VIN may recur in grafted skin used to cover surgical defects (Cox et al 1986).

Great care should be taken in the histological examination of specimens removed for the diagnosis or treatment of VIN. Unexpected stromal invasion may be found in up to 20% of patients in whom resected vulval skin is subjected to serial blocking (Chafe et al 1988); whilst in most cases this represents only very superficial stromal invasion (Fig. 6.8), it should be remembered that invasion of only the most minor degree may, in the vulva, be associated with lymph node metastases and even death (DiPaola et al 1975, Parker et al 1975, Yazigi et al 1978, Barnes et al 1980, Kolstad et al 1982, Buckley & Fox 1988, Atamdede & Hoogerland 1989).

Management is also affected by spread of the VIN to the perineal skin, peri-anal region, and the anal canal. This occurs in 14–35% of patients in whom the posterior part of the vulva is involved (Schlaerth et al 1984).

All types of VIN extend into the pilosebaceous units (Abell & Gosling 1961, Abell 1965, Mene & Buckley 1985, Baggish et al 1989, Shatz et al 1989), and treatment must be sufficient to eradicate this component as well as the surface lesion. Estimates of the depth of tissue destruction required vary from 1 mm in non-hairy skin to 5 mm in hair-bearing skin.

Patients with HPV-associated lesions and younger patients have a greater tendency to have multifocal disease in the vulva and intraepithelial or invasive neoplasia elsewhere in the lower genital tract, particularly the vagina and cervix. Lesions in these latter sites often significantly affect the choice of treatment (Rueda-Leverone et al 1987, Bornstein et al 1988, Planner & Hobbs 1988, Spitzer et al 1989).

PAGET'S DISEASE

A consideration of vulval intraepithelial neoplasia would not be complete without a mention of Paget's disease. Paget's disease of the vulva results from the presence, in the vulval epidermis and skin appendages, of secretory, glandular, adenocarcinoma cells (Roth et al 1977, Jones et al 1979, Ordonez et al 1987). The majority of cases are adenocarcinomas in situ and are of unknown aetiology.

In contrast with Paget's disease of the breast, in only 20–30% of cases will an underlying invasive neoplasm be detected (Buckley & Fox 1988) and this may be in the skin adnexa, Bartholin's gland, urinary tract or anorectal area. A picture similar to Paget's disease may also be encountered in metastatic carcinoma.

Paget's cells are generally regarded as representing an aberrant differentiation from a multipotential basal layer cell derived from the embryonic germinative layer of the epidermis (Medenica & Sahihi 1972, Friedrich & Wilkinson 1982, Salazar & Gonzalez-Angulo 1984, Guarner et al 1989). It has been suggested, however, that the cells may be derived from sweat glands but be of similar appearance (Koss & Brockunier 1969, Boehm & Morris 1971, Demopoulos 1971, Belcher 1972, Ferenczy & Richart 1972, Neilson & Woodruff 1972, Jones et al 1979, Webb & Beswick 1983, Kariniemi et al 1984, Mazoujian et al 1984, Moll & Moll 1985, Nagle et al 1985).

Recognition of Paget's disease

Identification of Paget's cells can often be made on routine histological sections. The cells are large, round or oval, and have copious pale cytoplasm and a vesicular, pale, oval or round nucleus which may be hyperchromatic, particularly when it lies peripherally and is indented. This imparts a signet-

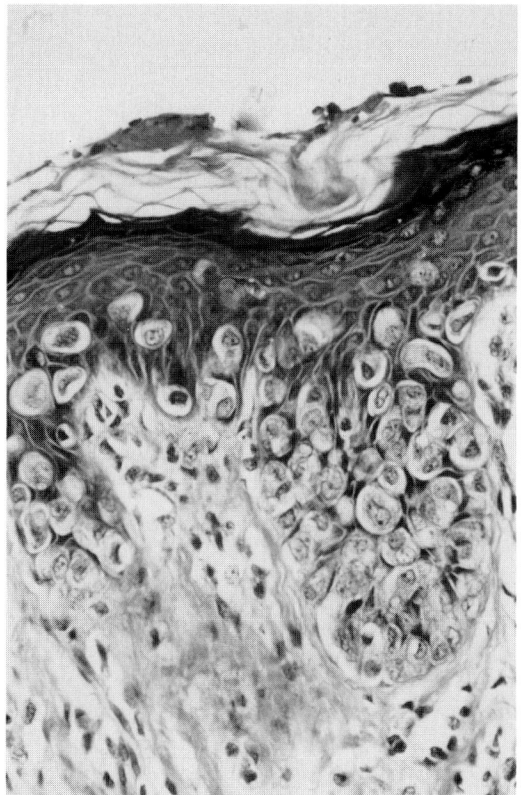

Fig. 6.9 Paget's disease. In the basal layers of this mildly hyperkeratotic squamous epithelium there are nests of large cells with pale cytoplasm and vesicular nuclei; similar individual cells lie higher in the epithelium. H & E, × 370.

ring form to the cells. Nucleoli may be prominent and mitoses are not uncommon (Jones et al 1979). The tumour cells lie singly or form clusters and nests, with or without tubule formation, in the basal and parabasal layers of the epithelium (Fig. 6.9); they may extend to the epidermal surface where they may be identified in cytological preparations (Dennerstein 1988). The cells are often seen in the outer root sheaths of hair follicles, in eccrine and apocrine sweat gland ducts and in sebaceous glands. When they cannot be recognized with certainty, it is important to remember that Paget's cells, although adenocarcinomatous, frequently contain only a trace of neutral and acid mucopolysaccharides, and in some cases only a small proportion of the tumour cells contain mucin.

It may be necessary to distinguish Paget's cells from those of Bowenoid VIN or atypical melanocytes, which they may closely resemble. The presence of intracytoplasmic melanin is insufficient evidence on which to exclude Paget's disease, because a trace of melanin may be found in Paget's cells when the skin is heavily pigmented. The detection of cytokeratins of different molecular weights may be a help in this respect because Paget's cells stain positively for 54 kD cytokeratin, whilst the atypical cells in Bowenoid VIN and superficial spreading melanoma do not (Shah et al 1987). Paget's cells also stain positively with epithelial membrane antigen and carcinoembryonic antigen, whilst approximately 60% react positively with gross cystic disease fluid protein, a marker of apocrine differentiation (Guarner et al 1989). A proportion of the cells also exhibit c-*erb*-B2 oncogene over-expression, but to a lesser degree than do the cells of mammary Paget's disease (Keatings et al 1990).

Pathological factors in prognosis and management

Paget's disease frequently extends beyond the clinically apparent margins and it is useful to undertake intraoperative frozen section examination of resection margins to ensure adequate excision (Stacy et al 1986). However, even when resection skin margins have been free from malignancy (Bergen et al 1989), recurrence has been reported not only in residual vulval skin but also in skin grafted from other areas of the body (de Jonge & Knobel 1988). It is also important to examine the adequacy of excision at the deep margin because of the tendency of the cells to involve the pilosebaceous units. Clearly the presence of an invasive carcinoma necessitates radical therapy.

REFERENCES

Abell M R 1965 Intraepithelial carcinomas of epidermis and squamous mucosa of vulva and perineum. Surgical Clinics of North America 45: 1179–1198
Abell M R, Gosling J R G 1961 Intraepithelial and infiltrative carcinoma of the vulva: Bowen's type. Cancer 14: 318–329
Andreasson B, Bock J E 1985 Intraepithelial neoplasia in the vulvar region. Gynecologic Oncology 21: 300–305
Atamdede F, Hoogerland D 1989 Regional lymph node recurrence following local excision for microinvasive vulvar carcinoma. Gynecologic Oncology 34: 125–128
Baggish M S, Sze E H, Adelson M D, Cohn G, Oates R P 1989 Quantitative evaluation of the skin and accessory appendages in vulvar carcinoma in situ. Obstetrics and Gynecology 74: 169–174
Barnes A E, Crissman J D, Schellhas H F, Azoury R S 1980 Microinvasive carcinoma of the vulva: a clinicopathologic evaluation. Obstetrics and Gynecology 56: 234–238
Beckmann A M, Kiviat N B, Daling J R, Sherman K J, McDougall J K 1988 Human papillomavirus type 16 in multifocal neoplasia of the female genital tract. International Journal of Gynecological Pathology 7: 39–47
Belcher R W 1972 Extramammary Paget's disease. Enzyme histochemical and electron microscopic study. Archives of Pathology 94: 59–64
Bender H G, Degen K W, Beck L 1988 Human papilloma virus findings in the perimeter of vulvo-vaginal malignancies. European Journal of Gynaecological Oncology 9: 287–290
Benedet J L, Murphy K J 1982 Squamous carcinoma in situ of the vulva. Gynecologic Oncology 14: 213–219
Bergen S, DiSaia P J, Liao S Y, Berman M L 1989 Conservative magagement of extramammary Paget's disease of the vulva. Gynecologic Oncology 33: 151–156
Bergeron C, Naghashfar Z, Canaan C, Shah K, Fu Y, Ferenczy A 1987 Human papillomavirus type 16 in intraepithelial neoplasia (bowenoid papulosis) coexistent invasive carcinoma of the vulva. International Journal of Gynecological Pathology 6: 1–11

Bermejo A, Bermejo M D, Roman P, Botella R, Bagan J V 1990 Lichen planus with simultaneous involvement of the oral cavity and genitalia. Oral Surgery, Oral Medicine, Oral Pathology 69: 209–216

Bernstein S G, Kovacs B R, Townsend D E, Morrow C P 1983 Vulvar carcinoma in situ. Obstetrics and Gynecology 61: 304–307

Bhawan J 1980 Multicentric pigmented Bowen's disease: a clinically benign squamous carcinoma in situ. Gynecologic Oncology 10: 201–205

Boehm B, Morris J McL 1971 Paget's disease and apocrine gland carcinoma of the vulva. Obstetrics and Gynecology 38: 185–192

Bornstein J, Kaufman R H, Adam E, Adler-Storthz K 1988 Multicentre intraepithelial neoplasia involving the vulva. Clinical features and association with human papillomavirus and herpes simplex virus. Cancer 62: 1601–1604

Buckley C H, Fox H 1988 Epithelial tumours of the vulva. In: Ridley C M (ed) The vulva. Churchill Livingstone, Edinburgh

Buckley C H, Butler E B, Fox H 1982 Cervical intraepithelial neoplasia. Journal of Clinical Pathology 35: 1–13

Buckley C H, Butler E B, Fox H 1984 Vulval intraepithelial neoplasia and microinvasive carcinoma of the vulva. Journal of Clinical Pathology 37: 1201–1211

Buscema J, Woodruff J D 1980 Progressive histobiologic alterations in the development of vulvar cancer. Report of five cases. American Journal of Obstetrics and Gynecology 138: 146–150

Buscema J, Woodruff J D, Parmley T H, Genadry R 1980 Carcinoma in situ of the vulva. Obstetrics and Gynecology 55: 225–230

Caglar H, Tamer S, Hreshchyshn M M 1982 Vulvar intraepithelial neoplasia. Obstetrics and Gynecology 60: 346–349

Chafe W, Richards A, Morgan L, Wilkinson E 1988 Unrecognized invasive carcinoma in vulvar intraepithelial neoplasia (VIN). Gynecologic Oncology 31: 154–165

Collins C G, Roman-Lopez J J, Lee F Y L 1970 Intraepithelial carcinoma of the vulva. American Journal of Obstetrics and Gynecology 108: 1187–1191

Cox S M, Kaufman R H, Kaplan A 1986 Recurrent carcinoma in situ of the vulva in a skin graft. American Journal of Obstetrics and Gynecology 155: 177–179

Crum C P 1982a Vulvar intrepithelial neoplasia: the concept and its application. Human Pathology 13: 187–189

Crum C P, Fu Y S, Levine R U, Richart R M, Townsend D E, Fenoglio C M 1982b Intraepithelial squamous lesions of the vulva: biologic and histologic criteria for the distinction of condylomas from vulvar intraepithelial neoplasia. American Journal of Obstetrics and Gynecology 144: 77–83

Daling J R, Chu J, Weiss N S, Emel L, Tamini H K 1984 The association of condylomata acuminata and squamous carcinoma of the vulva. British Journal of Cancer 50: 533–535

de Jonge E T, Knobel J 1988 Recurrent Paget's disease of the vulva after simple vulvectomy and skin grafting. A case report. South African Medical Journal 9: 46–47

Demopoulos R I 1971 Fine structure of the extramammary Paget's cell. Cancer 27: 1202–1210

Dennerstein G J 1988 Cytology of the vulva. Journal of Reproductive Medicine 33: 703–704

de Oliveira J M, Saliero V 1986 Involucrin expression in vulvar lesions. Journal of Reproductive Medicine 31: 828–830

Di Paola G R, Gomez-Rueda N, Arrighi L 1975 Relevance of microinvasion in carcinoma of the vulva. Obstetrics and Gynecology 45: 647–649

Di Paola G R, Rueda-Leverone N G, Belardi M G, Vighi S 1982 Vulvar carcinoma in situ: a report of 28 cases. Gynecologic Oncology 14: 236–242

Edwards L 1989 Vulvar lichen planus. Archives of Dermatology 125: 1677–1680

Ferenczy A, Richart R M 1972 Ultrastructure of perineal Paget's disease. Cancer 29: 1141–1149

Fiorica J V, Cavanagh D, Marsden D E, Shepherd J H, Ruffolo E H, Songster C L 1988 Carcinoma in situ of the vulva: 24 years experience in southwest Florida. Southern Medical Journal 81: 589–593

Forney J P, Morrow CP, Townsend D E, DiSaia J P 1977 Management of carcinoma in situ of the vulva. American Journal of Obstetrics and Gynecology 127: 801–806

Friedrich E G 1976 New nomenclature for vulvar disease. Report of the committee on terminology. Obstetrics and Gynecology 47: 122–124

Friedrich E G, Wilkinson E J 1982 The vulva. In: Blaustein A (ed) Pathology of the female genital tract, 2nd edn. Springer-Verlag, New York

Friedrich E G, Wilkinson E J, Fu Y S 1980 Carcinoma in situ of the vulva: a continuing challenge. American Journal of Obstetrics and Gynecology 136: 830–843

Fu Y S, Reagan J W, Townsend D E, Kaufman R H, Richart R M, Wentz W B 1981 Nuclear DNA study of vulvar intraepithelial and invasive squamous neoplasms. Obstetrics and Gynecology 57: 643–652

Gardner H L, Kaufman R H 1969 Benign diseases of the vulva and vagina. C V Mosby, St Louis

Guarner J, Cohen C, DeRose P B 1989 Histogenesis of extramammary and mammary Paget cells. An immunohistochemical study. American Journal of Dermatopathology 11: 313–318

Gupta J, Pilotti S, Shah K V, De Palo G, Rilke F 1987 Human papillomavirus-associated early vulvar neoplasia investigated by in situ hybridization. American Journal of Surgical Pathology 11: 430–434

Hewitt J 1986 Histologic criteria for lichen sclerosus of the vulva. Journal of Reproductive Medicine 31: 781–787

Husseinzadeh N, Newman N J, Wesseler T A 1989 Vulvar intraepithelial neoplasia: a clinicopathological study of carcinoma in situ of the vulva. Gynecologic Oncology 33: 157–163

Jeffcoate T N A, Woodcock A S 1961 Premalignant conditions of the vulva, with particular reference to chronic epithelial dystrophies. British Journal of Medicine 2: 127–134

Jones R W, McClean M R 1986 Carcinoma of the vulva: a review of 31 treated and five untreated cases. Obstetrics and Gynecology 68: 499–503

Jones R E Jr, Austin C, Ackerman A B 1979 Extramammary Paget's disease. A critical re-examination. American Journal of Dermatopathology 1: 101–132

Kariniemi A-L, Forsman L, Wahlström T, Vesterinen E, Andersson L 1984 Expression of differentiation antigens in mammary and extramammary Paget's disease. British Journal of Dermatology 110: 203–210

Keatings L, Sinclair J, Wright C et al 1990 c-erbB-2 oncoprotein expression in mammary and extramammary Paget's disease: an immunohistochemical study. Histopathology 17: 243–247

Kimura S, Hirai A, Harada R, Nagashima M 1978 So-called multicentric pigmented Bowen's disease. Dermatologica 157: 229–237

Kolstad P, Iversen T, Abeler V, Aalders J 1982 Microinvasive carcinoma of the vulva-definition and treatment problems. Clinical Oncology 1: 355–362

Koss L G, Brockunier A Jr 1969 Ultrastructural aspects of Paget's disease of the vulva. Archives of Pathology 87: 592–600

Kovi J, Tillman R L, Lee S M 1974 Malignant transformation of condyloma acuminatum. A light microscopic and ultrastructural study. American Journal of Clinical Pathology 61: 702–710

Mazoujian G, Pinkus G S, Haagensen D E Jr 1984 Extramammary Paget's disease—Evidence for an apocrine origin. An immunoperoxidase study of gross cystic disease fluid protein-15, carcino-embryonic antigen, and keratin proteins. American Journal of Surgical Pathology 8: 43–50

Medenica M, Sahihi T 1972 Ultrastructural study of a case of extramammary Paget's disease of the vulva. Archives of Dermatology 105: 236–243

Mene A, Buckley C H 1985 Involvement of the vulval skin appendages by intraepithelial neoplasia. British Journal of Obstetrics and Gynaecology 92: 634–638

Moll I, Moll R 1985 Cells of extramammary Paget's disease express cytokeratins different from those of epidermal cells. Dermatology 84: 3–8

Nagle R B, Lucas D O, McDaniel K M, Clark V A, Schmalzel G M 1985 New evidence linking mammary and extramammary cells to a common cell phenotype. American Journal of Clinical Pathology 83: 431–438

Neilson D, Woodruff J D 1972 Electron microscopy in in situ and invasive vulvar Paget's disease. American Journal of Obstetrics and Gynecology 113: 719–732

Nuovo G J, Friedman D, Richart R M 1990 In situ hybridization analysis of human papillomavirus DNA segregation patterns in lesions of the femal genital tract. Gynecologic Oncology 36: 256–262

Obalek S, Jablonska S, Beaudenon S, Walczak L, Orth G 1986 Bowenoid papulosis of the male and female genitalia: risk of cervical neoplasia. Journal of the American Academy of Dermatology 14: 433–444

Ordonez N G, Awalt H, Mackay B 1987 Mammary and extramammary Paget's disease. An immunocytochemical and ultrastructural study. Cancer 59: 1173–1183

Parker R T, Duncan I, Rampone J, Creasman W 1975 Operating management of early invasive epidermoid carcinoma of the vulva. American Journal of Obstetrics and Gynecology 123: 349–354

Pelisse M, Orth G, Croissant O et al 1985 Données anatomocliniques et virologiques dans vingt cas de maladie de Bowen vulvaire. Annales de Dermatologie et de Vénérologie 112: 749–750

Penn I 1986 Cancers of the anogenital region in renal transplant recipients. Analysis of 65 cases. Cancer 58: 611–616

Planner R S, Hobbs J B 1988 Intraepithelial and invasive neoplasia of the vulva in association with human papillomavirus infection. Journal of Reproductive Medicine 33: 503–509

Planner R S, Andersen H E, Hobbs J B, Williams R A, Fogarty L F, Hudson P J 1987 Multifocal invasive carcinoma of the vulva in a 25-year-old woman with Bowenoid papulosis. Australian and New Zealand Journal of Obstetrics and Gynaecology 27: 291–295

Powell L C Jr, Dinh T V, Rajaraman E V, Dillard E A Jr, Yandell R B, To T 1986 Carcinoma in situ of the vulva. A clinicopathologic study of 50 cases. Journal of Reproductive Medicine 31: 808–814

Ragnarsson B, Raabe N, Willems J, Pettersson F 1987 Carcinoma in situ of the vulva. Acta Oncologica 26: 277–280

Reid R, Fu Y S, Herschman B R et al 1984 Genital warts and cervical cancer. VI. The relationship between aneuploid and polyploid cervical lesions. American Journal of Obstetrics and Gynecology 150: 189–199

Reid R, Greenberg M, Jenson A B et al 1987 Sexually transmitted papillomaviral infections. I. The anatomic distribution and pathologic grade of neoplastic lesions associated with different viral types. American Journal of Obstetrics and Gynecology 156: 212–222

Ridley C M 1988 General dermatological conditions and dermatoses of the vulva. In: Ridley C M (ed) The vulva. Churchill Livingstone, Edinburgh

Rodke G, Friedrich E G Jr, Wilkinson E J 1988 Malignant potential of mixed vulvar dystrophy (lichen sclerosus associated with squamous cell hyperplasia). Journal of Reproductive Medicine 33: 545–550

Roth L M, Lees S C, Ehrlich C E 1977 Paget's disease of the vulva. A histogenic study of five cases including ultrastructural observations and review of the literature. American Journal of Surgical Pathology 1: 193–206

Rueda-Leverone N G, Di Paola G R, Meiss R P, Vighi S G, Llamosas F 1987 Association of human papillomavirus infection and vulvar intraepithelial neoplasia: a morphological and immunohistochemical study of 30 cases. Gynecologic Oncology 26: 331–339

Salazar H, Gonzalez-Angulo A 1984 Ultrastructural diagnosis in gynaecological pathology. Clinics in Obstetrics and Gynaecology 11: 25–77

Schlaerth J B, Morrow C P, Nalick R H, Gaddis O 1984 Anal involvement by carcinoma in situ of the perineum in women. Obstetrics and Gynecology 64: 406–411

Shah K D, Tabibzadeh S S, Gerber M A 1987 Immunohistochemical distinction of Paget's disease from Bowen's disease and superficial spreading melanoma with the use of monoclonal cytokeratin antibodies. American Journal of Pathology 88: 689–695; 89: 572 (erratum)

Shatz P, Bergeron C, Wilkinson E J, Arseneau J, Ferenczy A 1989 Vulvar intraepithelial neoplasia and skin appendage involvement. Obstetrics and Gynecology 74: 769–774

Soper D E, Patterson J W, Hurt W G, Fantl J A, Blaylock W K 1988 Lichen planus of the vulva. Obstetrics and Gynecology 72: 74–76

Spitzer M, Krumholz B A, Seltzer V L 1989 The multicentric nature of disease related to human papillomavirus infection of the female genital tract. Obstetrics and Gynecology 73: 303–307

Stacy D, Burrell M O, Franklin E W 1986 Extramammary Paget's disease of the vulva and anus: use of intraoperative frozen-section margins. American Journal of Obstetrics and Gynecology 155: 519–523

Twiggs L B, Okagaki T, Clark B, Fukushima M, Ostrow R, Faras A 1988 A clinical, histopathologic, and molecular biologic investigation of vulvar intraepithelial neoplasia. International Journal of Gynecological Pathology 7: 48–55

Wade T R, Kopf A W, Ackerman A B 1979 Bowenoid papulosis of the genitalia. Archives of Dermatology 115: 306–308

Webb J B, Beswick I P 1983 Eccrine hidradenocarcinoma of the vulva with Paget's disease. Case report with review of the literature. British Journal of Obstetrics and Gynaecology 90: 90–95

Wilkinson E J, Kneale B, Lynch P J 1986 Report of the ISSVD terminology committee. Journal of Reproductive Medicine 31: 973–974

Yazigi R, Piver M S, Tsukada Y 1978 Microinvasive carcinoma of the vulva. Obstetrics and Gynecology 51: 368–370

Zur Hausen H 1982 Human genital cancer: synergism between two virus infections or synergism between a virus infection and initiating events? Lancet ii: 1370–1372

7. Malignant melanoma and related lesions of the lower female genital tract

T. P. Rollason

INTRODUCTION

Understanding of melanocytic lesions of the vulva, vagina and cervix can only be considered, at best, to have advanced at the same rate as understanding of pigmented skin lesions generally. This chapter will firstly review previous work on these lesions, and will attempt to put this work into the context of modern understanding of pigmented lesions of the skin generally, and secondly will indicate those areas where recent advances have occurred with specific regard to the lower female genital tract.

The chapter will concentrate on pigmented melanocytic lesions, but these should be put into context. Friedrich (1983) compared the incidence of various pigmented lesions on the vulva in his clinical practice and found that lentigo simplex was the commonest (36%) followed by pigmented squamous cell carcinoma in situ (22%), benign melanocytic naevi (21%), 'reactive hyperpigmentation' (10%), pigmented basal cell papilloma (5%) and pigmented basal cell carcinoma (1%). Lichen simplex can also lead to pigmentation of the genitalia, and haemosiderin deposition may be heavy in lichen sclerosus, plasma cell vulvitis and urethral and vaginal prolapse (Ridley 1988). Urethral prolapse in particular may mimic malignant melanoma (Beilby & Ridley 1987). Melanocyte proliferation, and even malignant melanoma, has also been described in association with condylomata acuminata (Blessing et al 1989), though these may be no more than chance occurrences.

In contrast to the vulva, pigmented lesions of the vagina and cervix other than malignant melanoma (itself a rarity) appear to be extremely rare. Most reports are of blue naevi. In the past, bismuth salts have lead to mucosal pigmentation, which may include the vagina (Weiner 1940), and anti-malarials can also lead to mucosal pigmentation (Lutterloh and Shallenberger 1946).

LENTIGO SIMPLEX, 'MELANOSIS' AND RELATED CONDITIONS

The term 'melanosis' is ill defined and, on the vulva, has been used to mean simple patchy hyperpigmentation, hyperpigmentation with elongation of dermal papillae and lentigo simplex, and even pigmentation due to inorganic salts. Patchy and diffuse melanin pigmentation of the vulva has been stated to be common (Beilby & Ridley 1987). However, although Jones (1979) found patches of hyperpigmentation due to a local basal increase in melanin deposition, on 80% of vulvas of white women on post-mortem histological examination only 0.5% were *macroscopically* evident. No cause for this hyperpigmentation was found, and, in these cases, no lentiginous alteration was seen in dermal papillae, which could be up to 7 mm diameter. Jackson (1984) also described cases of extensive 'melanosis' of the vulva due to increased basal layer melanin pigmentation and deposition of melanin in melanophages in the upper dermis; no history of previous irradiation, inflammation or drug therapy was noted. Sison-Torre and Ackerman (quoted in Ridley 1988) have described extensive hyperpigmentation of the vulva due to lesions similar to lentigo simplex; again the aetiology was obscure.

Cases of 'melanosis' of the vagina have also been described (Grunberger 1973, Tsukuda 1976). These were simply cases of melanin pigmentation by vaginal melanocytes. Vaginal intraepithelial melanocytes are poorly studied but have been found in 3% of normal vaginas (Nigogosyan et al 1964) in varying distribution and numbers. Occasional cases of extensive vaginal melanin pigmentation have been seen after pelvic irradiation (Nigogosyan et al 1964, Tsukuda 1976). Norris and Taylor (1966) described two different pigmented lesions of the vagina, one resembling lentigo simplex and the other consisting of melanin-containing cells in the subepithelial tissues, which they termed 'melanosis' (further highlighting the deficiencies in the use of this term); no heterotopic tissues were present.

BENIGN MELANOCYTIC NAEVI

It has been commonly stated that most melanocytic naevi occurring on the female genitalia are junctional in type, but whilst some workers have found junctional and compound naevi to occur disproportionately frequently on the vulva others have disagreed (Christensen et al 1987). In the Birmingham Histopathology Data Pool, the relative proportions of the common types of naevus are the same as for the skin generally (Table 7.1). Some of these

Table 7.1   Types of vulval and total naevi in females (Birmingham Histopathology Data Pool figures)

	Intradermal		Compound		Junctional	
	No.	Mean age (years)	No.	Mean age (years)	No.	Mean age (years)
Vulva	14	49.0	7	28.7	0	—
All sites	770	28.7	349	27.7	65	21.6

discrepancies in published data may be due to inclusion of lesions on the mucocutaneous surfaces in some studies but not in others. Naevi occurring on these surfaces do appear to be most frequently junctional and uncommonly intradermal (Kendall Pierson 1987).

Pack et al (1952), in a clinical study of 1000 patients, found that vulvar naevi made up only 0.1% of all naevi studied (14 609 in total). Other workers have also commented on the relative preponderance of naevi on light-exposed skin (Green et al 1985) and their infrequent occurrence in the 'bathing suit areas'. The Birmingham figures for females (Table 7.1) again do not directly support these comments—only 1.7% of naevi were coded in females as arising on the skin of the perineum and vulva (21 of 1184), but as this area is approximately 2% of the total body area no evidence for a reduced incidence at this site emerges. In fact due to the alternative methods of coding vulval lesions in the Birmingham system, which is SNOP-based (Standard Nomenclature of Pathology), these figures are undoubtedly an underestimate of total vulval naevi.

Data on benign melanocytic naevi of the vagina is lacking but it is likely that any occurring here would be junctional, as on other mucous membranes. Nicholson (1936) reported a case of 'epidermal heteromorphosis' in the upper vagina. This was histologically described as an area of 1 cm in diameter, containing epidermal structures and including two well-described melanocytic naevi, one of which was clearly illustrated. Blue naevi in the vagina have been very rarely described. Rodriguez & Ackerman (1968), in a review of 45 cellular blue naevi and 147 blue naevi, found one cellular blue naevus involving the cervix, vagina and hymenal ring. Tobon & Murphy (1977) also reported a single blue naevus of the apex of the vagina in an elderly woman.

Cervical blue naevi are well described, with 50 cases in the world literature up to 1985 (Patel & Bhagavan 1985); indeed, the cervix appears to be the most common extracutaneous site for these lesions. They are usually found incidentally in hysterectomy specimens and are exclusively endocervical. There appears to be a preponderance of cases in postmenopausal women, which cannot be explained solely on the basis of relative frequency of hysterectomy in this group. No specific features differentiate blue naevi of the cervix from those of the skin generally. No cellular blue naevi confined to the cervix have been reported.

To date, the benign but histologically atypical and worrying pigmented spindle cell naevus (Sagebiel et al 1984) has not been described in the lower female genital tract and appears to involve predominantly the extremities. Spitz naevi have occasionally been described on the vulva in isolated form (Nodl quoted in Janovski & Douglas 1972, Hulagu & Erez 1973). The agminate (clustered) form (Capetanakis 1975) has not been specifically described in the lower female genital tract, but a few cases have been described involving all skin sites (Wallace 1974) and it has been illustrated on the upper inner thigh (Burket 1979).

PRECURSOR LESIONS OF MALIGNANT MELANOMA

Malignant melanoma at any site may arise either in 'normal' skin or in a pre-existing melanocytic naevus. It is generally accepted that the risk of development of malignant melanoma in a purely intradermal naevus or blue naevus is very low, though cases do appear to occur in both instances (Chung et al 1975). The component which appears to confer malignant potential is the junctional element.

During the natural history of a typical intradermal naevus, melanocytes proliferate at the dermoepidermal junction and, at the 4–6 mm stage of radial growth, begin to pass into the dermis. This is followed by loss of cells from the dermoepidermal junction and progressive differentiation of the dermal naevus cells towards a more 'neural' appearance (Briggs 1985, Green et al 1985). The pattern of the radial growth phase of naevi has been separated by Clark et al (1984) into two types: lentiginous, characterized by increase in number of simple melanocytes in the basal layer of the epidermis, and nested, characterized by small clusters of melanocytes at the tips of the rete ridges.

The nature of the changes constituting *atypical* melanocytic proliferation is still contentious and the use of the term 'dysplasia' in this context and that of a 'dysplastic naevus' has been vigorously criticized (Ackerman & Mihara 1985, Ackerman 1988).

Clark et al (1984) also separated the emergence of atypical proliferation in the intradermal radial melanocyte growth phase into two patterns: lentiginous melanocytic dysplasia, composed of melanocytes with large hyperchromatic nuclei and scanty artefactually vacuolated cytoplasm, and epithelioid melanocytic dysplasia (Fig 7.1), comprising larger melanocytes with more cytoplasm and lighter stained nuclei. These abnormal proliferated cells form small nests which are atypical in site, being unconfined to the tips of the rete.

Along with the alterations described above, changes in the epidermis such as acanthosis, hyper- and parakeratosis and pseudoepitheliomatous hyperplasia may occur with atypical melanocytic proliferations. The dermis also may be affected with widening of the papillary dermis focally in relation to the abnormal melanocytes in the overlying epidermis, telangiectasia and a patchy lymphocytic infiltrate. Fine 'lamellar' or eosinophilic fibrosis may be seen beneath the rete. Free melanin and melanin-laden macrophages may be prominent. Granulomas and germinal follicles, occasionally seen adjacent to invasive melanomas, are not recorded. The changes described in the preceding sections are those also described in both the familial and sporadic cases of 'dysplastic naevus' (Elder et al 1981), which may be junctional or compound in type.

The final result of the atypical melanocyte proliferation noted above is the development of malignant melanoma in situ, followed by invasive malignant melanoma. The criteria for separating atypical melanocytic hyperplasia

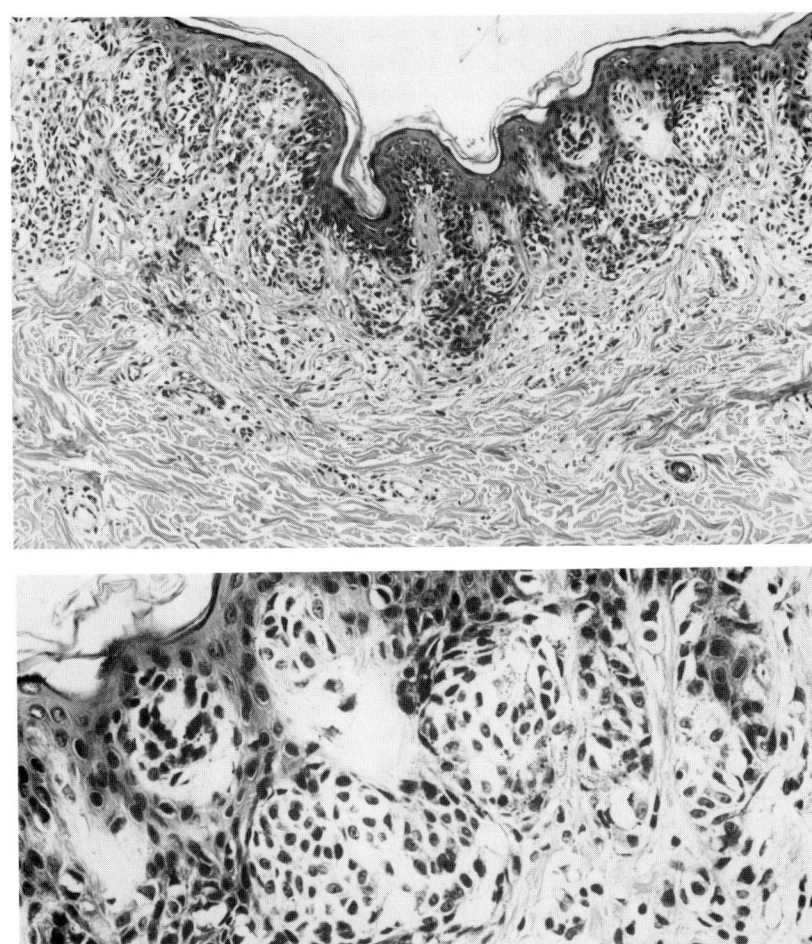

Fig. 7.1 Atypical melanocyte proliferation showing nests of melanocytes not confined to the tips of the rete ridges (epithelioid melanocytic 'dysplasia'). A patchy lymphocytic infiltrate is seen in the dermis and there is fine lamellar fibrosis beneath the rete.

from malignant melanoma in situ are, at present, ill defined. Most regard upward migration of solitary, or more significantly nested, melanocytes as the major differentiating feature. It appears that a similar pattern of radial migration followed by upward intraepithelial migration of melanocytes occurs in malignant melanomas arising de novo. Perhaps one third of malignant melanomas have adjacent melanocytic atypical proliferations, which may show a combination of patterns (Cook & Robertson 1985).

The proportion of malignant melanomas that arise in naevi has been extensively debated (Ackerman & Mihara 1985), but no conclusions have been reached. With regard specifically to the vulva, no cases of melanoma arising in congenital naevi are on record (Kendall Pierson 1987) and no systematic study of the existence of remnants of pre-existing acquired naevi in cases of malignant melanoma of the vulva is available. Studies at other sites have found such elements in between 10 and 30% of cases (Crucioli & Stilwell 1982, Lopansri & Mihm 1979).

Leaving aside the familial dysplastic naevus syndrome and simple morphological evidence from the histology of melanomas, evidence associating naevi with the later development of melanoma comes from population studies of the frequency of occurrence of naevi and melanomas in different individuals. Patients with cutaneous melanoma have greater numbers of naevi on the body than controls (Roush 1988), and 'excess' body naevi appear to confer approximately a three-fold increase in risk, but evidence of a linear correlation with increasing numbers of naevi is inconclusive. Employing the figures indicated previously (p. 121) Pack et al (1952) argued that as melanomas of the male and female genitalia make up 2.8% of all melanomas and only 0.1% of naevi occur on the genitalia, then naevi here must have a much greater malignant potential than on the skin generally. This is not borne out by figures from the Birmingham Histopathology Data Pool and West Midlands Regional Cancer Registry, where 1.7% of naevi were coded as originating in the skin of the perineal area and vulva (Table 7.1) and 0.7 and 2.2% of melanomas were coded as arising here. The discrepancy in the tumour incidences between the two sources is explainable, as indicated previously, by the ability to code vulval melanomas under several different SNOP codes. However, this under-representation in the Birmingham Histopathology Data Pool figures data may reasonably be expected to apply equally to naevi and melanomas, and relative incidences would therefore not be affected. Why Pack et al found such a low incidence of naevi on the vulva is difficult to determine, though perhaps reticence about thorough examination of this site played a part, as the study findings were based on clinical examination.

These studies on relative incidence of naevi and melanoma do not, of course, offer evidence of direct transformation, which is generally no more than anecdotal. Some further evidence can however be derived from types of naevi at different sites. In this regard, it is of interest that the Birmingham data on malignant melanoma (Table 7.2) confirmed the usually noted preponderance of these tumours on the trunk of men and lower legs of women (Macartney et al 1980), but both of these sites (more particularly the lower leg) showed a disproportionate number of junctional and compound naevi compared to intradermal naevi in both sexes. This might be offered as some minor further supportive evidence that naevi per se confer malignant risk. It might of course equally be argued that it is some genetic or environmental (e.g. sunlight) effect on these areas that confers the risk for

Table 7.2   Percentage distribution of naevi and melanomas (Birmingham Histopathology Data Pool figures)

	Intradermal		Compound		Junctional		Melanomas:		
	M	F	M	F	M	F	M	F	M:F ratio
Head and neck	73	62	32	31	18	26 ⎫	32	28	0.5:1.0
Upper limbs	6	7	6	12	5	11 ⎭			
Trunk	19	27	48	46	36	31	41	17	1.0:1.0
Lower limbs	2	4	14	11	41	32	27	55	0.2:1.0

M, male; F, female. (Modified, with permission from Macartney et al 1980.)

both melanoma and naevi with a junctional component. These figures also apply to naevi removed, and are therefore unlikely to represent the pattern of 'unremarkable' naevi at any site.

ATYPICAL VULVAL MELANOCYTIC NAEVI

A proportion of vulval naevi in premenopausal women and adolescents may show atypical features (Friedman & Ackerman 1981). These include a wide lateral extent, large pleomorphic epithelioid (or sometimes spindled) intraepidermal melanocytes with abundant eosinophilic cytoplasm and prominent nucleoli, variably sized superficial, intradermal melanocyte nests, and confluence of intra-epithelial melanocyte clusters on adjacent rete ridges. The lesions tend, however, to show overall symmetry, with cellular maturation in the deep dermis and little or no transepithelial migration of single cells or cell nests. Adnexal structures are often involved, and an inflammatory cell infiltrate may be seen in the dermis. The nature, and premalignant potential, of these naevi is still unclear. They may constitute an uncommon variant of 'dysplastic' naevus (if the existence of this entity is accepted) in that the histological appearances described are very similar, but Christensen et al (1987) have argued against this, having found, in a study of 59 naevi on the vulva, only one 'dysplastic' naevus. Christensen et al felt that this indicated no increased occurrence of these lesions at this site compared with the torso, where they regarded 7% of naevi as 'dysplastic'. They found three 'unusual' naevi which they felt were the same lesions described by the previously mentioned authors. These showed the features indicated above but only mild lentiginous melanocytic hyperplasia and mild atypia of melanocytes was seen, of insufficient degree to regard them as 'dysplastic'. None was seen on the trunk. These reports apart, no data exist on 'dysplastic' naevi or atypical melanocytic proliferations with specific reference to the lower female genital tract.

MALIGNANT MELANOMA

Incidence

Malignant melanoma of the vulva is generally considered to make up

Table 7.3   Incidences of malignant melanoma in women (West Midlands Regional Cancer Registry figures)

Sites	Time period	No. of cases (5 years)	Annual incidence rates per 100 000	
			Crude	Age-standardized
Vulva	1971–75	8	0.061	0.037
	1976–80	12	0.092	0.057
	1981–85	14	0.108	0.064
All other skin sites	1961–65	279	2.319	1.832
	1966–70	354	2.839	2.251
	1971–75	419	3.246	2.557
	1976–80	517	3.945	3.074
	1981–85	807	6.241	4.805

between 4 and 10% of all vulval malignant neoplasms (Kendall Pierson 1987) and approximately 4% of all melanomas in females (Morrow & Rutledge 1972, Chung et al 1975, Morrow & Di Saia 1976, Silvers & Halperin 1978). Our own figures are rather different (Bradgate et al 1990); in the West Midlands Regional Cancer Registry data, it accounts for 2.2% of all melanomas in women and 3.6% of all vulval malignant tumours. Nevertheless, even here it is the second most common vulval malignant tumour after squamous cell carcinoma. Malignant melanoma of the skin in general has increased five to six-fold in some countries in the past 40 years and its incidence still appears to be rapidly rising (Jensen & Bolander 1980, Little et al 1980, Osterlind & Moller Jensen 1986). There is, as yet, no evidence of a similar increase in incidence of melanoma on the vulva or elsewhere in the lower female genital tract, though incidence figures for the West Midlands do show a slight increase in vulval melanoma rates over a 15 year period (Table 7.3).

Malignant melanoma of the vagina is rare. Chung et al (1980) cited 81 published cases and Lee et al (1984) found 106 cases in the literature up to 1984, but in a proportion of these the histological details are poor and metastases cannot be considered to have been excluded. Chung et al (1980) found that the tumour in their registry accounted for 0.8% of malignant melanomas in females and 2.8% of all malignant vaginal neoplasms. Others have cited similar or lower figures (Ariel 1981a, Hilborne & Fu 1987), but Iverson & Robins (1980) found seven vaginal melanomas in a series of 47 mucosal melanomas uncovered in a survey of 1050 melanomas at all sites. In their study, vaginal melanoma made up 5% of all primary vaginal tumours.

Cervical melanomas have been described very rarely; Ariel (1981a) quoted 15 cases from the literature up to 1981. He also found four reports of 'melanotic tumours' arising in the uterine fundus and, as the melanin-containing cells were usually associated with glandular elements, questioned whether these were components of malignant mixed mesodermal tumour or teratomas. In one case, a striking similarity to melanotic progonoma was noted.

Survival

Survival rates in cases of malignant melanoma of the vulva are generally accepted to be very low. The 5-year survival rates in different series have varied from 13 to 55% (Das Gupta & D'urso 1964, Yackel et al 1970, Morrow & Rutledge 1972, Chung et al 1975, Karlen et al 1975, Edington & Monaghan 1980, Ariel 1981b, Bouma et al 1982, Philips et al 1982, Podratz et al 1983, Benda et al 1986, Bradgate et al 1990). Late recurrences are also a well-recognized problem (Bouma et al 1982, Podratz et al 1983). In the series of Bradgate et al, age-adjusted 5-year survival was 35% but 10-year survival was only 22%.

Patients with vulval malignant melanoma tend to be considerably older than those with skin melanoma generally. Mean ages in the seventh decade are common in series of vulval melanoma: this contrasts with a mean age of 46 years in one series of cutaneous melanomas (Elias et al 1977). Age has been found by several workers to be an important prognostic determinant in cutaneous melanomas with the over-65 age-group faring considerably worse than the under 65s (Huvos et al 1974, Shaw et al 1980, Rampen et al 1980, Bradgate et al 1990). This age difference in survival goes some way to explaining the difference in survival between series when comparing skin melanoma generally to vulval melanoma. It may also have tended to exaggerate the poor outcome in vulval melanoma patients due to their limited residual life expectancy. Older patients tend also to present later, with thicker tumours (Bradgate et al 1990).

Prognostic determinants

Clinical stage

No surgical staging method specific to vulval melanoma exists, and all previous clinical staging has been performed using the vulval squamous carcinoma staging system. The pre-1989 system on which all studies to date are based was highly subjective in application and required separation of cases into Stage II or III on the basis of a 'clinical suspicion' of groin node involvement. The recently introduced modified staging system (Shepherd 1989) is an improvement in that it allows inclusion of histological information on lymph nodes, but it retains the separation of cases into Stage I and II on the basis of a tumour transverse diameter less than or greater than 2 cm, an anachronism which appears to be morbidly inherent to the relevant FIGO Committee.

These failings of the staging system for vulvar tumours are reflected in the findings in most studies on vulval melanoma relating stage to outcome.

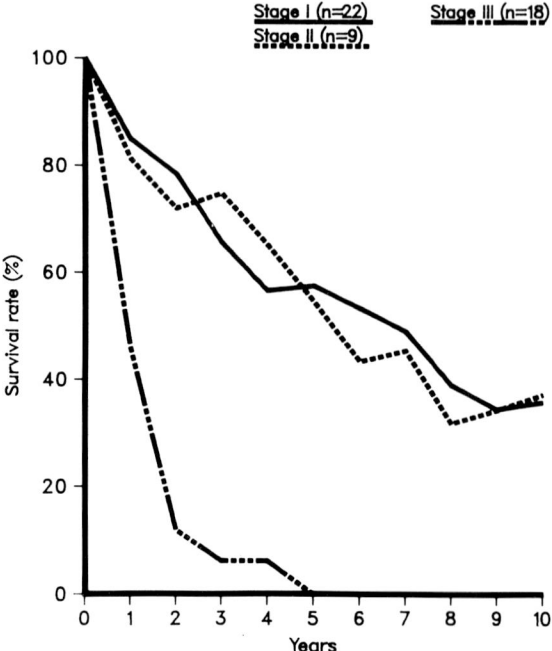

Fig. 7.2   Annual age-adjusted survival rates by stage for vulval malignant melanoma. (Reproduced with permission from Bradgate et al 1990.)

FIGO staging is consistently found to be important, but not when comparing Stage I with Stage II tumours (Podratz et al 1983, Bradgate et al 1990). As expected, the crude surface diameter measurements applied to the primary tumour have no discriminatory ability. The major prognostic difference is seen when comparing Stage I and II with Stage III and IV tumours (Bradgate et al 1990), with spread beyond the confines to the vulva therefore being the major indicator of poor outcome (Fig. 7.2). Although outcome for Stage III tumours has varied greatly in different series, with a few showing no survival difference to Stage I and II tumours (Philips et al 1982, Podratz et al 1983), most series have found a markedly poorer prognosis in Stage III cases (Morrow & Rutledge 1972, Jaramillo et al 1985, Bradgate et al 1990) and there is widespread acceptance that lymph node involvement is a major indication of poor outcome (Das Gupta & D'urso 1964, Yackel et al 1970, Morrow & Rutledge 1972, Edington & Monaghan 1970, Ariel 1981b). Bradgate et al (1990) found that 13% of cases with no clinical record of positive or suspicious nodes had histological node involvement, and other workers have recorded discrepancies in the region of 30% between clinical and histological findings (Das Gupta & D'urso 1964, Podratz et al 1983).

Although in most series of vulval melanoma groin node metastases have uniformly led to death within 5 years, occasional studies show long-term survivors in this group. Whether these patients can be identified at the time of primary therapy is unclear. Day et al (1981) found that, in skin melanomas generally, cases with nodal metastases could be divided into low-risk (5-year survival of 80%) and high-risk (17.5%) groups on the basis of the proportion of the removed nodes involved ($\geqslant 20\%$ involvement putting the patient in the high-risk group) and primary tumour thickness (> 3.5 mm leading to high risk). Clearly this should be attempted for vulval melanomas.

Depth of invasion

Survival of patients with cutaneous malignant melanomas has been found to correlate best with the histological staging methods which use level of invasion (Clark et al 1969) and tumour thickness (Breslow 1970). Several studies (Philips et al 1982, Podratz et al 1983, Jaramillo et al 1985, Johnson et al 1986, Beller et al 1986) have shown these methods to be of prognostic use in vulval melanomas. Others (Chung et al 1975) have introduced their own modifications specifically for vulval melanomas.

Many studies are hampered by small numbers but, using Clark's method, Podratz et al (1983) found that tumours confined to levels I and II had a 100% 5 year survival whereas those extending to level III or IV had a survival rate of 80% and those to level V a rate of only 28%. Chung (1975), using his own method, obtained survivals of 100% for level II, 40% for levels III and IV, and only 20% for level V.

The above results should not disguise the fact that it is, in practice, difficult to apply Clark's and similar techniques to tumours on the vulva. There are three reasons for this. Firstly, the junction of the papillary and reticular dermis is poorly defined or absent on the glabrous areas of the vulva. Secondly, the dermis may be very shallow in some areas with upward protrusions of adipose tissue, making even thin melanomas level IV or V (but see below for discussion on prognosis in thin, level IV melanomas). Thirdly, most vulval tumours are already Stage IV or worse at the time of presentation, giving this method little discriminatory ability if applied alone. For these reasons, if only one histological staging method is applied, the simpler method of measurement of the depth of the tumour from the granular cell layer of the overlying epidermis is to be preferred.

Using this simpler and more reproducible technique Podratz et al (1983), Philips et al (1982) and Jaramillo et al (1985) found that patients with vulval melanomas less than 0.76 mm deep all survived. Johnson et al (1986) found that maximum thickness amongst survivors was 1.3 mm. This was essentially supported by Bradgate et al (1990). Despite this overall agreement, it should be borne in mind that malignant melanoma remains an unpredictable disease when invasive; Bailet et al (1987) reported a vulval melanoma 0.75 mm thick (Clark's level II) that developed distant recurrences 2 years after treatment. It has been suggested that thin melanomas showing

Table 7.4   Survival comparison for vulval and other skin melanomas

	No. of cases	Mean age (years)	Mean thickness (mm)	Median survival (months)	5-year crude survival (%)
Vulva	28	58.5	6.1	50	43
Other skin sites	28	57.6	5.1	56	46

regressive changes have increased metastatic potential (Gromet et al 1978), though this would appear to have been more recently disproven (Kelly et al 1985a).

Some workers have felt that both of the above histological staging methods should be applied (Philips et al 1982, Podratz et al 1983), and this opinion has gained some support from recent reports on skin melanomas generally: there is evidence to suggest that Clark's level may give more prognostic information than depth in the thin, level IV melanoma. Kelly et al (1985b) found that melanomas in the 0.6–1.1 mm range, which arise in skin with a very shallow dermis and are Clark's level IV, carry a survival of only 59%, whereas the corresponding figures for similar depths but Clark's levels II and III were 97 and 94%. Somewhat similar findings in melanomas of the 'BANS' areas (upper neck, posterior arm, posterior neck and posterior scalp) had previously been reported by Day et al (1982a).

One gains the impression from the previously quoted papers that, in terms of prognosis, vulval melanomas appear to follow the same general rules as other skin melanomas. This goes against the historically expressed opinion that vulval melanomas have a particularly poor prognosis. This contention is not entirely unlikely, as melanomas of the trunk are believed to have a poorer prognosis that those on the limbs (Sondergaard & Shou 1985). The figures given in Table 7.4 utilize cases from the study of Bradgate et al (1990) matched for age, sex and depth of invasion against a group of skin melanomas from other sites: no differences in survival are seen, further evidence that prognosis depth for depth is similar to other skin melanomas.

Prognostic bands for depth measurements in vulval melanoma

As indicated above, Clark's level measurements in vulval melanoma are of limited practical value in the sense that most cases are level IV or more at the time of presentation. The same stricture can equally be applied to the depth measurement bands usually applied, as most melanomas at this site are more than 1.5 mm deep. In the series of Bradgate et al, for example, the three shallowest lesions were 0.9, 1.0 and 1.3 mm, but mean tumour thickness was 7.45 mm. Other workers have found even higher figures, e.g. 9.5 mm (Johnson et al 1986). One therefore must ask whether bands of greater overall thickness have prognostic usefulness in this tumour. Johnson et al (1986) showed that tumour thickness in vulval melanoma is inversely related to length of survival, and Day et al (1982b) indicated that, generally, skin melanomas that were more than 3.65 mm thick had a particularly poor

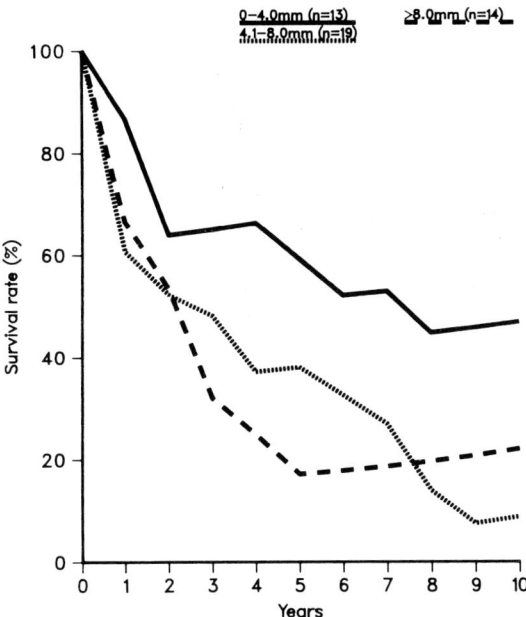

Fig. 7.3   Annual age-adjusted survival rates by tumour thickness for vulval malignant melanoma. (Reproduced with permission from Bradgate et al 1990.)

prognosis, though they felt that above this level no further prognostic information could be gained. Bradgate et al (1990) divided vulval melanomas into bands at 0.0–4.0, 4.1–8.0 and > 8 mm. Prognosis worsened significantly between bands (Fig. 7.3), with age-adjusted 5-year survivals of 59.3, 38.0 and 10.0%, respectively. Clearly these findings require further analysis, particularly with regard to melanomas at cutaneous sites other than the vulva.

Lesion type (growth pattern)

It is usual to divide melanomas into four histological types: superficial spreading, nodular, lentigo maligna and acral lentiginous (mucosal lentiginous). These types have been extensively described in standard texts and their basic differentiating characteristics will not be iterated here. It is, however, important to examine further the acral lentiginous (mucosal lentiginous) type of malignant melanoma. This term was originally introduced to describe a particular variant of malignant melanoma arising on the palms, soles and around and beneath the finger and toenails. It is said to account for approximately 8–10% of melanomas in the white population but to be the most common type in blacks and orientals (Kerl et al 1981). Tumour growth has been described by some as being characteristically rapid, with very poor prognosis (Fleming et al 1975, Coleman et al 1980), but depth for depth outcome is probably similar to other types (Jimbow et al

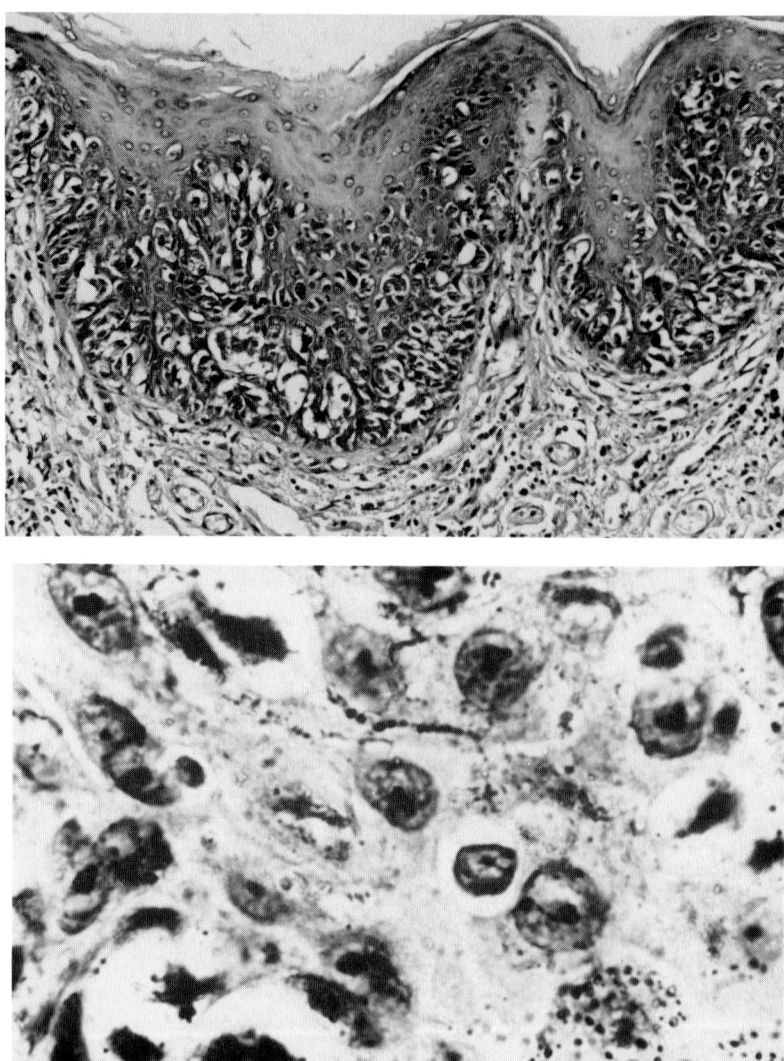

Fig. 7.4 The intraepithelial marginal component of this invasive vulval malignant melanoma shows a mucosal lentiginous pattern. Small cell groups showing cytoplasmic retraction and spindle cell differentiation are seen, together with single cells, extending along the dermoepidermal junction (upper). Dendritic melanocytes are clearly seen on Masson–Fontana staining (lower).

1984). In contrast to superficial spreading melanoma, this melanoma type is distinguished by nests of epidermal cells showing spindle cell differentiation and cytoplasmic retraction (Fig. 7.4 upper). Single melanoma cells extend along the dermoepidermal junction and some of these show dendritic processes, with finely granular melanin pigment extending up into the epidermis (Fig. 7.4 lower). There is no Pagetoid spread. It has been stated

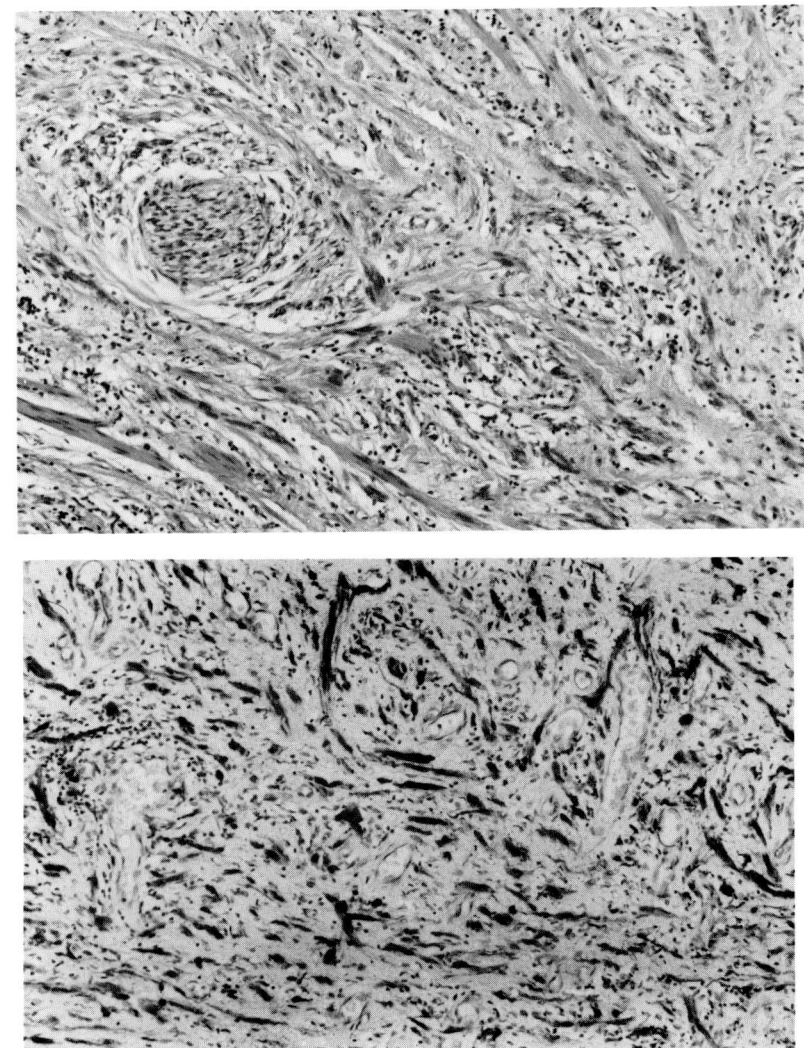

Fig. 7.5 A neurotropic vaginal malignant melanoma showing a dense desmoplastic response and ensheathing of a small nerve (upper). Immunoperoxidase staining utilizing anti-S100 antibody shows that the background spindle cells are predominantly malignant melanocytes (lower).

that this pattern of growth is the commonest occurring on mucosal membranes and at mucocutaneous junctions, including the vaginal and vulvovestibular mucocutaneous region (Kendall Pierson 1987).

In past series, most workers have found that vulval malignant melanomas are of superficial spreading type in 60–70% of cases, but some have found that nodular tumours predominate (Bouma et al 1982, Johnson et al 1986). A recent paper at variance with both of the above findings, however, is that of Benda et al (1986). They judged that 10 of 16 malignant melanomas of the vulva were of the mucosal lentiginous type. All of these occurred on 'mucous membrane', as did all three nodular melanomas seen, whereas all of the superficial spreading tumours occurred on 'skin'. This melanoma variant was described as long ago as 1974 on the vulva (Chung et al 1975), in a series where it was judged to make up nine of 34 reviewed cases, but few other vulval studies to date have commented on its occurrence. Johnson et al (1986) found that one of two acral or mucosal lentiginous melanomas, occurring in a series of 19 skin melanomas, was on the labium majus. Ronan et al (1990) found that two of 14 melanomas of the female genitalia were of mucosal lentiginous type, but both were vaginal. The vulval tumours were all superficial spreading or nodular. Clearly, further studies are necessary to clarify these findings.

A further melanoma variant, described previously only once on the vulva (Warner et al 1982) but again seen commonly in Benda's series (1986), is the so-called neurotropic melanoma. Almost one-third of Benda's cases were of the neutropic variety. Neurotropism has in the past generally been associated with lentigo maligna and acral lentiginous melanoma (Reed & Leonard 1979, Elder et al 1980). This melanoma variant shows a florid desmoplastic response and is marked by a striking tendency to track along peripheral nerves (Fig. 7.5). Whilst it is said to be very difficult to eradicate surgically, this did not appear to be particularly the case in Benda's series. A clearer definition of what degree of perineural spread is necessary for the diagnosis of 'neurotropic' melanoma is imperative if this term is to be shown to have any prognostic importance.

Some workers have reported a poorer prognosis in nodular malignant melanomas of the vulva (Podratz et al 1983, Johnson et al 1986): others have found no difference in prognosis between different types (Bradgate et al 1990), and Chung et al (1975) even found a poorer prognosis in superficial spreading melanoma. It appears likely that the poorer prognosis noted was a function of tumour thickness, with nodular melanomas tending to present at a greater thickness than other types (Johnson et al 1986, Bradgate et al 1990). This appears to be the reason for the poorer prognosis of polypoid melanomas at other skin sites also (McGovern et al 1983) and, allowing for thickness, prognosis for polypoid vulval melanoma appears to be no different from other variants (Bradgate et al 1990).

Cell type

The invasive component of malignant melanomas is usually composed predominantly of epithelioid or spindle cells or shows a balance of these two cell types. Uncommonly, other cell types may predominate, for example balloon cells and multinucleate cells. Most workers have found no association between survival and cell type in vulval melanoma (Chung et al 1975,

Podratz et al 1983, Johnson et al 1986). This is in keeping with the usual findings in skin melanomas overall, only four of 43 papers surveyed by Vollmer (1989) finding cell type to be of prognostic significance. However, Bradgate et al (1990) found a distinctly poorer survival for epithelioid melanomas of the vulva compared with other types (15% age-adjusted 5-year survival for epithelioid versus 43 and 49% for mixed and spindle cell). In this series, cell type appeared closely related to mitotic rate, and multivariate analysis suggested that these were not independent variables; epithelioid tumours had high rates of mitosis. It is of interest that epithelioid differentiation is associated with a poorer prognosis in choroid melanomas as well.

Other prognostic factors

Mitotic rate has been thought to be prognostically important in vulval melanomas by only a few workers (Johnson et al 1986, Bradgate et al 1990). In cutaneous melanomas generally, the position is complicated, with more series finding mitotic rate insignificant than significant (Vollmer 1989). As only Bradgate et al (1990) have looked at its effect in vulval melanoma by multivariate analysis, further studies are clearly required.

Tumour ulceration has been found by many workers to be an important prognostic indicator in cutaneous malignant melanomas (Balch et al 1980,

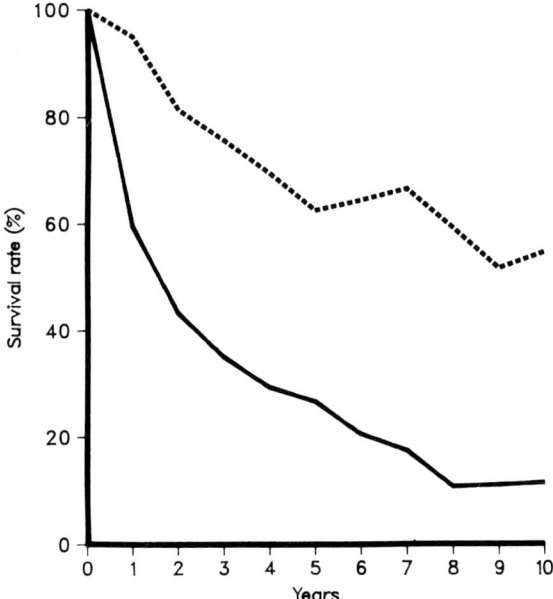

Fig. 7.6 Annual age-adjusted survival rates for ulcerated ($n = 35$; solid line) and non-ulcerated ($n = 13$; dotted line) malignant melanoma of the vulva. (Reproduced with permission from Bradgate et al 1990.)

McGovern et al 1982, Vollmer 1989) but not the majority. The adverse effect of ulceration on prognosis in skin melanomas is still apparent after adjusting for tumour thickness and appears to indicate a biologically more aggressive tumour (Balch et al 1980). This finding also appears to hold true for vulval melanomas specifically (Fig. 7.6), in which an association between ulceration and high mitotic rate is also evident (Bradgate et al 1990).

The significance in prognosis of site of melanoma on the vulva is the source of some confusion in the literature, as indeed is the relative incidence at different sites. Most series report a predilection for the labia minora and clitoris (Chung et al 1975, Podratz et al 1983, Morrow and Rutledge 1972, Benda et al 1986, Johnson et al 1986, Bradgate et al 1990), but others show a balance of central and lateral tumours (Philips et al 1982, Jaramillo et al 1985). Some workers (Podratz et al 1983, Johnson et al 1986) have found a poorer prognosis for central tumours, in particular those involving the clitoris, but this has been suggested by others to be the case only if urethral or vaginal involvement is present (Morrow 1981).

Though it is felt by some workers to be the case for melanomas at other cutaneous sites (Huvos et al 1974, Day et al 1981), there is no convincing evidence that the degree of lymphocytic infiltrate has importance in prognosis in vulval melanomas. A prognostic role for pigmentation, cellular atypia and vascular invasion is, to date, not supported by any firm evidence.

Recently it has been suggested that ploidy may be an important prognostic indicator in cutaneous melanomas generally but this technique has not been applied to vulval melanomas as a group. Bines et al (1988) found that tumour thickness, a cell type that was non-epithelioid, ulceration and the presence of a vertical growth phase were all associated with aneuploidy but, surprisingly, melanomas of the extremities had higher incidences of aneuploidy than head, neck and trunk melanomas. Patients with aneuploid tumours had a lower 3- and 5-year disease-free survival and a higher incidence of recurrences than those with diploid tumours, and aneuploidy was the most significant unfavourable prognostic factor after adjustment for tumour thickness. Sondergaard et al (1983) and Bruckner et al (1985) also found that aneuploid tumours had a higher recurrence rate, though specific associations with histological features varied. It is clear, however, that aneuploidy cannot be used as a specific indicator of malignancy *per se*, as all of these workers found aneuploidy in benign melanocytic naevi, one in 25% of cases (Sondergaard et al 1983).

Multivariate analysis in malignant melanoma

Despite over 50 multifactorial analyses in studies of cutaneous malignant melanoma, great confusion still exists over which prognostic factors are of most importance (Vollmer 1989). Many studies have technical faults, and most are not directly comparable. Thickness appears in most studies as the major prognostic factor, and other factors show great variability, possibly because of complex interactions with tumour thickness (Kopf et al 1987, Vollmer 1989). Before any conclusions can be reached standardization of study methods is necessary.

In vulval melanomas Bradgate et al (1990) found that, using univariate analysis, age, stage, thickness, cell type and mitotic rate were all significant prognostically, but on multifactional analysis, after adjusting for stage, thickness was no longer significant. Mitotic rate also appeared closely related to cell type and presence or absence of ulceration. These findings underline the importance of this technique in future studies of melanoma if understanding of the way prognostic factors interact is to be improved.

Therapy in vulval melanoma

Primary therapy for malignant melanoma at any site remains surgical removal. There has been considerable debate as to the extent of skin that should be removed. Most workers have in the past accepted the need for 5 cm margins, but margins 3 cm or less from the edge of the lesion have been recommended more recently (Urist et al 1985, Veronesi et al 1988). The traditional view that regional lymph node dissection is required has also been challenged for Stage I melanoma (Elder et al 1985). For Stage I and II vulval melanomas specifically, the site, the overall poor prognosis and the ability to resect the inguinal nodes in continuity by a well-tested procedure might argue for the continuation of radical surgery. However, whether radical vulvectomy is necessary has been questioned for some years (Philips et al 1982, Podratz et al 1983, Jaramillo et al 1985, Buckley & Fox 1988); Davidson et al (1987) found no benefit from radical or simple vulvectomy when compared to local excision, either in local control, disease-free interval or patient survival. Bradgate et al (1990) also found no significant difference in survival with different surgical treatment options, though there was a slightly better survival at 5 years after radical vulvectomy. Local excision alone in this series was compatible in some women with long-term survival, even occasionally in those with thick lesions. At present the conclusion must be that the minimum surgery required for Stage I and II vulval melanoma is wide local excision, with margins of a minimum of 3 cm on each side (where possible). Further prospective studies on outcome are clearly necessary before definitive guidelines can be issued.

Malignant melanoma of the vagina and cervix

Vagina

Most women with vaginal melanoma present with bleeding. The tumour shows a predilection for the lower third of the vagina, and great variation in size and colour is seen. About 20% have metastases when first seen (Ariel 1981b) and the prognosis appears to be extremely poor with perhaps only 5–20% surviving 5 years (Chung et al 1980, Lee et al 1984). Most studies

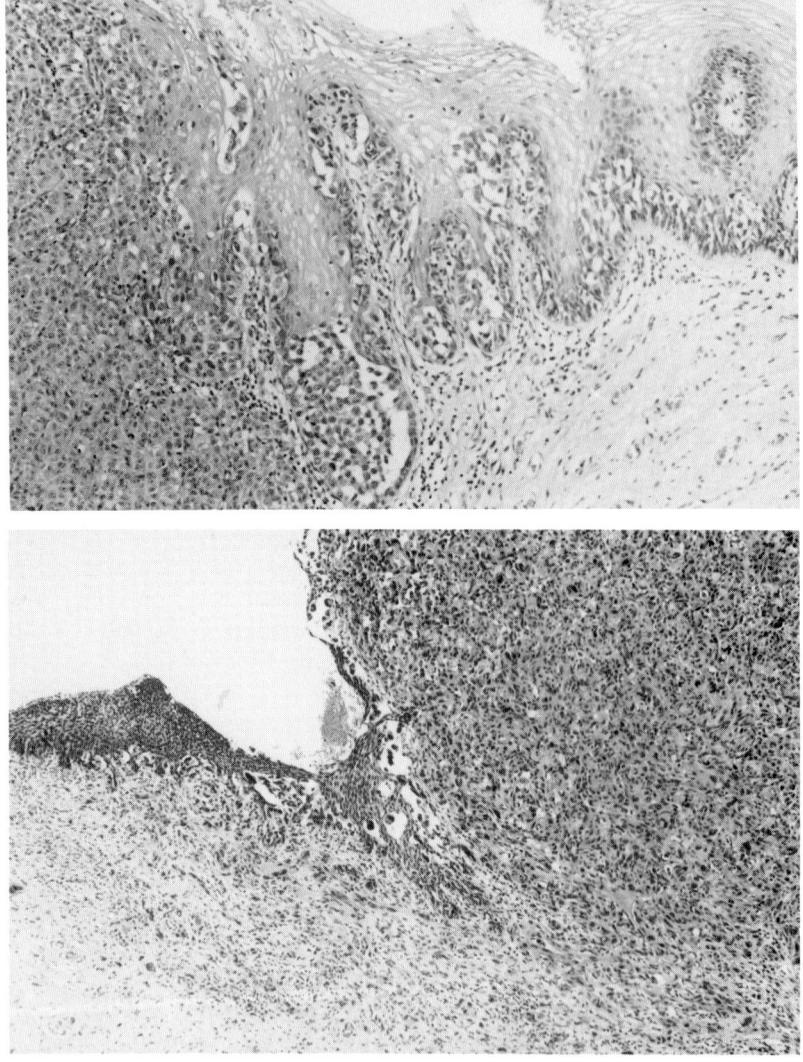

Fig. 7.7 Both of these widely separate intravaginal metastatic deposits from a recurrent vaginal malignant melanoma show 'epidermotropism' and junctional activity mimicking primary malignant melanomas.

were performed prior to the popularization of the concept of mucosal lentiginous melanoma and although it has been stated that cell types and lesion types are similar to the skin (Hilborne and Fu 1987), Chung et al (1980) commented that the associated intraepithelial component did not, in any of their cases, fulfil the criteria for superficial spreading melanoma. They described the pattern as lentiginous in the great majority, and specifically related the pattern to mucosal lentiginous melanoma. Intraepithelial spread was noted to be widespread in their cases and this has also been commented on by other workers. Figure 7.7 is from such a case, where intravaginal satellites also showed striking 'epidermotropism'. Norris and Taylor (1966) also indicated that the lentiginous pattern predominates in vaginal melanoma; but Ronan et al (1990), in a more recent study, described only two of seven vaginal melanomas as of mucosal lentiginous type, with nodular tumours being the commonest.

In view of the rarity of melanomas in the vagina, every effort should be made to exclude metastatic disease and a junctional component should be searched for diligently. It seems likely that lesion thickness will provide the best prognostic information but, as is the case for vulval tumours, most vaginal melanomas are advanced and deeply infiltrative at presentation (Chung et al 1980). Most authors favour Wertheim's hysterectomy and vaginectomy as therapy, with ileo-inguinal lymph node dissection for those in the lower third of the vagina.

Cervix

Cervical melanoma here has been reported on only 13 occasions up to 1981 (Ariel 1981a). To that date, no patients had been cured of their disease, however radical the surgery (Ariel 1981a), but long-term survivors have been reported (Chung et al 1980).

SUMMARY

Malignant melanoma and other pigmented lesions of the lower female genital tract have in the past excited relatively little research interest, mainly due to their rarity and, in the case of malignant melanoma, extremely poor perceived prognosis. They have tended to be isolated as gynaecological problems rather than treated in the surgical mainstream with skin tumours generally. In view of the dramatic changes in incidence of malignant melanoma overall, and the improvements in therapy likely to arise from the consequent increased research interest in pigmented lesions of the skin, it is time that the lesions of the lower female genital tract were subjected to the same diagnostic and prognostic criteria applied to these lesions at other sites, so that women may benefit rapidly from changes in therapy and attitude. Despite the relative rarity of malignant melanoma on the vulva, if prognosis is to be improved, it is also imperative that women are educated to apply the same degree of suspicion to pigmented lesions here as to those elsewhere on the skin.

REFERENCES

Ackerman A B, Mihara I 1985 Dysplasia, dysplastic melanocytes, dysplastic nevi, the dysplastic nevus syndrome and the relation between dysplastic nevi and malignant melanomas. Human Pathology 16: 87–91

Ackerman A B 1988 What nevus is dysplastic, a syndrome and the commonest precursor of malignant melanoma? A riddle and an answer. Histopathology 13: 241–256

Ariel I M 1981a Malignant melanoma of the female genital system: A report of 48 patients and review of the literature. Journal of Surgical Oncology 16: 371–383

Ariel I M 1981b Malignant melanoma of the female genital system. In: Malignant melanoma. Appleton-Century-Crofts, New York, p 489–506

Bailet J W, Figge D C, Tamimi H K 1987 Malignant melanoma of the vulva. A case report of distal recurrence in a patient with a superficially invasive primary lesion. Obstetrics and Gynecology 70: 515–517

Balch C M, Wilkerson J A, Murad T M, Soong S J, Ingalls A L 1980 The prognostic significance of ulceration in cutaneous melanoma. Cancer 45: 3012–3017

Beilby J O W, Ridley C M 1987 Pathology of the vulva. In: Fox H (ed) Haines and Taylor. Obstetrical and gynaecological pathology, 3rd edn. Churchill Livingstone, London, p 64–145

Beller U, Demopoulos R I, Beckman E M 1986 Vulvovaginal melanoma: A clinicopathologic study. Journal of Reproductive Medicine 31: 315–319

Benda J A, Platz C E, Anderson B 1986 Malignant melanoma of the vulva. A clinical–pathologic review of 16 cases. International Journal of Gynecological Pathology 5: 202–216

Bines S D, Van Roenn J H, Kheir S M, Coon J S 1988 Flow cytometry in melanoma. In: Nathanson L (ed) Malignant melanoma: biology, diagnosis and therapy. Kluwer Academic, Boston, p 155–159

Blessing K, McLaren K M, Maloney D J, Porteus I, Hunter J A 1989 Melanocytic proliferation in condylomata acuminata. Acta Dermato-Venereologica (Stockholm) 69: 238–241

Bouma J, Weening J J, Elders A 1982 Malignant melanoma of the vulva. Report of 18 cases. European Journal of Obstetrics and Gynecology and Reproductive Biology 13: 237–251

Bradgate M G, Rollason T P, McConkey C, Powell J 1990 Malignant melanoma of the vulva: a clinico-pathological study of 50 women. British Journal of Obstetrics and Gynaecology 97: 124–133

Breslow A 1970 Thickness, cross sectional areas and depth of invasion in the prognosis of malignant melanoma. Annals of Surgery 172: 902–908

Briggs J C 1985 Melanoma precursor lesions and borderline melanomas. Histopathology 9: 1251–1262

Bruckner T, Hiddemann W, Nomann B et al 1985 Differential pattern of DNA aneuploidy in human malignancies. Pathology Research and Practice 179: 310–317

Buckley C H, Fox H 1988 Epithelial tumours of the vulva. In: Ridley C M (ed) The vulva. Churchill Livingstone, Edinburgh, p 263–333

Burket J M 1979 Multiple benign juvenile melanoma. Archives of Dermatology 115: 229

Capetanakis J 1975 Juvenile melanoma disseminatum. British Journal of Dermatology 92: 207–211

Christensen W N, Friedman K J, Woodruff J D, Hood A F 1987 Histological characteristics of vulvar nevocellular nevi. Journal of Cutaneous Pathology 14: 87–91

Chung A F, Woodruff J M, Lewis J L 1975 Malignant melanoma of the vulva. A report of 44 cases. Obstetrics and Gynecology 45: 638–646

Chung A F, Cassey M J, Flannery J T, Woodruff J M, Lewis J L Jr 1980 Malignant melanoma of the vagina—report of 19 cases. Obstetrics and Gynecology 55: 720–727

Clark W H Jr, From L, Bernardino E A, Mihm M C 1969 Histogenesis and biologic behaviour of primary human malignant melanoma of the skin. Cancer Research 29: 705–727

Clark W H Jr, Elder D E, Guerry D 4th, Epstein M N, Greene M H, Van Horn M 1984 A study of tumor progression: the precursor lesions of superficial spreading and nodular melanoma. Human Pathology 15: 1147–1165

Coleman W P III, Loria P R, Reed R J, Krementz E T 1980 Acral lentiginous melanoma. Archives of Dermatology 116: 773–776

Cook M G, Robertson I 1985 Melanocytic dysplasia and melanoma. Histopathology 9: 647–658

Crucioli V, Stilwell J 1982 The histogenesis of malignant melanoma in relation to pre-existing pigmented lesions. Journal of Cutaneous Pathology 9: 396–404

Das Gupta T, D'urso J 1964 Melanoma of the female genitalia. Surgery, Gynecology and Obstetrics 119: 1074–1078

Davidson T, Kissin M, Westbury G 1987 Vulvo-vaginal melanoma—should radical surgery be abandoned? British Journal of Obstetrics and Gynaecology 94: 473–476

Day C L Jr, Sober A J, Lew R A et al 1981 Malignant melanoma patients with positive nodes and relatively good prognoses: microstaging retains prognostic significance in clinical Stage I melanoma patients with metastases to regional nodes. Cancer 47: 955–962

Day C L, Mihm M C, Sober A J et al 1982a Prognostic factors for melanoma patients with lesions 0.76–1.69 mm in thickness. Annals of Surgery 195: 30–34

Day C L, Lew R A, Mihm M C et al 1982b A multivariate analysis of prognostic factors for melanoma patients with lesions ⩾3.65 mm in thickness. The importance of revealing alternative Cox models. Annals of Surgery 195: 44–49

Edington P T, Monaghan J M 1980 Malignant melanoma of the vulva and vagina. British Journal of Obstetrics and Gynaecology 87: 422–424

Elder D E, Jucovy P M, Tuthill R J, Clark W H 1980 The classification of malignant melanoma. American Journal of Dermatopathology 2: 315–320

Elder D E, Greene M H, Bondi E E, Clark W H Jr 1981 Acquired melanocytic nevi and melanoma. The dysplastic nevus syndrome. In: Ackerman A B (ed) Pathology of malignant melanoma. Masson, New York, p 185–215

Elder D E, Guerry D, VanHorn M et al 1985 The role of lymph node dissection for clinical Stage I malignant melanoma of intermediate thickness (1.51–3.99 mm). Cancer 56: 413–418

Elias E G, Didolkar M S, Goel I P, Formeister J F, Valenzuela L A, Pickren J L, Moore R H 1977 A clinicopathologic study of the prognostic factors in cutaneous malignant melanoma. Surgery, Gynecology and Obstetrics 144: 327–334

Fleming I D, Barnawell J R, Burlison P E, Rankin J S 1975 Skin cancer in black patients. Cancer 35: 600–605

Friedman R J, Ackerman A B 1981 Difficulties in the histological diagnosis of melanocytic nevi on the vulvae of premenopausal women. In: Ackerman A B (ed) Pathology of malignant melanoma. Masson, New York, p 119–127

Friedrich E G 1983 Dark Lesions. In: Vulvar disease, 2nd edn. W D Saunders, Philadelphia, p 149–165

Green M H, Clark W H Jr, Tucker M A et al 1985 Current concepts. Acquired precursors of cutaneous malignant melanoma. The familial dysplastic nevus syndrome. New England Journal of Medicine 312: 91–97

Gromet M A, Epstein W L, Blois M S 1978 The regressing thin malignant melanoma. A distinctive lesion with metastatic potential. Cancer 42: 2282–2292

Grunberger V 1973 Melanosis of the vagina. Wiener Klinische Wochenschrift 85: 681–682

Hilborne L H, Fu Y S 1987 Intraepithelial, invasive and metastatic neoplasms of the vagina. In: Wilkinson E J (ed) Pathology of the vulva and vagina. Churchill Livingstone, New York, p 181–207

Hulagu C, Erez S 1973 Juvenile melanoma of the clitoris. Journal of Obstetrics and Gynaecology of the British Commonwealth 80: 89–91

Huvos A G, Shah J P, Mike V 1974 Prognostic factors in cutaneous malignant melanoma. Human Pathology 5: 347–357

Iverson K, Robins E 1980 Mucosal malignant melanomas. American Journal of Surgery 139: 660–664

Jackson R 1984 Melanosis of the vulva. Journal of Dermatologic Surgery and Oncology 10: 119–121

Janovski N A, Douglas C P 1972 Disease of the vulva, 1st American edn. Harper and Row, Maryland, p 70

Jaramillo B A, Gansel P, Averette H E, Sevin B L, Lovecchio J L 1985 Malignant melanoma of the vulva. Obstetrics and Gynecology 66: 398–401

Jensen O M, Bolander A M 1980 Trends in malignant melanoma of the skin. World Health Statistics Quarterly 33: 3–26

Jimbow K, Takahashi H, Miura S, Ikeda S, Kukita A 1984 Biological behaviour and natural course of acral malignant melanoma. Clinical and histologic features and prognosis of palmoplantar, subungual and other acral malignant melanomas. American Journal of Dermatopathology 6 (suppl): 43–53

Johnson T L, Kumar N B, White C D, Morley G W 1986 Prognostic features of vulvar melanoma: A clinicopathologic analysis. International Journal of Gynecological Pathology 5: 110–118

Jones I S C 1979 An assessment of vulval pigmentation. New Zealand Medical Journal 89: 348–350

Karlen J R, Pivers M S, Barlow J J 1975 Melanoma of the vulva. Obstetrics and Gynecology 45: 181–185

Kelly J W, Sagebiel R W, Blois M S 1985a Regression in malignant melanoma. A histologic feature without independent prognostic significance. Cancer 56: 2287–2291

Kelly J W, Sagebiel R W, Clyman S, Blois M S 1985b Thin level IV melanoma: a subset in which level is the major prognostic indicator. Annals of Surgery 202: 98–103

Kendall Pierson K 1987 Malignant melanomas and pigmented lesions of the vulva. In: Wilkinson E J (ed) Pathology of the vulva and vagina. Churchill Livingstone, New York, p 155–179

Kerl H, Hodl S, Stettner H 1981 Acral lentiginous melanoma. In: Ackerman A B (ed) Pathology of malignant melanoma. Masson, New York, p 217–242

Kopf A W, Welkorian B, Frankel R E 1987 Thickness of malignant melanoma: global analysis of related factors. Journal of Dermatology, Surgery and Oncology 13: 345–390, 401–420

Lee R B, Buttoni L Jr, Dhru K, Tamimi H 1984 Malignant melanoma of the vagina: a case report of progression from pre-existing melanosis. Gynecological Oncology 19: 238–245

Little J H, Holt J, Davis N 1980 The changing epidemiology of malignant melanoma in Queensland. Medical Journal of Australia 1: 66–69

Lopansri S, Mihm M C Jr 1979 Clinical and pathological correlation of malignant melanoma. Journal of Cutaneous Pathology 6: 180–194

Lutterloh C H, Shallenberger P L 1946 Unusual pigmentation developing after prolonged suppressive therapy with quinacrine hydrochloride. Archives of Dermatology and Syphilology 53: 349–354

Macartney J C, Rollason T P, Codling B W 1980 Use of a histopathological data pool for epidemiological analysis. Journal of Clinical Pathology 33: 351–355

McGovern V J, Shaw H M, Milton G W, McCarthy W H 1982 Ulceration and prognosis in cutaneous malignant melanoma. Histopathology 6: 399–407

McGovern V J, Shaw H M, Milton G W 1983 Prognostic significance of a polypoid configuration in malignant melanoma. Histopathology 7: 663–672

Morrow C P 1981 Melanoma of the female genital tract. In: Coppleson M (ed) Gynaecologic oncology. Churchill Livingstone, Edinburgh, p 784

Morrow C P, DiSaia P J 1976 Malignant melanoma of the female genitalia: A clinical analysis. Obstetric and Gynecological Survey 31: 233–271

Morrow C P, Rutledge F N 1972 Melanoma of the vulva. Obstetrics and Gynecology 39: 745–752

Nicholson G W 1936 An epidermal heteromorphosis of the vaginal vault. Journal of Pathology 43: 209–221

Nigogosyan G, De Le Pava S, Pickren J W 1964 Melanoblast in vaginal mucosa: origin for primary malignant melanoma. Cancer 17: 912–913

Norris H J, Taylor S B 1966 Melanomas of the vagina. American Journal of Clinical Pathology 46: 420–426

Osterlind A, Moller Jensen O 1986 Trends in incidence of malignant melanoma of the skin in Denmark 1943–1982. Recent Results in Cancer Research 102: 8–17

Pack G T, Lenson N, Gerber D M 1952 Regional distribution of moles and melanomas. Archives of Surgery 65: 862–870

Patel D S, Bhagavan B S 1985 Blue nevus of the uterine cervix. Human Pathology 16: 79–86

Philips G L, Twiggs L B, Okagaki T 1982 Vulvar melanoma: A microstaging study. Gynecological Oncology 14: 80–88

Podratz K C, Gaffey T A, Symmonds R E, Johansen K L, O'Brien P C 1983 Melanoma of the vulva: An update. Gynecological Oncology 16: 153–168

Rampen F H, Van Houten W A, Hop W C J 1980 Incisional procedures and prognosis in malignant melanoma. Clinical and Experimental Dermatology 5: 313–320

Reed R J, Leonard D D 1979 Neurotropic melanoma: A variant of desmoplastic melanoma. American Journal of Surgical Pathology 3: 301–311

Ridley C M 1988 General dermatological conditions and dermatoses of the vulva. In: The vulva. Churchill Livingstone, London, p 138–211

Rodriguez H A, Ackerman L V 1968 Cellular blue nevus: clinicopathologic study of 45 cases. Cancer 21: 393–405

Ronan S G, Eng A M, Briele H A, Walker M J, Das Gupta T K 1990 Malignant melanoma of the female genitalia. Journal of the American Academy of Dermatology 22: 428–435

Roush G C 1988 Abnormal nevi, excess total nevi, and melanoma: an epidemiological perspective. In: Nathanson L (ed) Malignant melanoma: biology, diagnosis and therapy. Kluwer, Boston, p 85–100

Sagebiel R W, Chinn B K, Egbert B M 1984 Pigmented spindle cell nevus. Clinical and histologic review of 90 cases. American Journal of Surgical Pathology 8: 645–653

Shaw H M, McGovern V J, Milton G W, Farago G A, McCarthy W H 1980 Malignant melanoma: Influence of site of lesion and age of patient in the female superiority in survival. Cancer 46: 2731–2735

Shepherd J 1989 Revised FIGO staging for gynaecological cancer. British Journal of Obstetrics and Gynaecology 8: 889–892

Silvers D H, Halperin A J 1978 Cutaneous and vulvar melanoma—an update. Clinical Obstetrics and Gynecology 21: 1117–1118

Sondergaard K, Larsen J K, Moller U, Christensen I J, Hou Jensen K 1983 DNA ploidy characteristics of human malignant melanoma analysed by flow cytometry and compared with histology and clinical course. Virchows Archiv. B. Cell Pathology 42: 43–52

Sondergaard K, Schou G 1985 Survival with primary malignant melanoma evaluated from 2012 cases. Virchows Archiv. A. Pathological Anatomy and Histopathology 406: 179–195

Tobon H, Murphy A I 1977 Benign blue nevus of the vagina. Cancer 40: 3174–3176

Tsukuda Y 1976 Benign melanosis of the vagina and cervix. American Journal of Obstetrics and Gynecology 124: 211–212

Urist M M, Balch C M, Soong S-J, Shaw H M, Milton G W, Maddox W A 1985 The influence of surgical margins and prognostic factors predicting the risk of local recurrence in 3445 patients with primary cutaneous melanoma. Cancer 55: 1398–1402

Veronesi U, Cascinelli N, Adamus J et al 1988 Thin Stage I primary cutaneous malignant melanoma. Comparison of excision with margins of 1 or 3 cm. New England Journal of Medicine 318: 1159–1162

Vollmer R T 1989 In: Rosen P P, Fechner R E (eds) Pathology annual part 1. Appleton and Lance, Norwalk, Connecticut, p 383–407

Wallace H J 1974 Eruptive juvenile melanomata. British Journal of Dermatology 91 (suppl 10): 37–38

Warner T F C S, Hafez G R, Buchler D A 1982 Neurotropic melanoma of the vulva. Cancer 49: 999–1004

Weiner K 1940 Vaginal melanosis caused by bismuth therapy and carcinoma of the cervix. Archives of Dermatology 42: 23–29

Yackel D B, Symmonds R E, Kempers R D 1970 Melanoma of the vulva. Obstetrics and Gynecology 35: 625–632

8. Microinvasive carcinoma of the lower female genital tract

David Lowe

INTRODUCTION

In the lower female genital tract, when a neoplasm ceases to remain in situ and becomes invasive or arises as an invasive carcinoma de novo it almost immediately gains, at least in theory, the capacity to metastasize to lymph nodes draining the area. In the cervix, and probably the vulva, lymphatic channels are found less than 0.5 mm below the surface epithelium (Averette et al 1976). The further the tumour extends into the underlying connective tissues in any direction, the more likely it will be to encounter vascular spaces, and so the chance of the tumour metastasizing increases in a continuous fashion. There are no anatomical divisions in the lower female genital tract, as there are in the stomach or large bowel, on which a classification of the extent of invasion could logically be based. To define a depth of invasion that is not associated with metastases, and that can be treated conservatively with local surgery, one must therefore be pragmatic rather than dogmatic (van Nagell et al 1983); and to be generally applicable the diagnosis cannot be so stringent that only a very small number of cases fall within it.

Assessment of a superficially invasive carcinoma in the lower female genital tract presents two problems to the diagnostic histopathologist: whether the tumour is invasive in the first place and, if it is, whether it is microinvasive. The first problem is not infrequent. It arises in cases in which the depth of stromal invasion is very small, when an inflammatory cell infiltrate obscures the margins of the in situ and invasive components, and when the suspicion of tangential sectioning raises the possibility that apparently invasive tumour may be simply cross-cutting or crypt involvement by cervical intraepithelial neoplasia (CIN). The second problem is more difficult: the concept of microinvasive squamous cell carcinoma of the cervix is established but its definition is not settled, and there is no accepted definition of microinvasive carcinoma in relation to cervical adenocarcinoma or carcinoma of the vulva and vagina.

The first use of the term microinvasive carcinoma is attributed to Mestwerdt (1947). In his initial paper, the term was applied to invasive cervical carcinomas that could be diagnosed only by microscopy rather than to carcinomas that had a specific depth of invasion, but he subsequently took the depth of 5 mm as the maximum extent of stromal invasion of these tumours (Mestwerdt 1953). This distance was probably an arbitrary choice and a reflection of the use of the metric system rather than because it was known to be clinically or prognostically important at that time (Burghardt 1984, Greer et al 1990).

The separation of microinvasive carcinoma from the general group of invasive cervical carcinomas was an attempt to identify a group of patients with invasive carcinoma who had a good prognosis and who could be treated relatively conservatively. For this separation to be acceptable in practice, the diagnosis of microinvasive carcinoma must be definable, usable and reproducible by pathologists, and important to clinicians in terms of management and prognosis.

MICROINVASIVE CARCINOMA OF THE CERVIX

More than 18 different terms have been applied to superficially invasive carcinoma of cervix (Nelson et al 1975), the most commonly used being microinvasive carcinoma. The depth of stromal invasion is an important indicator of behaviour in microinvasive carcinoma of the cervix but is not the only one. There is a relation between the size (in three dimensions) of a tumour and the tendency to develop lymph node metastases, as well as simply with the single dimension of depth of invasion (Burghardt & Holzer 1977).

Between 4 and 7% of cases of CIN are associated with superficial stromal invasion (Savage 1972), but this figure may be somewhat high, for there is evidence that microinvasive carcinoma of the cervix may be overdiagnosed. In a study of 936 cases originally classified as microinvasive carcinoma, only 530 (57%) met the criteria of FIGO Stage Ia (see below) and over-diagnosis was considerably commoner than under-diagnosis (Ebeling et al 1989). When there has been a cervical biopsy shortly before a further excision such as a cone biopsy or hysterectomy, care must be taken in the interpretation of the area from which the biopsy was taken. Groups of normal, inflamed, or metaplastic squamous cells can become enclosed by stroma as part of the healing process and may appear atypical because of the reaction to the inflammation caused by the first biopsy.

Depth of invasion

The FIGO classification of staging of cervical carcinoma does not use the term 'microinvasive carcinoma', though in many studies the FIGO Stage Ia has been taken as synonymous (Petterson 1988, Shepherd 1989). The FIGO report states that 'diagnosis of both of Stage Ia1 and Ia2 should be based on microscopical examination of removed tissues, preferably a cone, which must include the entire lesion'. Stage Ia1 is given as having 'minimal microscopically evident stromal invasion'. The lower limit of Stage Ia2 is that it can be measured macroscopically (even if dots have to be placed on the slide prior to measurement), and the upper limit is that the tumour must not invade more than 5 mm from the base of the epithelium in which it arises and must not have a horizontal spread of more than 7 mm. There is therefore the dichotomy that the diagnosis of Stage Ia requires microscopy, but the distinction between stages Ia1 and Ia2 rests on the pathologist's ability to measure the tumour macroscopically. The smallest depth of invasion that can be measured macroscopically is not addressed in the classification and will depend on several factors, such as how basophilic the tumour cells are (which will affect the contrast with the eosinophilia of the stroma around them and make the tumour more or les macroscopically evident), how the tumour is measured (gradations on plastic rulers are usually coarser than on metal ones), and how good the eyesight of the pathologist is. Once the diagnosis of Stage Ia2 is made, the tumour is measured under the microscope.

In many centres in the UK and elsewhere in the world, the maximum depth of stromal invasion of a carcinoma in Stage Ia1 is taken to be 1 mm (Kolstad 1989). This is measured microscopically by the pathologist reporting the case, using a Vernier scale or electronic methods; it attempts to conform with the letter of the FIGO staging method and is usable and reproducible. An important caveat is that emphasized by the FIGO definition: the biopsy should include the entire lesion. A diagnosis of microinvasive carcinoma cannot be made confidently if the tumour extends to an excision margin of the specimen, as the full extent of invasion cannot be assessed. It has been stated that microinvasive carcinoma can be diagnosed only by a cone biopsy specimen (Benson & Norris 1977), but modern biopsy techniques can produce quite large specimens that can encompass the whole of a tumour, and this requirement need not be absolute (Prendiville et al 1986).

Tumours that have invaded 1 mm or less are almost always focal rather than confluent, and are curable by cone excision or simple hysterectomy (Ruch et al 1976). To be sure that lymph node metastasis is very unlikely, some workers require that in addition there should be no vascular invasion (Averette et al 1976). A case of a tumour that invaded the stroma to a depth of only 0.8 mm and had metastasized to pelvic lymph nodes has been described, but in this there was a suggestion of vascular invasion (Collins et al 1989).

A tumour invasion depth of more than 5 mm from the base of the epithelium in which the tumour appears to originate is taken as the division between Stages Ia2 and Ib. Involvement of vascular spaces does not affect the staging, but the FIGO group working on the classification of early invasive carcinoma of the cervix recommended that the presence or absence of any vascular invasion should be recorded on the histology report. Patients with tumours that invaded up to 5 mm had lymph node metastases in 1–2% of cases (Averette et al 1976, Puente Gonzalez et al 1977, Ito et al 1986, Monaghan 1988, Dinh et al 1989, Tsukamoto et al 1989).

In several large studies of patients with microinvasive carcinoma of the cervix, none of the patients with invasive tumour of less than 3 mm and no vascular space involvement had metastases (van Nagell et al 1983, Tsukamoto et al 1989). The Committee on Nomenclature of the Society of Gynecologic Oncologists has proposed that 3 mm be adopted as the cut-off for micro-invasion; this should be measured from the base of the epithelium and there should, in addition, be no vascular space invasion (Seski et al 1977). The same definition has been adopted by the Japanese Society of Obstetrics and Gynecology and the Japanese Society of Pathology (Noda et al 1979). The base of the epithelium to which measurements are made is not specified in the definition, which makes it difficult to apply. In addition, it has been pointed out that when a depth of 3 mm invasion is taken as the maximum invasion of microinvasive carcinoma, some patients would suffer un-necessarily severe operations (Kolstad 1989).

The FIGO choice of 5 mm invasion depth and 7 mm horizontal tumour spread may not have been based in the first instance on data that supported its adoption (Greer et al 1990), but the risk of lymph node metastases in tumours invading 3 mm or less is less than 1%, against 8% for tumours invading 3–5 mm (Simon et al 1986). The FIGO staging is the one in general use and on which clinical management in most centres is based.

Tumour volume

Burghardt and others have emphasized that the volume of an invasive carcinoma is important, rather than the depth alone (Burghardt & Holzer 1977, Burghardt 1984), and some workers have suggested that volume is the most important prognostic factor (Patanaphan et al 1986). Measurements of volume from histological sections is difficult; the formula

volume = thickness × horizontal spread × $1\frac{1}{2}$ times the horizontal spread

gives a practical result, though this is often an overestimate of the true tumour volume as the tumour is measured as a notional cuboid (Burghardt 1984). The measurement of depth is made from the surface of the tumour. By this method, no tumour that measured less than 420 mm^3 and did not have vascular invasion was found to have metastases (Burghardt & Holzer 1977); carcinoma of less than 500 mm^3 that invaded to a depth of less than 3 mm with no vascular invasion was found to be unlikely to have metastasized (Bremond et al 1985). More recently, to be confident that metastasis is very unlikely, it has been recommended that the volume of poorly differentiated tumours should not be over 300 mm^3, and that of well-differentiated tumours should not be over 500 mm^3 (Burghardt et al 1988).

Differentiation of tumour cells

Tumour differentiation has been found to be related to depth of invasion by some workers: the greater the depth of invasion, the greater the prevalence of well-differentiated carcinoma (Sedlis et al 1979). Others have suggested that for microinvasive carcinoma, conventional grading methods are not useful and refer to the proportion of differentiated tumour (i.e. eosinophilic, large, polyhedral cells) to undifferentiated tumour (i.e. basophilic, small, spindle-shaped and round cells) (Sedlis et al 1987).

Growth pattern and ulceration

Exophytic tumour growth has been found by some workers (Patanaphan et al 1986) but not by others (Sedlis et al 1987) to have an independent effect on prognosis. Tumours that invade in a confluent fashion rather than as separate strands of tumour cells are associated with a relatively poor prognosis, but this may simply represent the stage of invasion that the tumour has reached (Averette et al 1976).

Previous biopsy can cause problems in assessing the depth of invasion of a tumour. If a volume of tumour tissue has been removed from the centre of a lesion, the remaining tumour measured on a subsequent cone biopsy may appear artificially shallow, and a misdiagnosis of Stage Ia1 may be made (Greer et al 1990). If a tumour is found to be ulcerated, a history of previous biopsy at the site should be sought.

Stromal reaction to tumour

The earliest stromal reactions around very early invasion are oedema, increased vascularity and lymphocytic infiltration (Averette et al 1976). In some tumours there may be a tendency later to develop an eosinophil infiltrate (Lowe 1988), and the degree of stromal oedema increases with the depth of invasion (Sedlis et al 1979).

Vascular invasion

Vascular invasion by tumour cells can be very difficult to distinguish from shrinkage artefact, and in some cases immunostaining for Factor VIII may be helpful. There should be definite evidence of involvement of a vascular space by tumour before this is accepted as true vascular invasion, so that over-diagnosis does not occur. Vascular invasion alone does not indicate that lymph node invasion is likely: in one series more than half of the 30 patients with microinvasive carcinoma studied had vascular invasion but none had metastatic tumour in lymph nodes (Roche & Norris 1975).

Markers of invasive carcinoma

There have been no reports of worthwhile markers that indicate that progression from CIN 3 to invasive carcinoma has occurred. Blood group isoantigens (Stendahl et al 1987), epidermal growth factor receptor (Ueda 1989), *ras* oncogene (Sagae et al 1990), involucrin (Sassoon et al 1985), tritium uptake (Schubert et al 1983), and Langerhans' cells (Hachisuga et al 1989) have been found to differ in amount or number in the different grades of CIN, microinvasive carcinoma and deeply invasive carcinoma, but none has been found to be of diagnostic use. There is evidence that in microinvasive carcinoma there is inversion of the ratio of CD4 and CD8 lymphocytes and reduction of cell-mediated immunity (Castello et al 1986) but, again, this cannot be used for diagnosis.

Histological features

Microinvasive carcinoma of the cervix usually starts in an area of CIN 3. The infiltrating tongue of cells is initially unifocal and in continuity with the overlying CIN 3; the contour of the lower levels of the surface epithelium or crypts involved with CIN 3 becomes irregular and ill defined; the basement membrane is inconspicuous, and gaps can be demonstrated by electron microscopy and with immunostains for collagen (though in practical terms neither of these procedures is useful for diagnosis) (Kudo et al 1990).

The invading cells tend to be more eosinophilic and larger than those of CIN 3, as in superficial vulval carcinoma, and this tendency increases with the depth of invasion (Sedlis et al 1979). There is also disruption of the polarity of the nuclei in the invasive cells, and development of large obvious nucleoli and bizarre cell forms (Savage 1972). The margins of the epithelium in areas of very early invasion lose their rounded contour and become scalloped. The adjacent stroma develops increasing desmoplasia. Invasive tumour cells have cytoplasmic protrusions like the pseudopodia of amoebae, with large numbers of microfilaments lying in the axis of the direction of the protrusion (Kudo et al 1990). In areas in which the basement membrane has disappeared one can find cytoplasmic vesicles of 70–90 nm in diameter; these are not found in neoplastic cells that have remained in situ.

Later, the points of invasion become multifocal, and confluent anastomosing cords of invading cells develop; this is especially likely when depth of invasion of the tumour cells exceeds 3 mm (Averette et al 1976). The number of mitoses increases with confluence of the tumour cells. The surface epithelium usually remains intact, but this depends on whether the tumour is exophytic or not, exophytic tumours having a greater tendency to ulcerate.

Histopathology reports on a case of microinvasive carcinoma of the cervix should include information on:

- The depth of invasion, measured from the highest stromal extension
- The thickness of the tumour measured from the surface
- The greatest diameter of the tumour in the sections available, and, in a cone biopsy specimen, the extent of the circumference involved by microinvasive carcinoma and CIN
- The growth pattern and differentiation of the tumour
- Whether there is vascular space involvement
- The type and severity of the stromal reaction if there is one
- The proximity of the tumour to the surgical excision margins.

'MICROINVASIVE' ADENOCARCINOMA OF THE CERVIX

There is no agreement about what constitutes a microinvasive adeno-carcinoma of endocervix. Some workers have taken the definition to be very superficial extension of the tumour into the endocervical stroma, without measurement of a distance (Tase et al 1989). Others have taken it to be the same as the Society of Gynecologic Oncologists' definition of microinvasive squamous cell carcinoma of cervix (Zuna 1984, Ayer et al 1988) or that of FIGO stage I (Qizilbash 1975). One group classified tumours with invasion limited to the most superficial 2 mm of the endocervical stroma as microinvasive (Betsill & Clark 1986, Clark & Betsill 1986); by this definition, superficially invasive adenocarcinoma behaved in the same way as in situ adenocarcinoma. To date, the number of reported cases with this condition is small (Barnes et al 1980, Sweetnam et al 1981, Evans & Monaghan 1985) (see also p. 123).

'MICROINVASIVE' CARCINOMA OF THE VAGINA

There have been occasional reports on the question of whether there should be a category of microinvasive carcinoma of vagina. In a well-argued paper, in which the authors stated that they did not intend to define criteria for the diagnosis or therapy of microinvasive carcinoma of the vagina, Peters et al (1955) took a depth of invasion of 2.5 mm from the surface of the epithelium as the cut-off for microinvasive tumours, and required that there should be no vascular space involvement. Eddy et al (1990) used the same measure-ments in their study, and found that patients treated with radiotherapy had a good prognosis. The superficially invasive carcinomas were almost all in the upper third of the vagina. No significant differences were found between patients with microinvasive and deeply invasive carcinoma in regard to clinical details.

Some workers have reported that patients with superficially invasive vaginal carcinoma have a median age 10 years younger than patients with FIGO Stage I carcinoma (Peters et al 1985), though the number of cases was small. As with superficially invasive vulval carcinoma, there appear to be no clinical or prognostic differences that clearly distinguish between tumours invading less than 2.5 mm and those that invade more deeply, and there is no good justification at present for defining a category of microinvasive carcinoma of vagina.

The histological features of superficially invasive carcinoma of the vagina are similar to those of the cervix. In very early cases, a stromal reaction of oedema, lymphocyte infiltration and developing fibrosis may be present before maturational changes in the epithelium become apparent (Wilkinson 1987).

'MICROINVASIVE' CARCINOMA OF THE VULVA

Microinvasive carcinoma of the vulva is a concept that appeals because of the analogy with cervical neoplasia, but there is no generally accepted definition of the condition or even of the name that should be given to it. Some workers use the term early invasive carcinoma, but this suggests that the tumour has been present for only a short time, and for indolent, well-differentiated tumours this might not be the case. Superficially invasive carcinoma is a purely descriptive term that has found wide acceptance (Buscema et al 1981, Dvoretsky et al 1984). The International Society for the Study of Vulvar Disease (ISSVD) considered that the term micro-invasive carcinoma should not be applied to the vulva as it was 'misleading and dangerous', and that Stage Ia cancer of vulva should be used instead (Kneale et al 1984). This is defined as a solitary lesion with a maximum diameter of 2 cm and a maximum depth of invasion of 1 mm. The depth of invasion should be measured from the dermoepidermal junction of the most superficial overlying dermal papilla to the deepest aspect of the invasive tumour cells.

Similarly, the FIGO staging classification does not include the term microinvasive carcinoma; to be in Stage I, the most superficial tumours must measure not more than 2 cm in diameter and there must be no palpable lymph nodes (T1N0M0) (Petterson 1988).

The risk factors for the progression of vulval intraepithelial neoplasia (VIN) to superficially invasive carcinoma of vulva include age, immune status, number of separate lesions and site of the lesions. Patients who are over the age of 60 years, are immunosuppressed, have multifocal VIN (especially VIN 3), and have carcinoma in situ in the midline (affecting the clitoral area or the perineum), all have a statistically increased risk of developing invasive carcinoma of the vulva (Buscema et al 1980, Jones & McLean 1986, Sedlis et al 1987). There are no firm data on whether ploidy or an association with human papillomavirus infection in carcinoma in situ of the vulva have any value in predicting the likelihood of development of invasive carcinoma (Bernstein et al 1983) (see also p. 111). The recurrence rate of VIN is 25% (Andreasson & Bock 1985), which is much higher than the rate of development of invasive carcinoma: VIN 3 progresses to invasive carcinoma in only 2–8% of cases (Buscema et al 1980, Andreasson & Bock 1985).

Superficially invasive carcinoma of the vulva is commonest on the labium majus, followed by the labium minus, area of clitoris and perineum, in descending order of frequency. Tumours arise more commonly on the right than the left; there is no apparent reason for this (Kunschner et al 1978).

The predictors for metastasis of vulval carcinoma include more than simply the depth of tumour cell invasion. Tumour size, histological grade and growth pattern, vascular space involvement, site (whether centrally located on the clitoris or perineum rather than laterally on a labium) and clinical suspicion of involvement of inguinal lymph nodes have also been shown to be related to prognosis (Sedlis et al 1987).

Depth of invasion

For the depth of invasion of a carcinoma to be useful as a diagnostic parameter there has to be agreement on the points from which measurements are taken, and consistency in the clinical and prognostic correlations of different assessors' results. Study of the significance of depth of invasion in vulval carcinoma has been hampered by lack of both of these. Even when the points of reference are established, measurement of distance in histological sections can be difficult. Calder et al (1990) found that there were significant differences in measurements among observers when an eye-piece graticule, a microscope-stage Vernier scale and a projection system were used for measuring the thickness of melanomas, and the same problem almost certainly applies to measurements of vulval, vaginal and cervical carcinomas.

Where should measurements of tumour invasion be made from, and where to? *Depth* has been used in different reports to refer variously to the greatest distance from an invasive tumour cell to the site of origin of the invasive tumour, the nearest basement membrane of non-invasive epithelium,

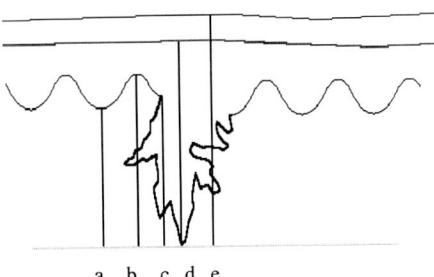

a   b   c   d   e

Fig. 8.1 Distance from the deepest invasive tumour cell to: a, basement membrane of the epithelium of the nearest adjacent rete ridge (irrespective of whether or not this is neoplastic epithelium); b, basement membrane over the most superficial dermal papilla adjacent to the invasive tumour; c, basement membrane of the non-invasive epithelium from which the invasive tumour apparently arises; d, granular cell layer of the epidermis over the tumour; e, surface of the tumour. (Modified from Wilkinson 1987 with permission of the publishers.)

and the distance that the tumour has invaded in the direction of the deep underlying tissues. For superficially invasive vulval carcinoma, the points from which invasion could be measured are illustrated in Figure 8.1. Each of these has conceptual and practical problems.

The optimal point from which invasion should be measured is difficult to determine, but the measurement should primarily represent the extent of dermal invasion of the tumour so that this can be correlated with prognosis. In most cases measurement b on Figure 8.1, from the top of the highest adjacent dermal papilla, gives the closest approximation of the distance that malignant cells have invaded the dermis, but in tumours that have invaded only a very short distance from the bottom of a rete ridge this measurement can appreciably overestimate the extent of dermal invasion.

Measurements made from the surface of the tumour take into account exophytic tumour growth as well as extent of dermal spread. A problem with this is that measurement of the full thickness of a tumour will in many cases also include the thickness of the keratin or parakeratin overlying it, and in well-differentiated vulval carcinomas this can be 200 μm or more thick (Fig. 8.2). There is no good evidence that this has a bearing on prognosis other than in relation to the differentiation of the tumour. Variations in keratin thickness can introduce a considerable proportional error in the measurement of tumours, especially well-differentiated tumours

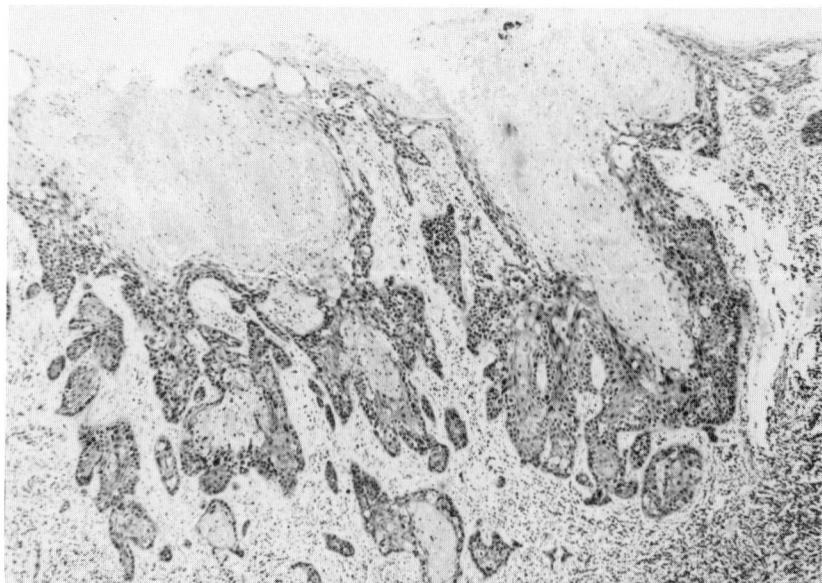

Fig. 8.2 Early invasive carcinoma of vulva over which there is extensive parakeratin formation. In many areas the surface layers of the parakeratin have been lost. Measurements made from the surface of the tumour in these cases are therefore unreliable.

less than 1000 µm thick (unpublished observations). Measuring from the granular cell layer, where this is present, avoids this error.

In our practice, we use interactive computed image analysis on vulval carcinomas and measure from the deepest invasive tumour cell to:

- The point of origin of the invasive cells from non-invasive epithelium, where this can be established with confidence (Fig. 8.2) or to
- The top of the most superficial adjacent dermal papilla, irrespective of the presence of neoplasia in the overlying epithelium and to
- The top of the lesion, from the granular cell layer when there is one, and from the surface of the tumour when it is non-keratinized, parakeratotic, eroded or ulcerated.

The first measurement gives the most accurate indication of the extent of dermal spread of the tumour cells but can be applied in only the small proportion of cases in which the tumour is very superficially invasive. The other two measurements are usable in almost all cases. As suggested by Wilkinson (1987), the first two measurements are referred to as the depth of invasion and the third as the thickness of tumour.

There is no depth of invasion that reliably delimits cases in which one can rely on there being no chance of lymph node metastases. In one study, 49% of all vulval tumours had invaded the dermis to a depth of less than 5 mm and about 20% of patients with these superficial tumours had lymph node metastases (Sedlis et al 1987). With a depth of invasion of 3 mm, the percentage of patients with lymph node metastases fell to zero (Chu et al 1982), though in other series occasional cases appear; a report of lymph node metastases in a patient with vulval carcinoma that invaded only 0.72 mm into the dermis has recently been published (Atamdede & Hoogerland 1989). In general terms, tumours that have invaded the dermis to a depth of 1 mm or less and do not have vascular invasion are very unlikely to metastasize.

Diameter of the tumour

Measurement of the diameter of the tumour has become an important part of the assessment of vulval carcinoma. It forms part of the definition of the FIGO staging of Stage I vulval cancer (Petterson 1988) and is related to the incidence of nodal metastasis (Donaldson et al 1981). The diameter of only the invasive tumour is measured, and not the VIN or atypical epithelium adjacent to it.

There appears to be little difference in likelihood of lymph node metastases if a carcinoma is 1 or 2 cm in diameter, provided that the depth of invasion is 1 mm or less (Magrina et al 1979). When 2 cm is taken as the arbitrary cut-off diameter, the incidence of inguinal metastases is 5–10% (Parker et al 1975, Yazigi et al 1978). Patients with carcinomas up to 3 cm diameter generally have a good prognosis (Krupp et al 1975, Donaldson et al

1981), though in one series 18.9% of those with vulval carcinomas of 3 cm diameter or less had metastatic carcinoma in lymph nodes, and for patients with tumours between 3 and 5 cm diameter the figure can be anywhere between 9.4 and 72.4% (Magrina et al 1979, Donaldson et al 1981). Patients with tumours less than 1 cm diameter can develop metastases (Atamdede & Hoogerland 1989), and there is no reliable and clinically useful size below which the chance of metastatic spread can be assumed to be zero.

Volume of the tumour

Measurement of tumour volume is also considered to be prognostically important. The volume of a superficially invasive carcinoma has been found to be of greater prognostic value than the depth of invasion, and the term *microcarcinoma* has been proposed as an alternative to microinvasive carcinoma for these tumours in the cervix (Burghardt 1984).

The formula given by Wilkinson et al (1982) for tumour volume (V) is based on a tumour with an idealized 'truncated cone' shape rather than the cuboid defined by Burghardt (see above, p. 148). Taking r_1 as the radius of the lesion at its surface, r_2 as the radius at the deepest point of invasion, and D as the tumour thickness:

$$V = \frac{\pi D \, (r_1^2 + r_1 r_2 + r_2^2)}{3}.$$

If computer-linked measurements of area are available and the largest tumour area on the tissue sections can be measured (A_{max}), the volume of a tumour with a horizontal diameter of h is approximated by the formula

$$V = \frac{2 \times h \times A_{max}}{3}.$$

The volume of tumour associated with metastatic spread in the vulva is appreciably less than that found in the cervix. For all histological types, the upper limit of volume for tumours not associated with metastases is below 300 mm³ (Wilkinson 1987), appreciably less than the volume of 420 mm³ reported by Burghardt for cervical tumours (Toplis et al 1986).

Tumour cell differentiation and patterns of invasion

There is conflicting evidence on whether the histological grade of superficially invasive squamous cell carcinoma of the vulva has a bearing on prognosis. Many workers found that there was no correlation (Magrina et al 1979, Buscema et al 1981, Iverson et al 1981), but Chu et al (1982) found that the degree of differentiation correlated with depth of invasion, and Sedlis et al (1987) found that the differentiation of the tumour, assessed by the proportion of small, relatively basophilic cells to large eosinophilic cells, was closely related to the incidence of nodal spread.

Two main patterns of growth can be found in superficially invasive vulval carcinomas that have progressed beyond the very early focal stage: confluent, and diffuse or 'spray pattern' invasion. There is no established definition of these. The term confluent growth is used to refer to a carcinoma that has apparently arisen multifocally or over a broad face and that has formed a discrete, compact tumour mass by merging of the invasive strands. The term diffuse growth is used for tumours that extend as poorly defined cords, and sometimes single-cell lines, into the dermis in a radial fashion away from the apparent point of origin. The diffuse pattern of growth has been shown to be associated with a significant risk of lymph node metastases (Dinh et al 1989, LaPolla et al 1988). Tumours with confluent growth have usually invaded well beyond 1 mm into the dermis (Hoffman et al 1983, Wilkinson 1987); it may be that confluence is not an independent variable and is simply a feature of the duration and histological grade of the carcinoma. It may be impossible confidently to determine the grade of differentiation of very superficially invasive carcinomas as there may be too little tumour on which grading can be based.

Vascular space involvement

It is very unusual to see vascular space involvement in vulval carcinomas that have invaded less than 1 mm into the dermis (Wilkinson 1987). Some studies have suggested that there is no good association between the demonstration of vascular spread and lymph node metastases in super-ficially invasive tumours (Buscema et al 1981, Hacker et al 1983, Dvoretsky et al 1984), but this is not generally accepted (Sedlis et al 1987). In practical terms, there can be difficulties in establishing whether tumours that have invaded less than 5 mm have vascular spread because of artefactual shrinkage on fixation, and this may contribute to the confusion in the data on this feature (Buscema et al 1981).

Histopathological features

The earliest histological changes in a carcinoma that has progressed from in situ to invasive are subtle, but there are some features that are present with reasonable frequency. One of the first changes is that the squamous cells at the site of invasion become larger and more eosinophilic than the in situ cells, with loss of palisading at the dermoepidermal junction (Fig. 8.3). The nuclei in the invading tumour cells are widely spaced and usually lose the hyperchromatism of the nuclei of the in situ component (Fig. 8.4). Single

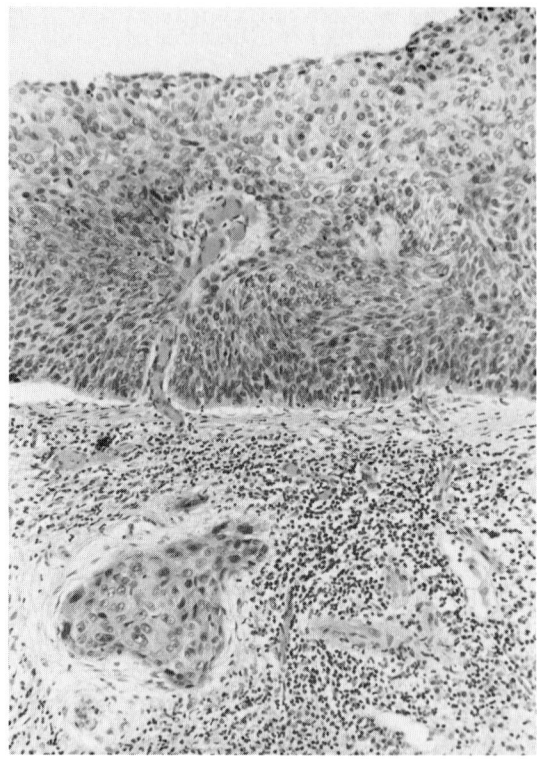

Fig. 8.3   The invasive tumour cells have more cytoplasm, and larger and more open nuclei, than the VIN 3 from which they arose. There is also local stromal oedema around the tumour cell islands and an infiltrate of lymphocytes and histiocytes.

squamous cells may be present in the stroma. There is often a chronic inflammatory cell infiltrate in the area of invasion, predominantly of lymphocytes with smaller numbers of histiocytes and occasional eosinophils. In difficult cases, a periodic acid–Schiff stain and immunostains for basement membrane are seldom helpful, and multiple serial sections are most useful.

The histopathology report on a case of invasive vulval carcinoma should include information on:

● The site of the tumour and the structures involved by it
● The depth of invasion measured from the highest dermal papilla, or from the site of invasion where this is obvious in very superficial tumours
● The thickness of the tumour
● The greatest diameter of the tumour on the histological sections available
● The growth pattern and differentiation of the tumour
● Whether there is involvement of vascular spaces
● The type and severity of the stromal reaction, if there is one

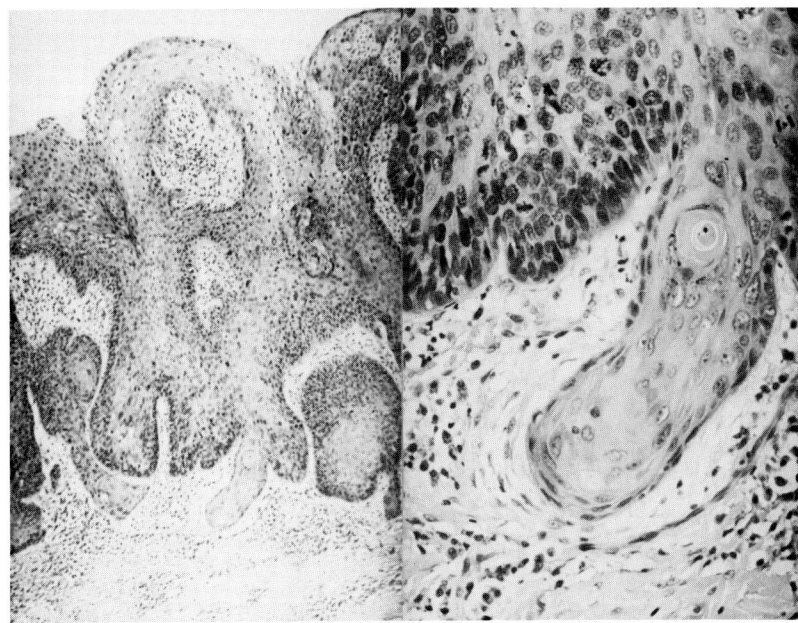

Fig. 8.4 The tongue of very superficially invasive tumour has become considerably more eosinophilic than the adjacent VIN, and the nuclei are larger and more vesicular than those in the in situ tumour.

- The proximity of the tumour to the excision margins
- Whether there is VIN or a vulval dermatosis in the non-neoplastic tissues adjacent to the tumour and in the contralateral vulva.

REFERENCES

Andreasson B, Bock J E 1985 Intraepithelial neoplasia in the vulvar region. Gynecologic Oncology 21: 300–305

Atamdede F, Hoogerland D 1989 Regional lymph node recurrence following local excision for microinvasive vulvar carcinoma. Gynecologic Oncology 34: 125–128

Averette H E, Nelson J H Jr, Ng A B, Hoskins W J, Boyce J G, Ford J H Jr 1976 Diagnosis and management of microinvasive (stage IA) carcinoma of the uterine cervix. Cancer 38: 414–425

Ayer B, Pacey F, Greenberg M 1988 The cytologic diagnosis of adenocarcinoma in situ of the cervix uteri and related lesions. II. Microinvasive adenocarcinoma. Acta Cytologica 32: 318–324

Barnes A E, Crissman J D, Schellhas H F, Azoury R S 1980 Microinvasive carcinoma of the vulva: a clinicopathologic evaluation. Obstetrics and Gynecology 56: 234–238

Benson W L, Norris H J 1977 A critical review of the frequency of lymph node metastasis and death from microinvasive carcinoma of the cervix. Obstetrics and Gynecology 49: 632–638

Bernstein S G, Kovacs B R, Townsend D E, Morrow C P 1983 Vulvar carcinoma in situ. Obstetrics and Gynecology 61: 304–307

Betsill W L Jr, Clark A H 1986 Early endocervical glandular neoplasia. I. Histomorphology and cytomorphology. Acta Cytologica 30: 115–126

Bremond A, Frappart L, Migaud C 1985 Study of 68 microinvasive carcinomas of the cervix uteri. Journal de Gynecologie, Obstetrique et Biologique de la Reproduction (Paris) 14: 1025–1031

Burghardt E 1984 Microinvasive carcinoma in gynaecological pathology. Clinics in Obstetrics and Gynaecology 11: 239–257

Burghardt E, Holzer E 1977 Diagnosis and treatment of microinvasive carcinoma of the cervix uteri. Obstetrics and Gynecology 49: 641–653

Burghardt E, Pickel H, Haas J, Lahousen M 1988 Objective results of the operative treatment of cervical cancer. Baillière's Clinics in Obstetrics and Gynaecology 2: 987–995

Buscema J, Stern J, Woodruff J D 1980a The significance of the histologic alterations adjacent to invasive vulvar carcinoma. American Journal of Obstetrics and Gynecology 137: 902–909

Buscema J, Stern J, Woodruff J D 1980b Progressive histobiologic alterations in the development of vulvar cancer. Report of five cases. American Journal of Obstetrics and Gynecology 138: 146–150

Buscema J, Stern J L, Woodruff J D 1981 Early invasive carcinoma of the vulva. American Journal of Obstetrics and Gynecology 140: 563–569

Calder C J, Campbell A P, Plastow S R 1990 Measurement techniques for melanoma: a statistical comparison. Journal of Clinical Pathology 43: 922–923

Castello G, Esposito G, Stellato G, Dalla Mora L, Abate G, Germano A 1986 Immunological abnormalities in patients with cervical carcinoma. Gynecologic Oncology 25: 61–64

Chu J, Tamimi H K, Ek M, Figge D C 1982 Stage I vulvar cancer: criteria for microinvasion. Obstetrics and Gynecology 59: 716–719

Clark A H, Betsill W L Jr 1986 Early endocervical glandular neoplasia. II. Morphometric analysis of the cells. Acta Cytologica 30: 127–134

Collins H S, Burke T W, Woodward J E, Spurlock J W, Heller P B 1989 Widespread lymph node metastases in a patient with microinvasive cervical carcinoma. Gynecologic Oncology 34: 219–221

Dinh T A, Dinh T V, Hannigan E V, Yandell R B, Dillard E A Jr Necessity for endocervical curettage in elderly women undergoing colposcopy. Journal of Reproductive Medicine 34: 621–624

Donaldson E S, Powell D E, Hanson M B, van Nagell J R Jr 1981 Prognostic parameters in invasive vulvar cancer. Gynecologic Oncology 11: 184–190

Dvoretsky P, Bonfiglio T, Helmkamp B F, Ramsey G, Chuang C, Beecham J B 1984 The pathology of superficially invasive, thin vulvar squamous cell carcinoma. International Journal of Gynecological Pathology 3: 331–342

Ebeling K, Bilek K, Johannsmeyer D et al 1989 Microinvasive stage Ia cancer of the uterine cervix—results of a multicenter clinic based analysis. Geburtshilfe und Frauenheilkunde 49: 776–781

Eddy G L, Singh K P, Gansler T S 1990 Superficially invasive carcinoma of the vagina following treatment for cervical cancer: a report of six cases. Gynecologic Oncology 36: 376–379

Evans A S, Monaghan J M 1985 Spontaneous resolution of cervical warty atypia: the relevance of clinical and nuclear DNA features: a prospective study. British Journal of Obstetrics and Gynaecology 92: 165–169

Greer B E, Figge D C, Tamimi H K, Cain J M, Lee R B 1990 Stage Ia2 squamous carcinoma of the cervix: difficult diagnosis and therapeutic dilemma. American Journal of Obstetrics and Gynecology 162: 1406–1411

Hachisuga T, Fukuda K, Hayashi Y, Iwasaka T, Sugimori H 1989 Immunohistochemical demonstration of histiocytes in normal ectocervical epithelium and epithelial lesions of the uterine cervix. Gynecologic Oncology 33: 273–278

Hacker N F, Nieberg R K, Berek J S et al 1983 Superficially invasive vulvar cancer with nodal metastases. Gynecologic Oncology 15: 65–77

Hoffman J S, Kumar N B, Morley G W 1983 Microinvasive squamous carcinoma of the vulva: search for a definition. Obstetrics and Gynecology 61: 615–618

Ito T, Yago H, Kuribayashi M, Ohsawa H 1986 Colposcopy in dysplasia, carcinoma in situ and microinvasive cancer of the cervix—systematic diagnosis. Nippon Sanka Fujinka Gakkai Zasshi 38: 168–176

Iverson T, Abeler V, Aadlers J 1981 Individualized treatment of stage I carcinoma of the vulva. Obstetrics and Gynecology 57: 84–89

Jones R W, McLean M R 1986 Carcinoma in situ of the vulva: a review of 31 treated and five untreated cases. Obstetrics and Gynecology 68: 499–503

Kneale B L et al 1984 Report of the ISSVD Task Force. Microinvasive cancer of the vulva: report of the International Society for the Study of Vulvar Disease Task Force. Proceedings of the 7th World Congress of the ISSVD. Journal of Reproductive Medicine 29: 454–456

Kolstad P 1989 Follow-up study of 232 patients with stage Ia1 and 411 patients with stage Ia2 squamous cell carcinoma of the cervix (microinvasive carcinoma). Gynecologic Oncology 33: 265–272

Krupp P J, Lee F Y L, Bohm J W, Batson H W K, Diem J E, Lemire J E 1975 Prognostic parameters and clinical staging criteria in epidermal carcinoma of the vulva. Obstetrics and Gynecology 46: 84–88

Kudo R, Sato T, Mizuuchi H 1990 Ultrastructural and immunohistochemical study of infiltration in microinvasive carcinoma of the uterine cervix. Gynecologic Oncology 36: 23–29

Kunschner A, Kanbour A I, David B 1978 Early vulvar carcinoma. American Journal of Obstetrics and Gynecology 132: 599–606

LaPolla J P, O'Neill C, Wetrich D 1988 Colposcopic management of abnormal cervical cytology in pregnancy. Journal of Reproductive Medicine 33: 301–306

Lowe D 1988 Carcinoma of the cervix with massive eosinophilia. British Journal of Obstetrics and Gynaecology 95: 393–401

Magrina J F, Webb M J, Gaffey T A, Symmonds R E 1979 Stage I squamous cell cancer of the vulva. American Journal of Obstetrics and Gynecology 134: 453–459

Mestwerdt G 1947 Probeexzision und Kolposcopie in des Fruhdiagnose des Portiokarcinoms. Zentralblatt für Gynakologie 4: 326–330

Mestwerdt G 1953 Atlas de Kolposkopie. Fischer, Jena

Monaghan J M 1988 Management decision using clinical and operative staging in cervical cancer. Clinics in Obstetrics and Gynaecology 2: 737–746

Nelson J H, Averette H E, Richart R M 1975 Detection, diagnostic evaluation and treatment of dysplasia and early carcinoma of the cervix. CA 25: 134–151

Noda K, Taki I, Takeuchi S et al 1979 A new proposal regarding criteria for Stage Ia cancer in the uterine cervix. The Joint Study Committee on Stage Ia Cancer in the Uterine Cervix. Gynecol Oncol 8: 353–369

Parker R T, Duncan I, Rampone J, Creasman W 1975 Operative management of early invasive epidermoid carcinoma of vulva. American Journal of Obstetrics and Gynecology 123: 349–355

Patanaphan V, Poussin-Rosillio H, Santa U V, Salazar O M 1986 Cancer of the uterine cervix Stage Ib—treatment results and prognostic factors. Cancer 57: 866–870

Peters W A, Kumar N B, Morley G W 1985 Microinvasive carcinoma of the vagina: a distinct clinical entity? American Journal of Obstetrics and Gynecology 153: 505–507

Petterson F 1988 Annual report on the results of treatment in gynaecological cancer. FIGO, Stockholm, vol 20

Prendiville W, Davies R, Berry P J 1986 A low voltage diathermy loop for taking cervical biopsies: a qualitative comparison with punch biopsy forceps. British Journal of Obstetrics and Gynaecology 93: 773–776

Puente Gonzalez H, Reyna Hinojosa R, Hinojosa Gonzalez S, Gonzalez Ramirez R, de Alba Lopez E 1977 Microinvasive carcinoma of the cervix and pregnancy. Diagnosis and treatment in 13 cases. Ginecologia e Obstetrica Mexico 42: 61–71

Qizilbash A H 1975 In-situ and microinvasive adenocarcinoma of the uterine cervix. A clinical, cytologic and histologic study of 14 cases. American Journal of Clinical Pathology 64: 155–170

Roche W D, Norris H J 1975 Microinvasive carcinoma of the cervix. The significance of lymphatic invasion and confluent patterns of stromal growth. Cancer 36: 180–186

Ruch R M, Pitcock J A, Ruch W A 1976 Microinvasive carcinoma of the cervix. American Journal of Obstetrics and Gynecology 125: 87–92

Sassoon A F, Said J W, Nash G, Shintaku I P, Banks Schlegel S 1985 Involucrin in intraepithelial and invasive squamous cell carcinomas of the cervix: an immunohistochemical study. Human Pathology 16: 467–470

Sagae S, Kudo R, Kuzumaki N et al 1990 Ras oncogene expression and progression in intraepithelial neoplasia of the uterine cervix. Cancer 66: 295–301

Savage E W 1972 Microinvasive carcinoma of the uterine cervix. American Journal of Clinical Pathology 113: 708–717

Schubert B, Kunz J, Banaschak A 1983 Labelling patterns of carcinomas of the cervix and their precancerous stages after 3H-thymidine incorporation. Acta Histochemica Supplement band (Jena) 27: 111–115

Sedlis A, Sall S, Tsukada Y, Park R, Mangan C, Shingleton H, Blessing J A 1979 Microinvasive carcinoma of the cervix uteri: a clinicopathologic study. American Journal of Obstetrics and Gynecology 133: 63–74

Sedlis A, Homesley H, Bundy B N et al 1987 Positive groin lymph nodes in superficial squamous cell vulvar cancer. A Gynecologic Oncology Group Study. American Journal of Obstetrics and Gynecology 156: 1159–1164

Seski J C, Abell M R, Morley G W 1977 Microinvasive squamous cell carcinoma of the cervix: definition, histological analysis, late results of treatment. Obstetrics and Gynecology 50: 410–414

Shepherd J H 1989 Revised FIGO staging for gynaecological cancer. British Journal of Obstetrics and Gynaecology 96: 889–892

Simon N L, Gore H, Shingleton H M, Soong S J, Orr J W, Hatch K D. 1986 Study of superficially invasive carcinoma of the cervix. Obstetrics and Gynecology 68: 19–24

Stendahl U, Lindgren A, Busch C 1987 Blood group isoantigen expression during tumour progression of cervical neoplasia. Anticancer Research 7: 1285–1286

Sweetnam P, Evans D M, Hibbard B M, Jones J M 1981 The Cardiff Cervical Cytology Study. Prevalence and epidemiology of cervical neoplasia. Journal of Epidemiology and Community Health 35: 83–90

Tase T, Okagaki T, Clark B A, Twiggs L B, Ostrow R S, Faras A J 1989 Human papillomavirus DNA in adenocarcinoma in situ, microinvasive adenocarcinoma of the uterine cervix, and coexisting cervical squamous intraepithelial neoplasia. International Journal of Gynecological Pathology 8: 8–17

Toplis P J, Casemore V, Hallam N, Charnock M 1986 Evaluation of colposcopy in the postmenopausal woman. British Journal of Obstetrics and Gynaecology 93: 843–851

Tsukamoto N, Kaku T, Matsukuma K et al 1989 The problem of stage Ia (FIGO, 1985) carcinoma of the uterine cervix. Gynecologic Oncology 34: 1–6

Ueda M 1989 Immunohistochemical studies on epidermal growth factor receptor in oncogenesis of uterine cervical cancer. Nippon Sanka Fujinka Gakkai Zasshi 41: 1401–1408

van Nagell J R Jr, Greenwell N, Powell D F, Donaldson E S, Hanson M B, Gay E C 1983 Microinvasive carcinoma of the cervix. American Journal of Obstetrics and Gynecology 145: 981–991

Wilkinson E J (ed) 1987 Pathology of the vulva and vagina. Churchill Livingstone, Edinburgh

Wilkinson E J, Rico M J, Pierson K K 1982 Microinvasive carcinoma of the vulva. International Journal of Gynecological Pathology 1: 29–39

Yazigi R, Piver M S, Tsukada Y 1978 Microinvasive carcinoma of the vulva. Obstetrics and Gynecology 51: 368–370

Zuna R E 1984 Association of condylomas with intraepithelial and microinvasive cervical neoplasia: histopathology of conization and hysterectomy specimens. International Journal of Gynecological Pathology 2: 364–372

9. Abnormalities of the glandular epithelium of the endocervix

L. J. R. Brown

INTRODUCTION

Interest in the ectocervix is such that the glandular epithelium receives scant attention and any abnormalities may be overlooked or misinterpreted. The incidence of cervical adenocarcinoma is increasing, and there are uncertainties about the causes and natural history of the early stages of the disease. This chapter covers developments in the understanding of pre-invasive and early-stage adenocarcinomas, highlights differences between neoplastic, infective and benign conditions, and dwells on some aspects of invasive lesions.

THE NORMAL CERVIX

In women of reproductive age the cervical canal is 27 mm long on average (range 18–35 mm), lined by a single layer of columnar epithelium which covers a series of clefts, ridges and, occasionally, villi (Hafez 1982). These structures are orientated obliquely to the cervical canal so that in histological sections they appear as a system of glands that reach a maximum depth of 7.8 mm (mean 3.4 mm) (Anderson & Hartley 1980). The epithelium is composed of two cell types: secretory cells that produce glycoproteins, and ciliated cells that move the mucus towards the vagina. The secretory cells go through a cycle of synthesis, secretion and exhaustion under β-adrenergic control (Whitaker et al 1989), and the nuclei, which are generally basally situated, may rise to occupy the middle of the cell when the secretion has been released (Hafez 1982). Acidic and neutral mucins are synthesized, though acidic mucins predominate, the composition changing with the menstrual cycle. Intracellular sialomucins increase relative to sulphomucins in pre- and peri-ovulatory phases of the menstrual cycle but fall after ovulation and in women outside the reproductive age-group, in whom sulphomucins predominate (Wakefield & Wells 1985, Gilks et al 1989a). Sialomucin-rich secretory product is copious and watery, well suited to sperm entry.

The endocervix plays a major role in preventing microbial contamination of the uterine cavity. Endocervical columnar cells contain vitamin B_{12} R-binder (a protein similar to gastric intrinsic factor), which has specific antibacterial activity (Kim et al 1988). The columnar cells also add secretory component to dimeric secretory type IgA produced by stromal plasma cells (Kutteh et al 1988).

BENIGN CONDITIONS

Viral infections

Bizarre multinucleate endocervical cells with polylobulated, mulberry-like, vesicular or deeply staining nuclei have been described and illustrated (Fox & Buckley 1983, Brown & Wells 1986). The similarity to the viral changes that are usually present in the ectocervix has prompted suggestions that herpes simplex or papillomaviruses may be the cause. Unfortunately the changes are seen only in one or two cells, frustrating attempts to detect viral sequences by in situ hybridization (personal observations). The role of papillomaviruses in glandular neoplasia is considered on page 87.

Epstein–Barr virus (EBV) has been detected by in situ hybridization in exfoliated cervical glandular epithelium (Sixbey et al 1986). A role for EBV in the development of cervical adenocarcinoma has been proposed (Young & Sixbey 1988), supported by the observation that seminal plasma seems to aid the transmission of EBV (Turner et al 1990). Nasopharyngeal carcinoma, which is known to be related to EBV infection, may coexist (Singh et al 1989).

Cytomegalovirus infection is more common than rare observations of enlarged 'owl's-eye' nuclei might suggest (Myerson et al 1984).

Hyperplasia of Gartner's duct (mesonephric remnant, Wolffian duct remnant)

Gartner's duct remnants are most commonly encountered incidentally as isolated vestigial acini; when they are hyperplastic there is a danger of confusion with adenocarcinoma. From the embryological position of Gartner's duct in the lateral portions of the cervix, hyperplastic remnants can ramify into any quadrant of the deep cervical wall and may surround a larger duct (Brown & Wells 1986). Small acini are lined by low cuboidal cells with clear cytoplasm housing spherical vesicular nuclei in a low nuclear-cytoplasmic ratio (Fig. 9.1). Glassy periodic acid–Schiff positive, diastase-resistant, intra-acinar secretion stains with Alcian blue at pH 2.5 and mucicarmine (Aryoud et al 1985, Lang & Dallenbach-Hellweg 1990).

In contrast to adenocarcinoma, there is no nuclear atypia, mitotic activity, papillae or complex branched glands, and no stromal oedema, inflammation or necrosis that might indicate invasion. Distinction from minimal deviation adenocarcinoma (adenoma malignum) may be difficult, especially in small biopsies, but the simple glandular profiles are the most helpful features

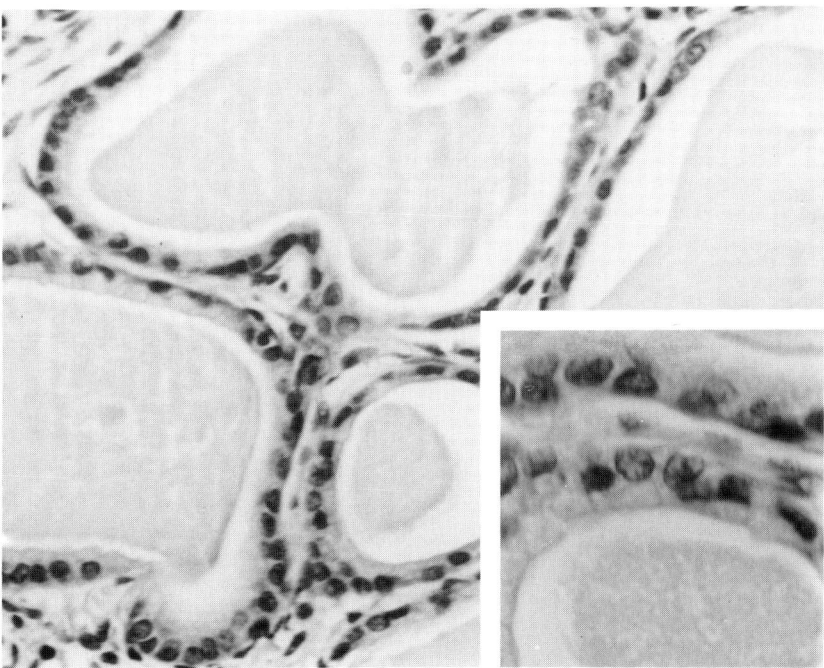

Fig. 9.1 Gartner's duct hyperplasia. The acini contain eosinophilic secretion and are lined by bland, low cuboidal cells (inset).

(Gilks et al 1989b). Usefully, Gartner's duct hyperplasia always stains negative for carcinoembryonic antigen, whilst most adenocarcinomas are carcinoembryonic antigen positive. Luminal reactivity with HMFG1 contrasts with the cytoplasmic reactivity of neoplastic glands (Brown et al 1987). Additionally, up to 30% of cases have intracytoplasmic vimentin, and cervical adenocarcinoma does not (Dabbs et al 1986, Lang & Dallenbach-Hellweg 1990). Electron microscopy shows a poorly developed secretory apparatus, prominent cytotelolysosomes and myelin figures similar to transitional epithelium, Brenner tumours and Walthard's rests. Hormonal imbalance has been postulated as an aetological factor by Lang & Dallenbach-Hellweg (1990), but these authors concede that their results were from an uncontrolled, selected series and need confirmation. No recurrences of Gartner's duct hyperplasia have been reported even when excision was incomplete (Shah et al 1980). However, mesonephric adenocarcinomas may rarely originate in areas of Gartner's duct hyperplasia (Buntine 1979).

Microglandular hyperplasia

Microglandular hyperplasia occurs in women of reproductive age in association with oral contraceptive use, hormonal replacement therapy, and

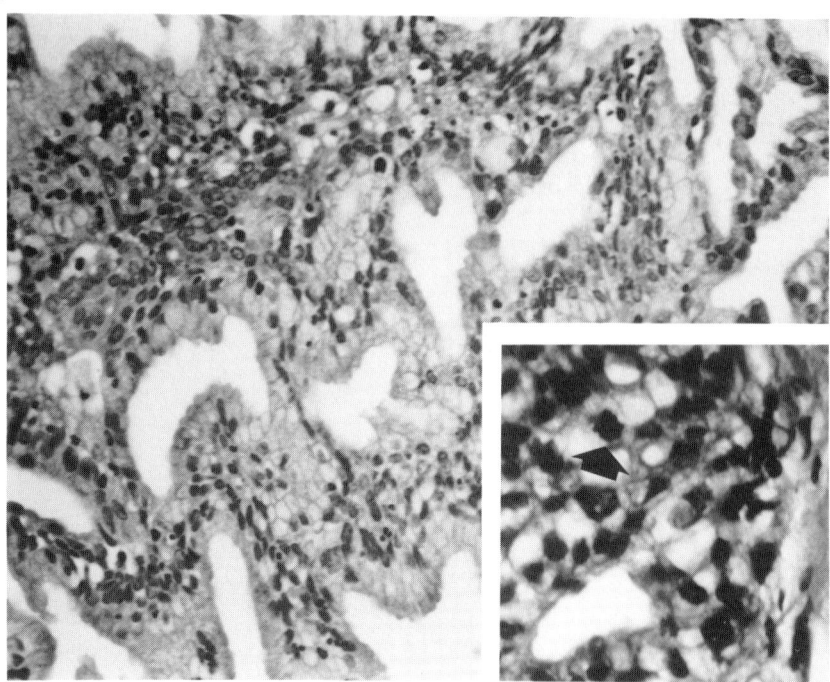

Fig. 9.2 Microglandular hyperplasia with areas of vacuolated cells, solid proliferations and rare mitoses (arrowed in inset).

pregnancy, in which it probably represents florid reserve cell hyperplasia with glandular differentiation. Nevertheless, the condition may occur outside these circumstances, and 6% of reported cases have been in post-menopausal women (Chumas et al 1985). This common, complex pro-liferation of small, tightly packed glands may form polypoid projections into the endocervical canal. The acini are lined by cuboidal, columnar or flattened epithelial cells which may be vacuolated and contain mucin. Stromal oedema and inflammation are common, and occasionally eosino-phils are numerous (Helmerhorst et al 1984). Attention to cytological detail and awareness of the condition avoids confusion of this entirely benign condition with adenocarcinoma.

Rarely, the bland nuclear features may be overshadowed by worrying atypical growth patterns such as solid areas, signet-ring cells, clear cells, stromal hyalinization, pseudoinfiltration, moderate nuclear atypia and occasional mitoses—fewer than one per 10 high-power fields (Young & Scully 1989b). In these cases the presence of associated areas of recognizable microglandular hyperplasia and absence of intracytoplasmic glycogen can aid the diagnosis (Fig. 9.2). Luminal reactivity with the antibodies HMFG1 and anti-CA125, with negative staining for carcinoembryonic antigen, also contrasts with the dense cytoplasmic reaction for all three in adenocarcinoma (Speers et al 1983, Brown et al 1987, Nambu et al 1988) and is inconsistent with the suggestion (Dallenbach-Hellweg 1984) that microglandular hyperplasia is a premalignant lesion. Furthermore, clinical studies have found that there is no particular relationship between microglandular hyperplasia and adenocarcinoma, and do not support a premalignant role of microglandular hyperplasia (Jones & Silverberg 1989).

Metaplasias

The Müllerian epithelium of the endocervical glands is capable of a variety of metaplastic changes. In tubal metaplasia the glands are lined by columnar or cuboidal cells that may be ciliated, secretory or inactive (Wells & Brown 1986). Small, dark, basal cells have been identified as T lymphocytes (Peters 1986), and to complete the similarity with the Fallopian tube this metaplastic epithelium also produces amylase (Bruns et al 1982). Previously published illustrations show the histology clearly (Wells & Brown 1986), but more often metaplasia is incomplete and hyperchromasia of the cells can lead to confusion with intraepithelial neoplasia (Jaworski et al 1988) (Fig. 9.3). Identical tubal metaplasia has been reported in the skin

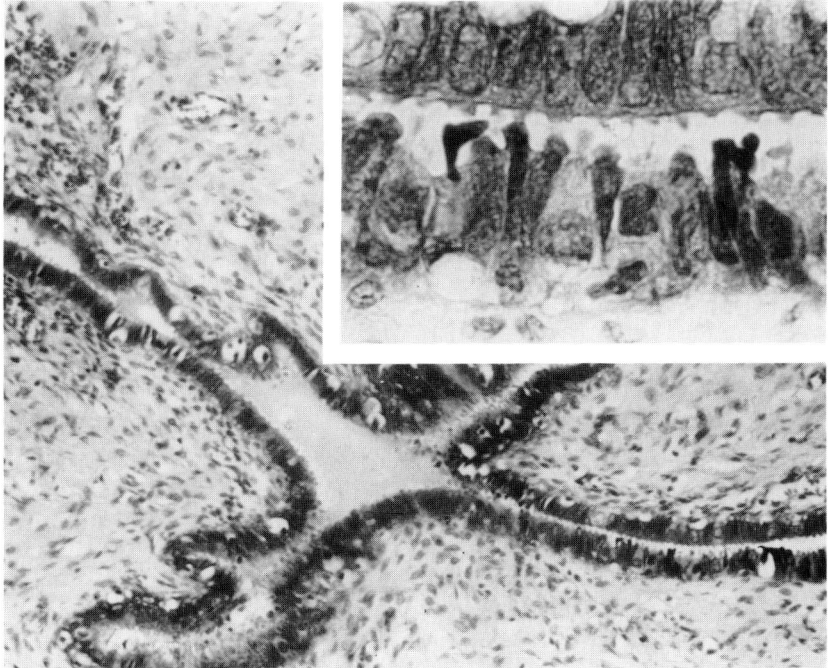

Fig. 9.3 Tubal metaplasia. At low power the epithelium has a worrying hyperchromatic appearance but the high power view (inset) reveals ciliated cells, mucus secreting columnar cells, dark intercalated cells and basal lymphocytes.

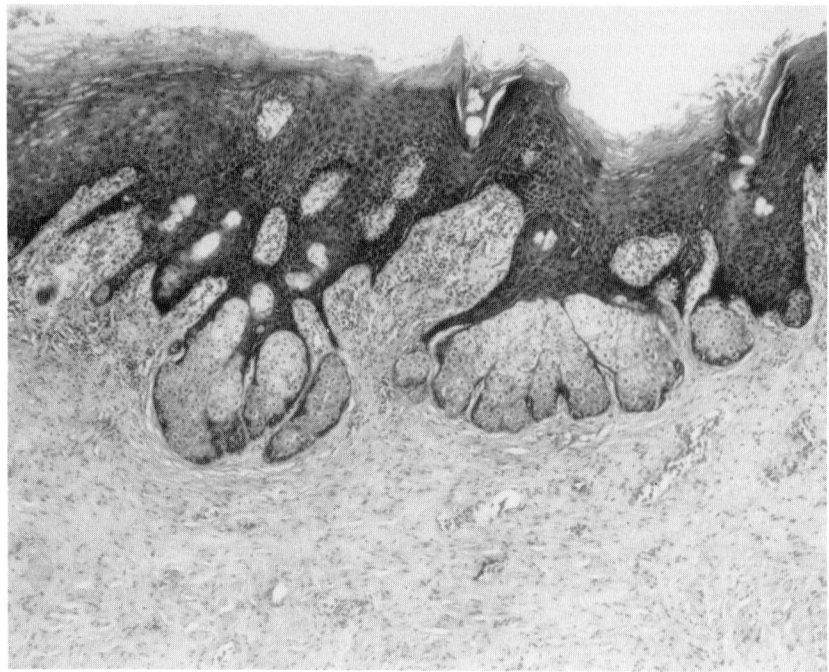

Fig. 9.4   Well-formed sebaceous glands in an area of ectocervical hyperkeratosis associated with stromal chronic inflammation.

(Varma et al 1991), indicating that Müllerian epithelia are not alone in this metaplastic capability.

Well-formed sebaceous glands (Fig. 9.4) arise from ectocervical epithelium probably related to trauma, surgery or prolonged inflammation (Fichera & Santanocito 1989).

Areas of intestinal metaplasia featuring goblet cells containing acidic mucins, absorptive cells and argentaffin cells (Trowell 1985) are rarely seen in normal cervices but are more common in cervical adenocarcinoma and adenocarcinoma in situ (Gloor & Ruzicka 1982, Ostor et al 1984, Jaworski et al 1988). Enteric-type cervical neoplasms may originate from areas of intestinal metaplasia (Fox et al 1988) (see below).

NEOPLASTIC CONDITIONS

Cervical glandular atypia (dysplasia, intraepithelial neoplasia)

The concept of glandular dysplasia (Bousfield et al 1980) has now been more closely defined and variously termed cervical glandular atypia (Brown & Wells 1986) and cervical intraepithelial glandular neoplasia (Gloor & Hurlimann 1986). These terms cover a spectrum of pre-malignant histo-

Table 9.1 Features of cervical glandular atypia

Increased nuclear size	Altered mucin production/histochemistry
Increased nuclear cytoplasmic ratio	Abnormal glandular profiles
Nuclear stratification	Outpouchings
More darkly staining nuclei	Intraluminal tufting
Nuclear pleomorphism	Papillary projections
Mitotic figures	Cytoplasmic reactivity for HMFG1
Abnormal chromatin pattern	

logical appearances from minor alterations of nuclear morphology and staining to changes indistinguishable from adenocarcinoma in situ. Overall, the features include changes of nuclear size, shape, staining and position, accompanied by aberrant glandular profiles, and are similar to columnar cell dysplasias of the gastrointestinal tract (Table 9.1). Two grading systems have been proposed, largely based on the degree of nuclear abnormality and stratification: low-grade (Fig. 9.5) and high-grade (Fig. 9.6) cervical glandular atypia; or cervical intraepithelial glandular neoplasia grades I, II and III. Grading columnar cell neoplasia is, however, notoriously difficult (Brown et al 1985). Morphometric characterization (Van Roon et al 1983) has been attempted. Nevertheless, the dividing line between low- and high-

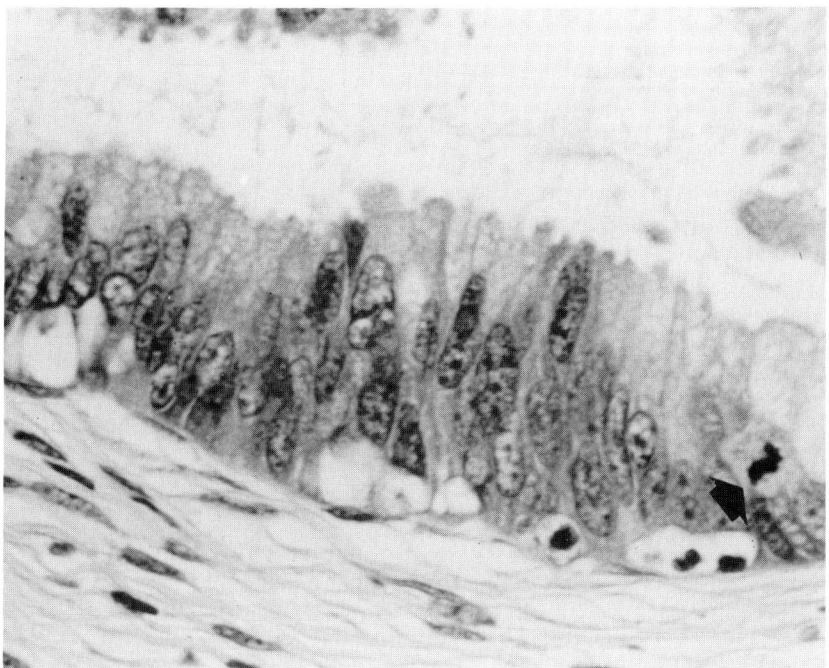

Fig. 9.5 Low-grade cervical glandular atypia. Note the mitosis (arrow), stratified nuclei, coarse irregular chromatin pattern and prominent, multiple nucleoli.

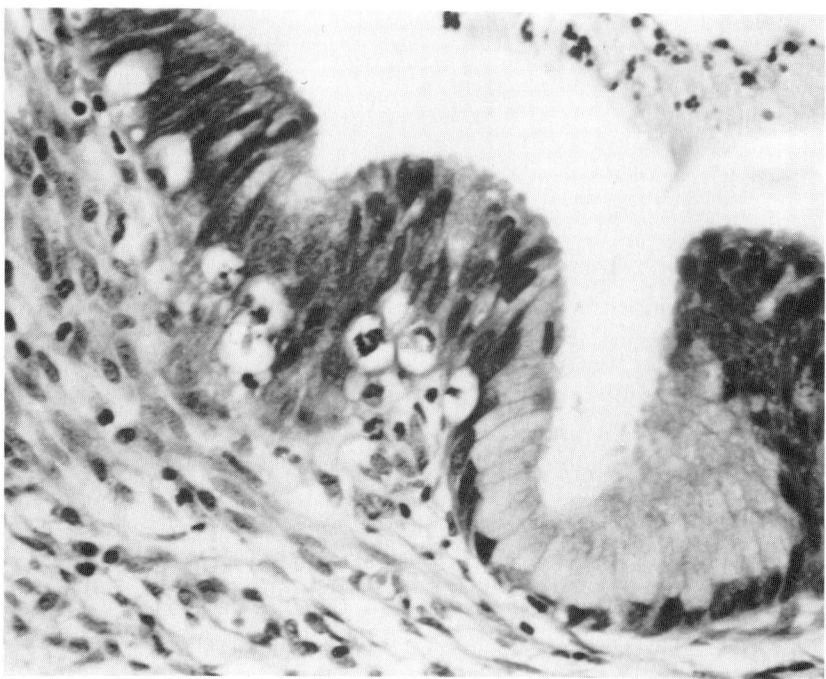

Fig. 9.6 High-grade cervical glandular atypia. There is an abrupt change from normal epithelium (lower right) to atypical epithelium in the upper left. Nuclei are stratified into the upper third of the epithelium and there is marked nuclear hyperchromasia.

grade glandular atypia is hazy and it can be difficult to distinguish high-grade lesions from adenocarcinoma in situ.

Gloor & Hurlimann (1986) subdivided the lesions into those showing cervical (type A) or enteric (type B) differentiation. There does not appear to be any prognostic or therapeutic difference between these cervical and intestinal variants, but the absence of sulphomucins in the intestinal type clearly differentiates them from the sulphomucin-containing normal glands (Wakefield & Wells 1985) and aids in diagnosis. Milk fat globule antigen recognized by the monoclonal antibody HMFG1 is present in the cytoplasm of cells from cases of glandular atypia, in contrast to the luminal distribution of the antigen in normal glands (Brown et al 1987).

As might be expected of a pre-malignant lesion, the distribution of cervical glandular atypia mirrors that of adenocarcinoma in situ, and, as in that lesion, there may be an abrupt change in a gland from normal to atypical epithelium (Fig. 9.6). Affected glands are found beneath the transformation zone and arranged in continuity or multifocally throughout the cervix, often high in the endocervical canal. A transitional zone of surrounding glands with glandular atypia may accompany adenocarcinoma in situ and invasive adenocarcinoma (Brown & Wells 1986, Rollason et al 1988), although there is no evidence of this zone in the absence of these histological changes (Cullimore et al 1989a).

Cervical glandular atypia is frequently associated with squamous intra-epithelial neoplasia and has been found associated with cervical intra-epithelial neoplasia (CIN) 3 in 15% of cases in one series (Brown & Wells 1986), adding weight to the theory of a common origin for squamous and glandular neoplasms from subcolumnar reserve cells in the transformation zone (Boon et al 1981a).

The mean age of patients with cervical glandular atypia has been quoted as 34.0–36.9 years (Gloor & Hurlimann 1986, Brown and Wells 1986), younger than the 35–39 years for adenocarcinoma in situ, 44 years for microinvasive and 49 or 57 years for deeply invasive adenocarcinoma (Bousfield et al 1980) (see below), supporting the concept of a pre-malignant lesion. Long-term follow-up studies have not been completed, but in one case where cervical glandular atypia accompanied an adenocarcinoma in situ, a lesion identical to cervical glandular atypia developed 5 years later in the vagina (Cullimore et al 1989b). If hysterectomy is not performed, minimum treatment should include a cone biopsy that is more than 25 mm in depth, with clear margins, followed by cytological surveillance for any disease which may remain (Luesley et al 1987).

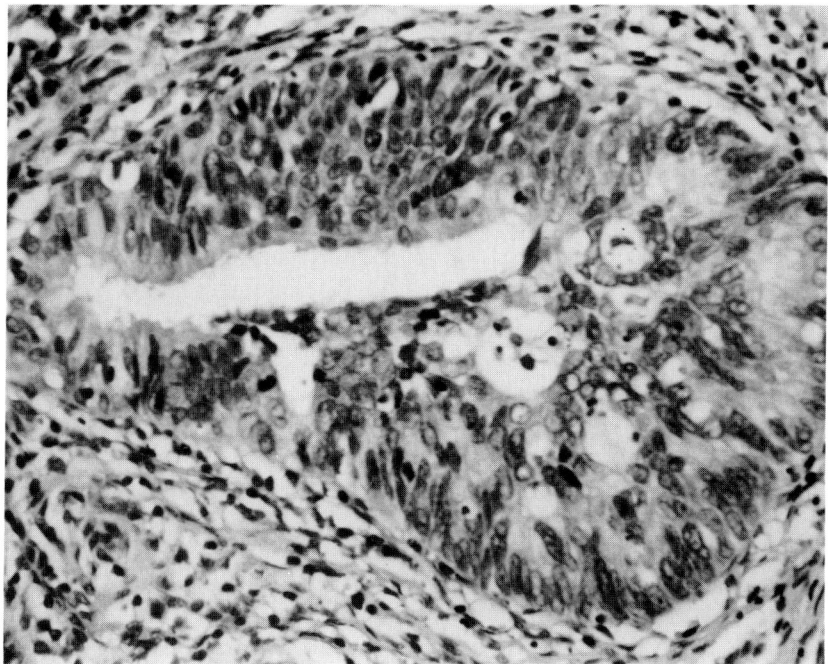

Fig. 9.7 In this example of adenocarcinoma in situ, the gland is lined by a mitotically active dysplastic epithelium exhibiting glandular and squamous (top) differentiation.

Adenocarcinoma in situ

Adenocarcinoma in situ occurs in women aged 35–39 years (Qizilbash 1975, Boon et al 1981, Ostor et al 1984, Bertrand et al 1987, Hopkins et al 1988, Andersen & Arffman 1989). These lesions are frequently overshadowed by the squamous intraepithelial or invasive malignancies with which they often coexist (Freidell & McKay 1953, Boon et al 1981b, Brown & Wells 1986, Jaworski et al 1988, Andersen & Arffmann 1989) and, if noticed, may be difficult to distinguish from invasive adenocarcinoma. Adenocarcinoma in situ may show a range of epithelial abnormalities, from severe dysplasia with grossly enlarged nuclei, marked mitotic activity and loss of polarity, to changes in which there is an abnormal nuclear–cytoplasmic ratio, nuclear stratification and increased mitotic activity which merge with the spectrum of changes of glandular atypia (Fig. 9.7) (Qizilbash 1975, Brown & Wells 1986). Intracellular mucin production is absent in the endometrioid type, although intestinal types with goblet cells, argentaffin cells and Paneth cells do occur. Rarely there may be serous, clear cell and adenosquamous variants (Gloor & Ruzicka 1982, Ostor et al 1984, Jaworski et al 1988, Andersen & Arffmann 1989). A basement membrane surrounds the glands; their profiles may be similar to the normal endocervical pattern, or may exhibit a more complex pattern of tunnel clusters, infolding, outpouching and intraluminal papillary projections. Within a single gland there may be one or more abrupt transitions to normal epithelium. Surrounding glands may feature the intermediate changes of cervical glandular intraepithelial neoplasia. (Brown & Wells 1986, Jaworski et al 1988).

The glands tend to be of fairly uniform size and have smooth borders with no solid areas or complex papillary formations (Fu et al 1987a). Affected glands extend no deeper than the level of surrounding normal glands, less than 4 mm from the surface epithelium (Anderson & Hartley 1980), but measuring depth of invasion is fraught with difficulty and one should rely on the stromal response of oedema, desmoplasia and inflammation to indicate invasion (Fu et al 1987a, Rollason et al 1989). Cytological similarities between adenocarcinoma in situ and adenocarcinoma have been highlighted by morphometry (Boon et al 1981b, Gloor & Ruzicka 1982, Van Roon et al 1983), but the measurements taken were highly selective and may have exaggerated the differences from normal tissues. Adenocarcinoma in situ has been subclassified as type I or II on the basis of nuclear morphology (Gloor & Ruzicka 1982); however, subsequent investigators have found no notable differences in behaviour or distribution, and the types commonly coexist (Ostor et al 1984, Tobon & Dave 1988).

Adenocarcinoma in situ usually affects only one quadrant of the cervix and appears to arise at the squamocolumnar junction, but lesions may be multifocal extending up to 30 mm along the endocervix (Christopherson et al 1979, Ostor et al 1984, Andersen & Arffmann 1989, Colgan & Lickrish 1990, Bertrand et al 1987). Excision may be incomplete when cones of tissue less than 25 mm in length are taken, and there may be skip lesions up the endocervical canal (Luesley et al 1987). Consequently, extensive sectioning is needed to detect adenocarcinoma in situ, and the diagnosis should not be made on a punch biopsy (Ostor et al 1984). The distribution of adeno-carcinoma in situ does not depend on the presence or extent of squamous neoplasia but may involve both the deep glands and surface epithelium of the endocervical canal (Colgan & Lickrish 1990, Jaworski et al 1988). Treatment by cone biopsy of at least 30 mm in depth may be adequate if the margins are clear (Ostor et al 1984, Bertrand et al 1987, Luesley et al 1987, Andersen & Arffmann 1989), but multifocal disease may not be eradicated and involved margins may reflect more aggressive disease necessitating hysterectomy (Noda et al 1983, Hopkins et al 1988).

If adenocarcinoma in situ is overlooked or undertreated, invasion may occur in 3 years (Boon et al 1981b), although progression usually takes 14 years on average (Christopherson et al 1979, Kashimura et al 1990). The cytological appearance is similar to invasive adenocarcinoma but without tumour diathesis (inflammatory cells and necrotic debris): surveillance may aid the initial diagnosis or be used in follow-up (Tobon & Dave 1988, Van Roon et al 1983, Ostor et al 1984). Colposcopy is usually unhelpful (Andersen & Arffmann 1989).

The frequent association between adenocarcinoma in situ and squamous neoplasia lends weight to the theory that both lesions develop from the subcolumnar reserve cell through a process of atypical reserve cell hyper-plasia (Boon et al 1981a), possibly under the influence of human papillo-mavirus (Tase et al 1988). Adenocarcinoma in situ has been reported with squamous carcinoma in a ratio of 1:239 (Christopherson et al 1979) and 1:25 (Boon et al 1981b), and with CIN 3 in a ratio of 1:105 (Brown & Wells 1986).

Early invasive adenocarcinoma

Immunostaining for laminin does not distinguish between in situ and invasive carcinoma, indicating that invasive glandular elements continue to produce a surrounding basement membrane (Vogel & Mendelsohn 1987, Toki et al 1990). Consequently, demonstrating early invasive lesions by a break in the basement membrane is inappropriate. Rarely, the earliest stages of stromal invasion appear squamoid with increased cytoplasmic eosino-philia similar to that of microinvasive epidermoid lesions (Matsukuma et al 1989, Rollason et al 1989), but this is not the usual pattern. Stromal oedema, an inflammatory cell reaction and a desmoplastic stromal response more commonly point to invasion by obvious glandular elements progressing proximally from the squamocolumnar junction (Noda et al 1983, Burghardt 1984, Buscema & Woodruff 1984, Teshima et al 1985, Matsukuma et al 1989). The diagnosis of microinvasive adenocarcinoma has been defined as a tumour volume of less than 500 mm^3 in experimental work (Burghardt 1984) but, in practice, a maximum depth of invasion less than 2 mm is more useful (Matsukuma et al 1989; see also Ch. 28). As in adenocarcinoma in situ, the lesions may be multifocal and cone biopsy excision may not be curative. Nevertheless, the prognosis following hysterectomy appears to be excellent (Burghardt 1984, Berek et al 1985, Teshima et al 1985).

Cytology can provide a 50% predictive accuracy of early invasion, based on the detection of small crowded cells, papillary groupings and syncytia of glandular cells in smears which may or may not show neoplastic features. There are, however, more cytological similarities than differences between frankly invasive and early invasive lesions (Betshill & Clark 1986), which may lead to over-treatment (Ayer et al 1988).

Adenocarcinoma

The incidence of adenocarcinoma of the cervix is increasing; it accounts for 3–34% of invasive cervical tumours. The wide variation in reported incidence may be due to a failure to recognize mucin in poorly differentiated lesions, but the increase in incidence appears to be real, independent of the reduction in incidence of squamous cell carcinomas (Ireland et al 1985, Peters et al 1986, Brand et al 1988, Webb & Sheehan 1989, Leminen et al 1990a). The incidence is disproportionately high in women younger than 40 years, but suggestions that this may be due to oral contraceptive use (Dallenbach-Helweg 1984) have found little support in experimental, clinical or epidemiological studies (Valente & Hanjani 1986, Peters et al 1986, Brown et al 1987, Devesa et al 1989, Goodman et al 1989, Jones & Silverberg 1989). The prognosis generally does not depend on the histological subtype (Shingleton et al 1981, Korhonen 1984, Hopkins et al 1988), although endometrioid types may do better (Saigo et al 1986). Tumour size, depth of invasion, stage, vascular permeation, lymph node involvement and differentiation are all related to prognosis: spread to lymph nodes is particularly sinister (Korhonen 1984, Hopkins et al 1988, Berek et al 1985, Saigo et al 1986). Morphology reveals an association between poor prognosis and enlarged, variably sized nuclei, which correlates with flow cytometric measurements of aneuploidy, triploidy and an above median S-phase fraction (Fu et al 1987b, Leminen et al 1990b). Nuclear organizer region counts do not help (Newbold et al 1990).

Most workers agree that adenocarcinoma has a worse outcome than squamous cell carcinoma (Tamimi & Figge 1982, Korhonen 1984, Silcocks et al 1987, Kleine et al 1989), although this is refuted by some studies (Ireland et al 1985, Kilgore et al 1988). When compared with squamous cell carcinoma epidemiologically, adenocarcinoma is associated with a higher socio-economic class, better education and a later age at first intercourse. This suggests that a different combination of oncogenic factors may be at work (Korhonen 1980, Horowitz et al 1988, Young & Sixbey 1988, Young et al 1991) although papillomaviruses have been incriminated in both lesions (Tase et al 1988).

Adenosquamous carcinomas

Mucin occurs in up to 35% of cervical tumours in the absence of glandular differentiation. Compared with mucin negative lesions, these tumours have been found to be associated with a higher incidence of lymph node metastases and a worse prognosis by some (Benda et al 1985, Ireland et al 1987, Buckley et al 1988) but not by all workers (Kilgore et al 1988). In women younger than 45 years the tumours are more likely to be mucin-positive, a feature that may be relevant to the poor prognosis in this age-group (Cook & Draper 1984, Shorrock et al 1990). Adenosquamous carcinoma appears to have a worse prognosis than either adenocarcinoma or squamous cell carcinoma (Fu et al 1982, Gallup et al 1985, Greer et al 1989), although some disagree (Hopkins et al 1988). Poor survival may be due in part to higher DNA ploidy and greater depth of invasion at presentation (Fu et al 1982a). Because of the implications for survival and treatment a diastase periodic acid–Schiff stain should be used for the diagnosis and classification of cervical carcinomas (Wells & Brown 1986).

Overtly glandular areas may be intimately mixed with squamous cell areas. Lesions with 5–80% glands are termed adenosquamous if predominantly squamous, and mucoepidermoid (Fig. 9.8) if mainly glandular

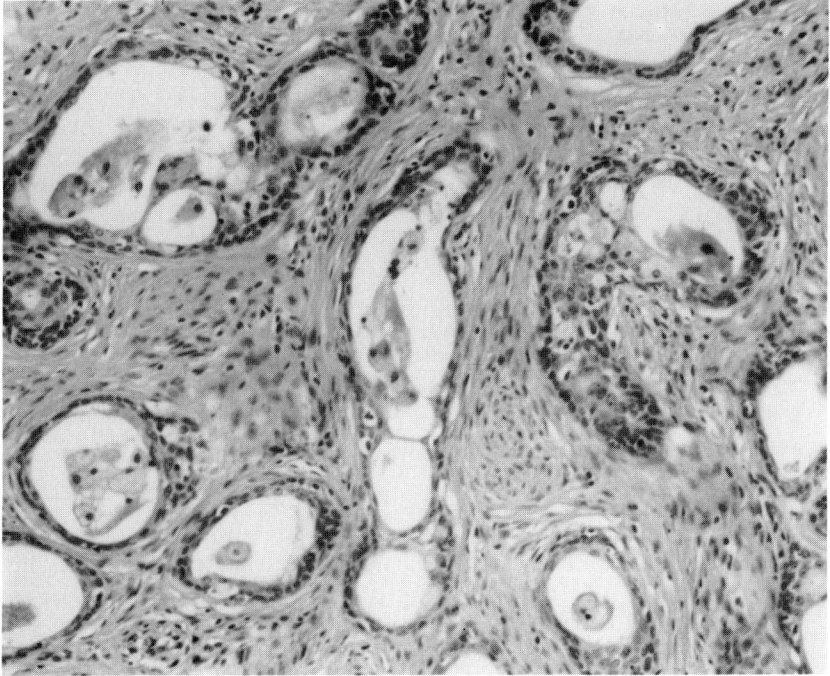

Fig. 9.8   The mucoepidermoid variant of adenosquamous carcinoma resembles the salivary gland lesion. The irregularly shaped acini are lined by peripheral layers of squamous cells with central accumulations of mucin secreting cells.

(Yajima et al 1984). Adenocarcinoma has greater than 80% glandular differentiation, squamous cell carcinoma less than 5%, and mixed tumours contain less than 5% glands but are mucin-positive. Because of the frequent coexistence of glandular and squamous neoplasms (Maier & Norris 1980, Choo & Naylor 1984), this regularly-seen differentiation along dual pathways has been taken as evidence of a common progenitor cell. Normally, differentiation from subcolumnar reserve cells in the trans-formation zone follows either glandular or squamous lines, depending on pH. Oncogenic agents such as viruses, with or without co-factors, may cause separate or mixed glandular and squamous differentiation (Boon et al 1981a, Tase et al 1988, Turner et al 1990). An alternative, less acceptable view holds that reserve cells form epidermoid tumours, columnar cells give rise to adenocarcinomas and neoplasias or both cell types may coexist to form mixed lesions (Yajima et al 1984).

'Glassy Cell' carcinoma

This has been singled out as a poorly differentiated variant of adeno-squamous carcinoma representing less than 1.5% of all cervical carcinomas. The cells are large with ground-glass cytoplasm, distinct cell walls, large nuclei and prominent nucleoli. The cytoplasm may contain sparse periodic acid–Schiff positive droplets, and the cell boundaries are highlighted by periodic acid–Schiff and eosin (Maier & Norris 1982, Zaino et al 1982, Tanaka et al 1984). The stroma is heavily inflamed with plasma cells and eosinophils, a dense eosinophil response possibly related to increased length of survival (Tamimi et al 1988). Generally the prognosis is poor with little response to radiotherapy, although good results have been claimed in early stage small lesions that can be detected cytologically (Pak et al 1983, Tanaka et al 1984, Nunez et al 1985, Randall et al 1986). Separate classification from poorly differentiated adenosquamous carcinomas is probably not justified (Maier & Norris 1982, Wells & Brown 1986), especially in view of the good ultrastructural evidence (Ulbright & Gersell 1983) of both glandular and squamous differentiation.

Minimal deviation adenocarcinoma (adenoma malignum)

This rare, extremely well-differentiated variant of adenocarcinoma has a poor prognosis only partly because it is difficult to diagnose on biopsy. Clinically, there may be a profuse mucoid discharge and the cervix is usually grossly enlarged. The tumour is composed of irregularly shaped glands, often with a claw-shaped or slit-like profile, lined by remarkably bland mucinous endocervical type epithelium which hardly appears different by conventional histology from normal cervical glandular epithelium (Kaku & Enjoji 1983, Kaminski & Norris 1983, Michael et al 1984, Gilks et al 1989b). Small focal areas of subtle cytological atypia may be present (Fig. 9.9) but

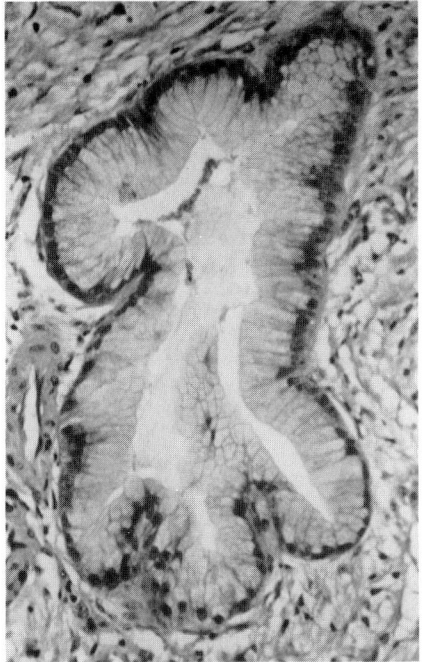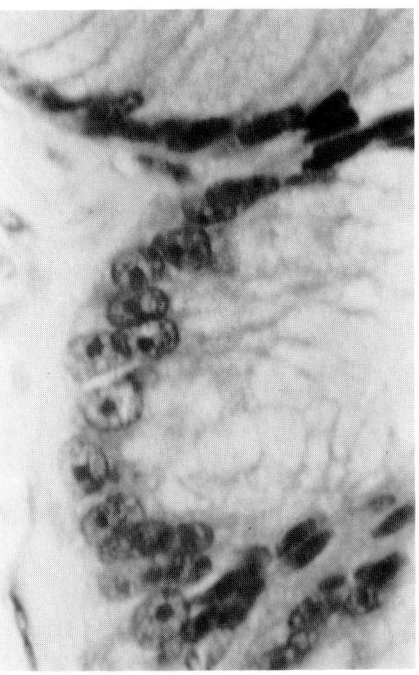

Fig. 9.9 Adenoma malignum. The low-power view (left) shows an abnormally shaped gland lined by deceptively normal appearing epithelium. Only at high power (right) can the slightly enlarged atypical nuclei with prominent nucleoli be appreciated.

Table 9.2 Features of adenoma malignum (modified from Michael et al 1984)

Abnormal gland pattern
    Haphazard proliferation of mucinous glands infiltrating the deep stroma and orientated in all directions
    Large glands with convoluted, claw-shaped outlines
    Small, slit-shaped glands with pointed ends
    Epithelial tufting or intraluminal papillary fronds: focal, rare
    Desmoplastic response and chronic inflammatory infiltrate in some cases
    Necrosis absent
    Single layer of columnar mucinous epithelium generally identical to that seen in normal endocervical glands
Cytologic abnormalities, focal and subtle
    Loss of nuclear polarity
    Nuclear enlargement and angular nuclear contours
    Large eosinophilic nucleoli
    Chromatin clumping and parachromatin clearing
Cytoplastic reactivity for
    Carcinoembryonic antigen
    Transferrin receptor
    HMFG1
Increased numbers of argyrophilic cells
Altered mucin histochemistry

the diagnosis is more apparent in deep (greater than 8 mm) cone biopsy or hysterectomy specimens in which the very deeply infiltrative nature of the lesion can be appreciated. Areas of vascular and perineural invasion and clearly malignant epithelial areas aid the diagnosis (Table 9.2), but without these pointers there is a danger of confusion with mesonephric (Gartner's duct) hyperplasia, adenomatoid hyperplasia (tunnel clusters) and deep Nabothian cysts (Gilks et al 1989b, Clement & Young 1989).

Positive cytoplasmic immunoreactivity for carcinoembryonic antigen, transferrin receptor and HMFG1, inappropriate expression of blood group antigens as well as increased staining for neutral mucins, sialomucins and a relative deficiency of sulphomucins, distinguish adenoma malignum from benign lesions (Bates et al 1985, Steeper & Wick 1986, Brown et al 1987, Mizuuchi et al 1987, Bulmer et al 1990). Unlike the more usual forms of well-differentiated adenocarcinoma, the basement membrane is fragmented, a feature which might help to explain the poor prognosis (Toki et al 1990). In the normal endocervix endocrine cells are rare, but argyrophilic cells containing serotonin, somatostatin, gastrin and pancreatic polypeptide are present in adenoma malignum, indicating a similarity to foregut-derived epithelium (Kaku & Enjoji 1983, Fetissof et al 1985, 1986).

Adenoma malignum is associated with the Peutz-Jeghers syndrome where in situ lesions have been detected (Fetissof et al 1985), and, although ovarian tumours are a feature of Peutz–Jeghers syndrome, accompanying ovarian tumours are also commonly seen outside this condition (Young & Scully 1988). In 26 cases of adenoma malignum (Gilks et al 1989b) there were 15 ovarian abnormalities including mucinous carcinomas and sex-cord tumours with annular tubules (in patients who did not have the Peutz–Jeghers syndrome), indicating a danger if the ovaries are conserved. One case featured bilateral sex cord tumours with annular tubules, bilateral mucinous ovarian tumours and adenoma malignum (Chen 1986). The reported mortality is approximately 60% by 7 years, with abdominopelvic recurrences in the first 2 years (Gilks et al 1989b). Deaths may occur up to 10 years after diagnosis, and long-term follow-up is necessary (Kaminski & Norris 1983).

Enteric tumours

Villous and tubulovillous adenomas of the cervix are rare lesions which probably originate in areas of intestinal metaplasia (Michael et al 1986, Fox et al 1988, Alvaro & Nogales 1988, Trowell 1985). Thin, finger-like papillary fronds are covered by stratified columnar epithelium (Fig. 9.10) which contains intestinal-like O-acetylated sialomucins and carcinoembryonic antigen. Normal mitoses may be seen and there is little nuclear atypia. Neuroendocrine cells are absent. Ultrastructurally, the presence of glycocalyceal bodies and microvillous core rootlets are additional markers of intestinal differentiation. As with intestinal tumours there may be an

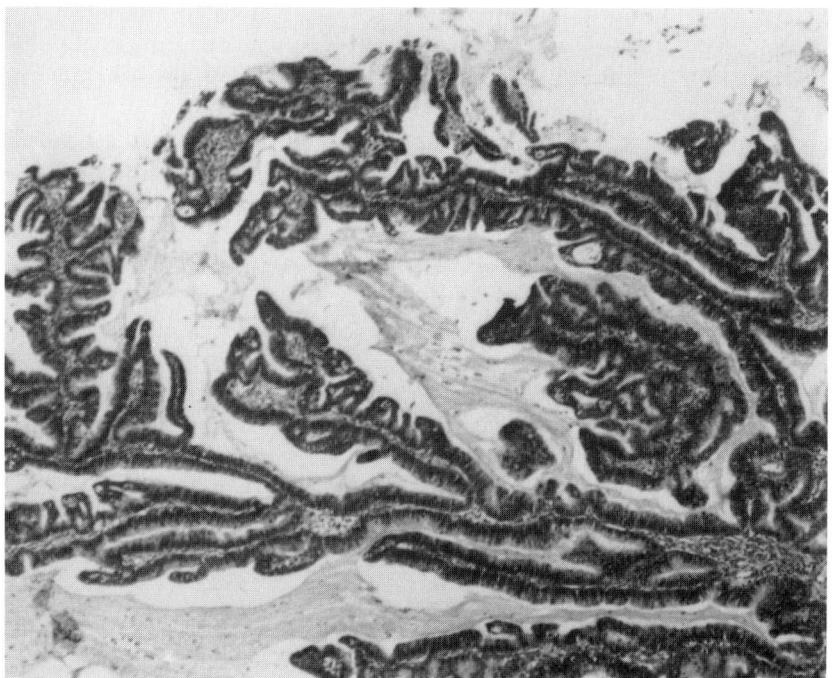

Fig. 9.10 Villous adenoma of the cervix. Long branching fronds are covered by dysplastic columnar epithelium identical to that seen in tumours of the bowel.

adjacent or underlying adenocarcinoma, although, unlike the bowel, there is no limiting muscularis mucosae to distinguish invasive from adenomatous lesions.

Young & Scully (1989a) concede there may be no distinction between villous adenomas with invasive components and villoglandular adeno-carcinomas and note an excellent prognosis. They suggest cone biopsy and close follow-up if there is less than 3 mm invasion, no vascular permeation and complete excision.

Intestinal differentiation in adenocarcinoma of the cervix with Paneth cells, argentaffin cells, goblet cells and a brush border has been recognized for 25 years (Azzopardi & Hou 1965), but very few cases have been reported. Similar changes may be seen in adenocarcinoma in situ (Gloor & Ruzicka 1982, Ostor et al 1984, Jaworski et al 1988) and a cervical adenocarcinoma documented by Fox et al (1988) contained goblet cells positive for O-acetylated sialomucin. Too few examples have been reported to establish whether enteric differentiation affects the prognosis.

Neuroendocrine tumours

Neuroendocrine cells are rare in normal glands, but argyrophilic cells may be seen in cervical adenocarcinomas, adenoma malignum, cervical glandular atypia, enteric tumours and areas of intestinal metaplasia (Scully et al 1984, Ueda et al 1984, Trowell 1985, Fetissof et al 1986, Barrett et al 1987, Chan et al 1990). Neuroendocrine tumours exhibit a range of differentiation, from small cell anaplastic, 'oat cell' carcinomas to well-differentiated carcinoids. All types may be associated with squamous or glandular neoplasia and may show histological or ultrastructural differentiation along squamous or glandular pathways (Yoshida et al 1984). This suggests that neuroendocrine tumours may also derive from a common stem cell (Mullins & Hilliard 1981, Groben et al 1985), possibly through a process of neuroendocrine cell hyperplasia (Chan et al 1990). Electron microscopy reveals neurosecretory granules whilst neurone-specific enolase, neurofilament protein and a diversity of polypeptides may be demonstrated histochemically. 'Oat cell' carcinomas of the cervix may secrete adrenocorticotrophic hormone and cause Cushing's syndrome, but carcinoid syndrome has not been reported (Scully et al 1984, Ibrahim et al 1984, Chan et al 1990). Neurosecretory granules in poorly differentiated adenocarcinomas are associated with a poor prognosis, and small cell neuroendocrine tumours are rapidly fatal. Carcinoids may metastasize and kill (Groben et al 1985, Barrett et al 1987).

Adenoid cystic carcinoma

Similar in some respects to adenoid cystic carcinoma of the respiratory tract and salivary glands, this is a more aggressive, often fatal tumour characterized by lymphatic spread, local recurrence and pulmonary meta-stases. Although usually seen in the sixth and seventh decades, several instances have been reported in patients below 40 years of age (King et al 1989). Small, dark, uniform cells with scanty cytoplasm, moderately pleomorphic nuclei and inconspicuous nucleoli form sheets, cribriform areas and variously sized nests around hyaline eosinophilic material (Van Dinh & Woodruff 1985). Areas of necrosis are common, whilst the mitotic activity may be impressive (from 10 to 90 mitoses per 10 high-power fields) (Ferry & Scully 1988). By electron microscopy the cystic spaces can be seen to contain basement membrane-like material and thus enclose stroma rather than intra-acinar secretion (Mazur & Battifora 1982). Immunohisto-chemistry demonstrates cytokeratins and actin, but the myoepithelial cells seen ultrastructually do not react consistently for S100 protein (Ferry & Scully 1988). Despite a superficial similarity to the adenoid variant of basal cell carcinoma, there are distinct histological differences; adenoid cystic carcinoma behaves in a far more aggressive fashion, although both types probably arise from the same subcolumnar reserve cells. There are sufficient differences in behaviour, ultrastructure and S100 reactivity to adenoid cystic carcinomas of other sites to warrant the appellation 'adenoid cystic' carcinoma (Ferry & Scully 1988).

Co-existent ovarian neoplasia

The association between endometrial adenocarcinoma and endometrioid tumours of the ovary is well recognized, but a significant proportion of cervical adenocarcinomas are associated with second primary tumours in the ovary. In a study of 161 cervical adenocarcinomas there were 25 examples of ovarian neoplasia (Kaminski & Norris 1984), of which six were malignant ovarian primaries (four endometrioid, one serous and one clear cell adenocarcinoma), eight were benign or borderline tumours and the remainder were metastatic from the cervix. Endometrioid tumours were most often present at both sites, but adenocarcinoma in situ and mucinous cervical adenocarcinomas can also often be synchronous with benign, borderline or malignant ovarian mucinous tumours, especially if the cervical tumour is an adenoma malignum. Associated mucinous meta-plasias of the Fallopian tubes and endometrium were noted in some cases, suggesting a field change in the Müllerian epithelium eventually leading to multicentric neoplasia (LiVolsi et al 1983, Young & Scully 1988). These studies are largely based on referral material and probably exaggerate the incidence; nevertheless, they emphasize the importance of adequate ovarian assessment in cases of cervical adenocarcinoma.

Spread from other primary adenocarcinomas

Distinguishing primary cervical adenocarcinoma from metastases may be difficult, the main area of confusion being distinction between endometrial adenocarcinoma and cervical endometrioid variants. Endometrial tumours may involve the cervix by spread along the endocervical canal or through the cervical stroma (Kadar et al 1982). The cervical tumours have been claimed to be more likely to demonstrate cytoplasmic mucin and carcinoembryonic antigen than their endometrial counterparts, which produce little mucin and react weakly for apical carcinoembryonic antigen (Fenoglio et al 1981, Cohen et al 1982). However, mucin staining may be unreliable and some cervical adenocarcinomas are negative for carcinoembryonic antigen, whilst apical and dense cytoplasmic reactivity for carcinoembryonic antigen can be present in both cervical and endometrial tumours (Cooper et al 1987, Maes et al 1988). Similarly, staining for lysosyme and secretory component is unlikely to be useful in an individual case (Patterson et al 1990). Vimentin positivity may help as it occurs rarely in cervical tumours but is present in 65% of endometrial adenocarcinomas (Dabbs et al 1986). Adjacent cervical glandular neoplasia or, alternatively, atypical endometrial hyperplasia may indicate the primary site, and it appears that routine histology offers as good a way as any in making a diagnosis. The fibrous stroma of cervical tumours is represented by a cellular endometrial-like stroma in endometrial primaries (Cohen et al 1982).

Metastases from the ovary are seen less frequently (Mazur et al 1984) and of the rare deposits from elsewhere, breast, bowel and stomach are the most common primaries (Zhang et al 1983, Cohan & Kaplan 1984).

SPECIAL TECHNIQUES

A variety of methods has been used to distinguish benign from malignant lesions and to gauge prognosis in adenocarcinoma.

Steroid receptors

Biochemical analyses of oestrogen and progestagen receptors reveal few differences between adenocarcinoma and squamous cell carcinoma. There is no correlation with grade, stage or type of tumour, although a relationship between positive receptor status and survival has been shown in pre-menopausal women (Potish et al 1986). Hunter et al (1987) found no relationship to the menopause and only a weak correlation between progesterone receptor presence and survival. Consequently, it is not surprising that in contrast to the breast, hormonal manipulations are not used in treatment.

Amylase

Studies on fixed tissue have shown that immunoreactive amylase is present in normal endocervical epithelium but that adenocarcinomas are negative (Hayashi et al 1986, Lee & Raju 1988). British workers (Griffin et al 1989) used a starch-film digestion technique and confirmed that fresh normal glands contained amylase which was reduced in the two examples of adenocarcinoma they examined. However, by immunohistochemistry on fixed tissue, the normal glands were negative but reserve cells were positive as were the examples of adenocarcinoma, adenocarcinoma in situ and cervical glandular atypia examined. The British group interpreted these discrepancies between the studies by invoking racial differences, but further work is clearly needed.

Tumour markers

Normal cervical glands do not contain carcinoembryonic antigen, but the majority of in situ and invasive adenocarcinomas, including adenoma malignum, exhibit dense cytoplasmic reactivity for the antigen (Hurlimann & Gloor 1984, Steeper & Wick 1986). CA19-9 recognizes an antigenic marker of intestinal differentiation: normal endocervical glands are negative but 56% of adenocarcinomas, 40% of early invasive adenocarcinomas and all of three cases of adenoma malignum were strongly positive (Nambu et al 1988). CA125 is ubiquitous in female genital tract epithelia and is distributed along the luminal aspect of endocervical cells. A cell surface antigen recognized by HMFG1 exhibits a similar distribution. Neoplastic glandular epithelia, including cervical glandular atypia, exhibit dense cytoplasmic reactivity for CA125 and with HMFG1. Areas of microglandular hyperplasia are negative for carcinoembryonic antigen and give luminal reactivity with HMFG1 and CA125 (Brown et al 1987, Nambu et al 1988). A ratio greater than 0.5 of (carcinoembryonic antigen + CA19–9)/CA125 in cervical mucus is said to be a marker of invasive adenocarcinoma (Fujii et al 1988).

REFERENCES

Alvaro T, Nogales F 1988 Villous adenoma and invasive adenocarcinoma of the cervix. International Journal of Gynecological Pathology 7: 96–97
Andersen E S, Arffmann E 1989 Adenocarcinoma in situ of the uterine cervix: A clinico-pathologic study of 36 cases. Gynecologic Oncology 35: 1–7
Anderson M C, Hartley R B 1980. Cervical crypt involvement by intraepithelial neoplasia. Obstetrics and Gynecology 55: 546–550
Ayer B, Pacey F, Greenberg M 1988 The cytologic diagnosis of adenocarcinoma in situ of the cervix uteri and related lesions. II microinvasive adenocarcinoma. Acta Cytologica 32: 318–324
Ayroud Y, Gelfand M M, Ferenczy A 1985 Florid mesonephric hyperplasia of the cervix: a report of a case with review of the literature. International Journal of Gynecological Pathology 4: 245–254
Azzopardi J G, Hou L T 1965 Intestinal metaplasia with argentaffin cells in cervical adenocarcinoma. Journal of Pathology and Bacteriology 90: 686–690
Barrett R J, Davos I, Leuchter R S, Lagasse L D 1987 Neuroendocrine features in poorly differentiated and undifferentiated carcinomas of the cervix. Cancer 60: 2325–2330
Bates C, Wells M, Kingston R, Bulmer J N, Bird C C 1985 Minimal deviation adenocarcinoma ('adenoma malignum') of the endocervix. A histochemical and immunohistochemical study of two cases. Journal of Pathology 145: 71A
Benda J A, Platz C E, Buchsbaum H, Lifshitz S 1985 Mucin production in defining mixed carcinoma of the uterine cervix: a clinicopathologic study. International Journal of Gynecological Pathology 4: 314–327
Berek J S, Hacker N F, Fu Y-S, Sokale J R, Leuchter R C, Lagasse L D 1985 Adenocarcinoma of the uterine cervix: histologic variables associated with lymph node metastasis and survival. Obstetrics and Gynecology 65: 46–52
Bertrand M, Lickrish G M, Colgan T J 1987 The anatomic distribution of cervical adenocarcinoma in situ: implications for treatment. American Journal of Obstetrics and Gynecology 157: 21–25
Betshill W L, Clark A H 1986 Early endocervical glandular neoplasia: I Histomorphology and cytomorphology. Acta Cytologica 30: 115–126
Boon M E, Kirk R S, Rietveld-Scheffers P E M 1981a The morphogenesis of adenocarcinoma of the cervix—a complex pathological entity. Histopathology 15: 565–577
Boon M E, Baak J P A, Kurver P J H, Overdiep S H, Verdonk G W 1981b Adenocarcinoma in situ of the cervix: an underdiagnosed lesion. Cancer 48: 768–773
Bousfield L, Pacey F, Young Q, Krumins I, Osborn R 1980 Expanded cytological criteria for the diagnosis of adenocarcinoma in situ and related lesions. Acta Cytologica 24: 283–296
Brand E, Berek J S, Hacker N F 1988 Controversies in the management of cervical adenocarcinoma. Obstetrics and Gynecology 71: 261–269
Brown L J R, Wells M 1986 Cervical glandular atypia associated with squamous intraepithelial neoplasia: a pre-malignant lesion? Journal of Clinical Pathology 39: 22–28
Brown L J R, Smeeton N C, Dixon M F 1985 Assessment of dysplasia in colorectal adenomas: an observer variation and morphometric study. Journal of Clinical Pathology 38: 174–179

Brown L J R, Griffin N R, Wells M 1987 Cytoplasmic reactivity with the monoclonal antibody HMFG1 as a marker of cervical glandular atypia. Journal of Pathology 151: 203–208

Bruns D E, Mills D E, Davory J 1982 Amylase in Fallopian tube and serous ovarian neoplasms. Immuno-histochemical localization. Archives of Pathology and Laboratory Medicine 106: 17–20

Buckley C H, Beards C S, Fox H, 1988 Pathological prognostic indicators in cervical cancer with particular reference to patients under the age of 40. British Journal of Obstetrics and Gynaecology 95: 47–56

Bulmer J N, Griffin N R, Bates C, Kingston R E, Wells M 1990 Minimal deviation adenocarcinoma (adenoma malignum) of the endocervix: a histochemical and immunohistochemical study of two cases. Gynecologic Oncology 36: 139–146

Buntine D W 1979 Adenocarcinoma of the uterine cervix of probable wolffian origin. Pathology 11: 713–718

Burghardt E 1984 Microinvasive carcinoma in gynaecological pathology. Clinics in Obstetrics and Gynaecology 11: 239–257

Buscema J, Woodruff J D 1984 The significance of neoplastic atypicalities in endocervical epithelium. Gynecologic Oncology 17: 356–362

Chan K C, Tsui W M S, Tung S T, Ching R C T 1990 Endocrine cell hyperplasia of the uterine cervix. A precursor of neuroendocrine carcinoma of the cervix? American Journal of Clinical Pathology 92: 825–830

Chen K T K 1986 Female genital tract tumors in Peutz–Jeghers syndrome. Human Pathology 17: 858–861

Choo Y C, Naylor B 1984 Coexistent squamous cell carcinoma and adenocarcinoma of the uterine cervix. Gynecologic Oncology 17: 168–174

Christopherson W M, Nealon N, Gray L A 1979 Noninvasive precursor lesions of adenocarcinoma and mixed adenosquamous carcinoma of the cervix uteri. Cancer 44: 975–983

Chumas J C, Nelson B, Mann W J, Chalas E, Kaplan C G 1985 Microglandular hyperplasia of the uterine cervix. Obstetrics and Gynecology 66: 406–409

Clement P B, Young R H 1989 Deep nabothian cysts of the uterine cervix. A possible source of confusion with minimal-deviation adenocarcinoma ('Adenoma malignum'). International Journal of Gynecological Pathology 8: 340–348

Cohan L, Kaplan A L 1984 Postmenopausal bleeding secondary to metastatic disease in the endocervix from carcinoma of the breast. Gynecologic Oncology 17: 133–136

Cohen C, Schulman G, Budgeon L R 1982 Endocervical and endometrial adenocarcinoma. An immunoperoxidase and histochemical study. American Journal of Surgical Pathology 6: 151–157

Colgan T J, Lickrish G M 1990 The topography and invasive potential of cervical adenocarcinoma in situ with and without associated squamous dysplasia. Gynecologic Oncology 36: 246–249

Cook G A, Draper G J 1984 Trends in cervical cancer and carcinoma in situ in Great Britain. British Journal of Cancer 50: 367–375

Cooper P, Russell G, Wilson D 1987 Adenocarcinoma of the cervix—a histochemical study. Histopathology 11: 1321–1330

Cullimore J E, Rollason T P, Marshall T 1989a Nuclear organiser regions in adenocarcinoma in situ of the endocervix. Journal of Clinical Pathology 42: 1276–1280

Cullimore J E, Luesley D M, Rollason T P, Waddell C, Wiliams D. R. 1989b A case of glandular intraepithelial neoplasia involving the cervix and vagina. Gynecologic Oncology 34: 249–252

Dabbs D J, Geisinger K R, Norris H T 1986 Intermediate filaments in endometrial and endocervical carcinomas. The American Journal of Surgical Pathology 10: 568–576

Dallenbach-Hellweg G 1984 On the origin and histological structure of adenocarcinoma of the endocervix in women under 50 years of age. Pathology Research and Practice 179: 38–50

Devesa S S, Young J L, Brinton L A, Fraumeni J F 1989 Recent trends in cervix uteri cancer. Cancer 64: 2184–2190

Fenoglio C M, Crum C P, Pascal R R, Richart R M 1981 Carinoembryonic antigen in gynecologic patients. II. Immunohistological expression. Diagnostic Gynecology and Obstetrics 3: 291–299

Ferry J A, Scully R E 1988 'Adenoid cystic' carcinoma and adenoid basal carcinoma of the uterine cervix. American Journal of Surgical Pathology 12: 134–144

Fetissof F, Berger G, Dubois M P, Philippe A, Lansac J, Jobard P 1985 Female genital tract and Peutz–Jeghers syndrome. An immunohistochemical study. International Journal of Gynecological Pathology 4: 219–229

Fetissof F, Dubois M P, Heitz P U, Lansac J, Arbeille-Brassart B, Jobard P 1986 Endocrine cells in the female genital tract. International Journal of Gynecological Pathology 5: 75–87

Fichera G, Santanocito A 1989 Pilo-sebaceous ectopy of the uterine cervix. Clinical Experimental Obstetrics and Gynaecology 16: 21–25

Fox H, Buckley C H 1983 In: Austin Gresham G (ed) Atlas of gynaecological pathology. Current histopathology. MTP Press, Lanaster, vol 5, p 39–40

Fox H, Wells M, Harris M, McWilliam L J, Anderson G S 1988 Enteric tumours of the lower female genital tract: a report of three cases. Histopathology 12: 167–176

Freidell G H, McKay D C 1953 Adenocarcinoma in situ of the endocervix. Cancer 6: 887–897

Fu Y S, Reagan J W, Fu A S, Janiga K E 1982a Adenocarcinoma and mixed carcinoma of the uterine: II. Prognostic value of nuclear DNA analysis. Cancer 49: 2571–2577

Fu Y S, Reagan J W, Hsiu J G, Storaasli J P, Wentz W B 1982b Adenocarcinoma and mixed carcinoma of the uterine cervix: a clinicopathologic study. Cancer 49: 2560–2570

Fu Y S, Berek J S, Hilborne L H 1987a Diagnostic problems of in situ and invasive adenocarcinoma of the uterine cervix. Applied Pathology 5: 47–56

Fu Y S, Hall T L, Berek J S, Hacker N F, Reagan J W 1987b Prognostic significance of DNA ploidy and morphometric analyses of adenocarcinoma of the uterine cervix. Analytical and Quantatitive Cytology and Histology 9: 17–24

Fujii S, Konishi I, Nambu Y et al 1988 Analysis of the levels of CA125, carcinoembryonic antigen and CA19-9 in the cervical mucus for a detection of cervical adenocarcinoma. Cancer 62: 541–547

Gallup D G, Harper R H, Stock R J 1985 Poor prognosis in patients with adenosquamous cell carcinoma of the cervix. Obstetrics and Gynecology 65: 416–422

Gilks C B, Reid P E, Clement P B, Owen D A 1989a Histochemical changes in cervical mucus-secreting epithelium during the normal menstrual cycle. Fertility and Sterility 51: 286–291

Gilks C B, Young R H, Aguirre P, DeLellis R A, Scully R E 1989b Adenoma malignum (minimal deviation adenocarcinoma) of the uterine cervix. A clinicopathological and immunohistochemical analysis of 26 cases. American Journal of Surgical Pathology 13: 717–729

Gloor E, Hurliman J 1986 Cervical intraepithelial glandular neoplasia (adenocarcinoma in situ and glandular dysplasia). Cancer 58: 1272–1280

Gloor E, Ruzicka J 1982 Morphology of adenocarcinoma in situ of the uterine cervix: a study of 14 cases. Cancer 49: 294–302

Goodman H M, Buttlar C A, Niloff J M et al 1989 Adenocarcinoma of the uterine cervix: prognostic factors and patterns of recurrence. Gynecologic Oncology 33: 241–247

Greer B E, Figge D C, Tamimi H K, Cain J M 1989 Stage 1B adenocarcinoma of the cervix treated by radical hysterectomy and pelvic node dissection. American Journal of Obstetrics and Gynecology 160: 1509–1541

Griffin N R, Wells M, Fox H 1989 Modulation of the antigenicity of amylase in cervical glandular atypia, adenocarcinoma in situ and invasive adenocarcinoma. Histopathology 15: 267–279

Groben P, Reddick R, Askin F 1985 The pathologic spectrum of small cell carcinoma of the cervix. International Journal of Gynecological Pathology 4: 42–57

Hafez E S E 1982 Structural and ultrastructural parameters of the uterine cervix. Obstetrical and Gynecological Survey 37: 507–516

Hayashi Y, Fukayama M, Koike M, Nakayama T 1986 Amylase in human lungs and the female genital tract. Histochemical and immunohistochemical localization. Histochemistry 85: 491–496

Helmerhorst T J M, Dijkhuizen G H, Veldhuizen R W, Stolk J G 1984 Microglandular hyperplasia—a complicating factor in the diagnosis of cervical intraepithelial neoplasia. European Journal of Obstetrics, Gynecology and Reproductive Biology 17: 53–59

Hopkins M P, Roberts J A, Schmidt R W 1988 Cervical adenocarcinoma in situ. Obstetrics and Gynecology 71: 842–844

Horowitz I R, Jacobson L P, Zucker P K, Currie J L, Rosenshein N B, 1988. Epidemiology of adenocarcinoma of the cervix. Gynecologic Oncology 31: 25–31

Hunter R E, Longcope C, Keough P 1987 Steroid hormone receptors in carcinoma of the cervix. Cancer 60: 392–396

Hurlimann J, Gloor E 1984 Adenocarcinoma in situ and invasive adenocarcinoma of the uterine cervix. An immunohistologic study with antibodies specific for several epithelial markers. Cancer 54: 103–109

Ibrahim N B N, Briggs J C, Corbishley C M 1984 Extrapulmonary oat cell carcinoma. Cancer 54: 1645–1661

Ireland D, Hardiman P L, Monaghan J M 1985 Adenocarcinoma of the uterine cervix: a study of 73 cases. Obstetrics and Gynecology 65: 82–85

Ireland D, Cole S, Kelly P, Monaghan J M 1987 Mucin production in cervical intraepithelial neoplasia and in stage 1b carcinoma of cervix with pelvic lymph node metastases. British Journal of Obstetrics and Gynaecology 94: 467–472

Jaworski R C, Jones A 1990 DNA ploidy in adenocarcinoma of the uterine cervix. Journal of Clinical Pathology 43: 435–436

Jaworski R C, Pacey N F, Greenberg M L, Osborne R A 1988 The histologic diagnosis of adenocarcinoma in situ and related lesions of the cervix uteri. Cancer 61: 1171–1181

Jones M W, Silverberg S G 1989 Cervical adenocarcinoma in young women. Possible relationship to microglandular hyperplasia and use of oral contraceptives. Obstetrics and Gynecology 73: 984–988

Kadar N R D, Kohorn E I, LiVolsi V A, Kapp D S 1982 Histologic variants of cervical involvement by endometrial carcinoma. Obstetrics and Gynecology 59: 85–92

Kaku T, Enjoji M 1983 Extremely well differentiated adenocarcinoma ('adenoma malignum') of the cervix. International Journal of Gynecological Pathology 2: 28–41

Kaminski P F, Norris H J 1983 Minimal deviation carcinoma ('adenoma malignum') of the cervix. International Journal of Gynecological Pathology 2: 141–152

Kaminski P F, Norris H J 1984 Coexistence of ovarian neoplasms and endocervical adenocarcinoma. Obstetrics and Gynecology 64: 553–556

Kashimura M, Shinohara M, Oikawa K, Hamasaki K, Sato H 1990 An adenocarcinoma in situ of the uterine cervix that developed into invasive adenocarcinoma after 5 years. Gynecologic Oncology 36: 128–133

Kilgore L C, Soong S-J, Gore H, Shingleton H M, Hatch K D, Partridge E E 1988 Analysis of prognostic features in adenocarcinoma of the cervix. Gynecologic Oncology 31: 137–148

Kim Y C, Kudo H, Ogawa K et al 1988 Vitamin B_{23} R-binder localization in the human uterus: an immunohistochemical study. American Journal of Obstetrics and Gynecology 159: 522–526

King L A, Talledo O E, Gallup D G, Melhus O, Otken L B 1989 Adenoid cystic carcinoma of the cervix in women under age 40. Gynecologic Oncology 32: 26–30

Kleine W, Ran K, Schwoeorer D, Pfleiderer A 1989 Prognosis of the adenocarcinoma of the cervix uteri: a comparative study. Gynecologic Oncology 35: 145–149

Korhonen M O 1984 Adenocarcinoma of the uterine cervix. Prognosis and prognostic significance of histology. Cancer 53: 1760–1763

Kutteh W H, Hatch K D, Blackwell R E, Mestecky J 1988 Secretory immune system of the female reproductive tract: 1. Immunoglobulin and secretory component-containing cells. Obstetrics and Gynecology 71: 56–60

Lang G, Dallenbach-Hellweg G 1990 The histogenetic origin of cervical mesonephric hyperplasia and mesonephric adenocarcinoma of the uterine cervix studied with immunohistochemical methods. International Journal of Gynecological Pathology 9: 145–147

Lee Y S, Raju G C 1988 The expression and localisation of amylase in normal and malignant glands of the endometrium and endocervix. Journal of Pathology 155: 201–205

Leminen A, Paavonen J, Forss M, Wahlstrom T, Vesterinen E 1990a Adenocarcinoma of the uterine cervix. Cancer 65: 53–59

Leminen A, Paavonen J, Vesterinen E et al 1990b Deoxyribonucleic acid flow cytometric analysis of cervical adenocarcinoma: Prognostic significance of deoxyribonucleic acid ploidy and S-phase fraction. American Journal of Obstetrics and Gynecology 162: 848–853

LiVolsi V A, Merino M J, Schwartz P E 1983 Coexistent endocervical adenocarcinoma and mucinous adenocarcinoma of ovary: a clinicopathologic study of four cases. International Journal of Gynecological Pathology 1: 391–402

Luesley D M, Jordan J A, Woodman C B J, Watson N, Williams D R, Waddell C 1987 A retrospective review of adenocarcinoma-in-situ and glandular atypia of the uterine cervix. British Journal of Obstetrics and Gynaecology 94: 699–707

Maes G, Fleuren G J, Bara J, Nap M 1988 The distribution of mucins, carcinoembryonic antigen and mucus associated antigens in endocervical and endometrial adenocarcinomas. International Journal of Gynecological Pathology 7: 112–122

Maier R C, Norris H J 1980 Co-existence of cervical intraepithelial neoplasia with primary adenocarcinoma of the endocervix. Obstetrics and Gynecology 56: 361–364

Maier R C, Norris H J 1982 Glassy cell carcinoma of the cervix. Obstetrics and Gynecology 60: 219–224

Matsukuma K, Tsukamoto N M, Tsunehisa K et al 1989 Early adenocarcinoma of the uterine cervix—its histologic and immunohistologic study. Gynecologic Oncology 35: 38–43

Mazur M T, Battifora H A 1982 Adenoid cystic carcinoma of the cervix. Ultrastructure, immunofluorescence and criteria for diagnosis. American Journal of Clinical Pathology 77: 494–500

Mazur M T, Hsueh S, Gersell D J 1984 Metastases to the female genital tract. Analysis of 32 cases. Cancer 53: 1978–1984

Michael H, Grawe L, Kraus F T 1984 Minimal deviation endocervical adenocarcinoma: clinical and histologic features, immunohistochemical staining for carcinoembryonic antigen and differentiation from confusing benign lesions. International Journal of Gynecological Pathology 3: 261–276

Michael H, Sutton G, Hall M T, Roth L M 1986 Villous adenoma of the uterine cervix associated with invasive adenocarcinoma. A histologic, ultrastructural and immunohistochemical study. International Journal of Gynecological Pathology 5: 163–169

Mizuuchi H, Kudo R, Tamura H et al 1987 Identification of transferrin receptor in cervical and endometrial tissues. Gynecologic Oncology 31: 292–300

Mullins J D, Hilliard G D 1981 Cervical carcinoid ('argyrophil cell' carcinoma) associated with an endocervical adenocarcinoma: a light and ultrastructural study. Cancer 47: 785–790

Myerson D, Hackman R C, Nelson J A, Ward D C, McDougall D K 1984 Widespread presence of histologically occult cytomegalovirus. Human Pathology 15: 430–439

Nambu Y, Fujii S, Konishi I, Nonogaki H, Mori T 1988 Immunohistochemical localizations of CA 125, carcinoembryonic antigen and CA 19-9 in normal neoplastic glandular cells of the uterine cervix. Cancer 62: 2580–2588

Newbold K M, Rollason T P, Luelsley D M, Ward K 1990 Nucleolar organiser regions and proliferative index in glandular and squamous carcinomas of the cervix. Journal of Clinical Pathology 43: 441–442

Noda K, Kimura K, Ikeda M, Teshima K 1983 Studies on the histogenesis of cervical adenocarcinoma. International Journal of Gynecological Pathology 1: 336–346

Nunez C, Abdul-Karim F W, Somrak T M 1985 Glassy cell carcinoma of the uterine cervix. Cytopathological and histopathological study of five cases. Acta Cytologica 29: 803–809

Ostor A G, Pagano R, Davoren R A, Fortune D W, Chanen W, Rome R 1984 Adenocarcinoma in situ of the cervix. International Journal of Gynecological Pathology 3: 179–190

Pak H Y, Yokota S B, Paladugu R R, Agliozzo C M 1983 Glassy cell carcinoma of the cervix. Cytologic and clinicopathologic analysis. Cancer 52: 307–312

Patterson A, Wilson B, Cooper P, Arends J W 1990 Lysozyme and secretory component in endocervical and endometrial adenocarcinoma. Histopathology 16: 515–516

Peters R K, Chao A, Mack T M, Thomas D, Bernstein L, Henderson B E 1986 Increased frequency of adenocarcinoma of the uterine cervix in young women in Los Angeles County. Journal of the National Cancer Institute 76: 423–428

Peters W M 1986 Nature of 'basal' and 'reserve' cells in oviductal and cervical epithelium in man. Journal of Clinical Pathology 39: 306–312

Potish R A, Twiggs L B, Adcock L L, Prem K A, Savage J E, Leung B S 1986 Prognostic importance of progesterone and estrogen receptors in cancer of the uterine cervix. Cancer 58: 1709–1713

Qizilbash A 1975 In situ and microinvasive adenocarcinoma of the uterine cervix. American Journal of Clinical Pathology 64: 155–170

Randall M E, Kim J, Mills S E, Hahn S S, Constable W C 1986 Uncommon variants of cervical carcinoma treated with radical irradiation. Cancer 57: 816–822

Rollason T P, Byrne P, Williams A, Brown G 1988 Expression of epithelial membrane and 3 fucosyl-N-acetyllactosamine antigens in cervix uteri with particular reference to adenocarcinoma in situ. Journal of Clinical Pathology 41: 547–552

Rollason T P, Gullimore J, Bradgate M G 1989 A suggested columnar cell morphological equivalent of squamous carcinoma in situ with early stromal invasion. International Journal of Gynecological Pathology 8: 230–236

Saigo P E, Cain J M, Kim W S, Gaynor J J, Johnson K, Lewis J L 1986 Prognostic factors in adenocarcinoma of the uterine cervix. Cancer 57: 1584–1593

Scully R E, Aguirre P, DeLellis R A 1984 Argyrophilia, serotonin and peptide hormones in the female genital tract and its tumours. International Journal of Gynecological Pathology 3: 51–70

Shah K H, Kurman R J, Scully R E, Norris H S 1980 Atypical hyperplasia of mesonephric remnants in the cervix. Laboratory Investigation 42: 149

Shingleton H M, Gore H, Bradley D H, Soong S J 1981 Adenocarcinoma of the cervix. I. Clinical evaluation and pathologic features. American Journal of Obstetrics and Gynecology 139: 799–814

Shorrock K, Johnson J, Johnson I R 1990 Epidemiological changes in cervical carcinoma with particular reference to mucin-secreting subtypes. Histopathology 17: 53–57

Silcocks P B S, Thornton-Jones H, Murphy M 1987 Squamous and adenocarcinoma of the uterine cervix: A comparison using routine data. British Journal of Cancer 55: 321–325

Singh P, Ilancheran A, Ratnan S S, Lim-Tan S K, O'Reilly A P 1989 Cervical adenocarcinoma in women with nasopharyngeal carcinoma. Cancer 64: 1152–1155

Sixbey J W, Lenon S M, Pagano J S 1986 A second site for Epstein–Barr virus shedding: the uterine cervix. Lancet ii: 1122–1124

Speers W C, Picaso L G, Silverberg S G 1983 Immunohistochemical localisation of carcinoembryonic antigen in microglandular hyperplasia and adenocarcinoma of the endocervix. American Journal of Clinical Pathology 79: 105–107

Steeper T A, Wick M R 1986 Minimal deviation adenocarcinoma of the uterine cervix ('adenoma malignum'). Cancer 58: 1131–1138

Szyfelbein W M, Young R H, Scully R E 1983 Adenoma malignum of the cervix: cytological findings. Acta Cytologica 26: 691–698

Tamimi H K, Figge D C 1982 Adenocarcinoma of the uterine cervix. Gynecologic Oncology 13: 335

Tamimi H K, Marit E K, Hesla J, Cain J M, Figge D C, Greer B E 1988 Glassy cell carcinoma of the cervix redefined. Obstetrics and Gynecology 71: 837–841

Tanaka T, Ohbayashi F, Shima H, Shimonaka G, Takahashi M 1984 Glassy cell carcinoma of the uterine cervix. Pathology Research and Practice 178: 389–394

Tase T, Okagaki T, Clark B A et al 1988. Human papillomavirus type and localization in adenocarcinoma and adenosquamous carcinoma of the uterine cervix. Cancer Research 48: 993–999

Teshima S, Shimosato Y, Kishi K, Kasamatsu T, Ohmi K, Uei Y. 1985 Early stage adenocarcinoma of the uterine cervix. Histopathologic analysis with consideration of histogenesis. Cancer 56: 167–172

Tobon H, Dave H 1988 Adenocarcinoma in situ of the cervix. Clinicopathologic observations of 11 cases. International Journal of Gynecological Pathology 7: 139–151

Toki N, Kaku T, Tsukamoto N et al 1990 Distribution of basement membrane antigens in the uterine cervical adenocarcinomas: an immunohistochemical study. Gynecologic Oncology 38: 17–21

Trowell J E 1985 Intestinal metaplasia with argentaffin cells in the uterine cervix. Histopathology 9: 551–559

Turner M J, White J O, Soutter W P 1990 Human seminal plasma inhibits the lymphocyte response to infection with Epstein–Barr virus. Gynecologic Oncology 37: 60–65

Ueda G, Yamasaki M, Inoue M et al 1984. Immunohistochemical demonstration of peptide hormones in cervical adenocarcinomas with argyophil cells. International Journal of Gynecological Pathology 2: 373–379

Ulbright T M, Gersell 1983 Glassy cell carcinoma of the uterine cervix. A light and electron microscopic study of five cases. Cancer 51: 2255–2263

Valente P T, Hanjani P 1986 Endocervical neoplasia in long-term users of oral contraceptives: clinical and pathological observations. Obstetrics and Gynecology 67: 695–704

Van Dinh T, Woodruff J D 1985 Adenoid cystic and adenoid basal cell carcinoma of the cervix. Obstetrics and Gynecology 65: 705–709

Van Roon E, Boon M E, Kurver P J H, Baak J P A 1983 The association between precancerous-columnar and squamous lesions of the cervix: a morphometric study. Histopathology 7: 887–896

Varma S K, Rayner S S, Brown L J R 1991 Cutaneous ciliated cyst: case report and literature review. Plastic and Reconstructive Surgery 86: 344–346

Vogel H P, Mendelsohn G 1987 Laminin immunostaining in hyperplastic, dysplastic and neoplastic lesions of the endometrium and uterine cervix. Obstetrics and Gynecology 69: 794–799

Wakefield E A, Wells M 1985 Histochemical study of endocervical glycoproteins throughout the normal menstrual cycle and adjacent to cervical intraepithelial neoplasia. International Journal of Gynecological Pathology 4: 230–239

Webb M J, Sheehan T M 1989 Invasive carcinoma of the cervix in young women. Australia and New Zealand Journal of Obstetrics and Gynaecology 29: 47–51

Wells M, Brown L J R 1986 Glandular lesions of the uterine cervix: the present state of our knowledge. Histopathology 10: 777–792

Whitaker E M, Nimmo A J, Morrison J F B, Griffin N R, Wells M 1989 The distribution of β-adrenoreceptors in the human cervix. Quarterly Journal of Experimental Physiology 74: 573–576

Yajima A, Fukuda M, Noda K 1984 Histopathological findings concerning the morphogenesis of mixed carcinoma of the uterine cervix. Gynecologic Oncology 18: 157–164

Yoshida A, Yoshida H, Fukunishi R, Inohara T 1984 Carcinoid tumour of the uterine cervix. A light and electron microscopic study. Virchows Archives 402: 331–336

Young F I, Ward L M, Brown L J R 1991 Absence of human papilloma virus in cervical adenocarcinoma by in-situ hybridisation. Histopathology 44: 340–341

Young L S, Sixbey J W 1988 Epstein-Barr virus and epithelial cells: a possible role for the virus in the development of cervical carcinoma. Cancer Surveys 7: 507–518

Young R H, Scully R E 1988 Mucinous ovarian tumours associated with mucinous adenocarcinomas of the cervix. International Journal of Gynecological Pathology 7: 99–111

Young R H, Scully R E 1989a Villoglandular papillary adenocarcinoma of the uterine cervix. A clinicopathological analysis of 13 cases. Cancer 63: 1773–1779

Young R H, Scully R E 1989b Atypical forms of microglandular hyperplasia of the cervix simulating carcinoma. American Journal of Surgical Pathology 13: 50–56

Zaino R J, Nahhas W A, Mortel R 1982 Glassy cell carcinoma of the uterine cervix. An ultrastructural study and review. Archives of Pathology and Laboratory Medicine 106: 250–254

Zhang Y C, Zhang P F, Wei Y H 1983 Metastatic carcinoma of the cervix uteri from the gastrointestinal tract. Gynecologic Oncology 15: 287–290

10. Pathophysiology of dysfunctional uterine bleeding

Brian L. Sheppard

INTRODUCTION

Dysfunctional uterine bleeding is one of the least understood of common gynaecological conditions even though it is responsible for a significant number of referrals to gynaecology clinics. It is generally defined as excessively heavy, prolonged or frequent bleeding of uterine origin which is not due to disease in the pelvis, endocrine or haematological disorders, or pregnancy. Most women with dysfunctional uterine bleeding have excessive menstrual bleeding, and this is a major clinical problem; it may lead to iron deficiency anaemia and ultimately necessitate hysterectomy. Studies have shown that 50–60% of women undergoing hysterectomy for excessive menstrual bleeding have no demonstrable pathological lesions and therefore may be classified as having dysfunctional uterine bleeding (Rybo 1982, Sheppard et al 1991).

Objective measurement of menstrual blood loss in representative populations has shown that the mean menstrual loss per period is about 30–40 ml. Menstrual blood loss above 80 ml per cycle is considered excessive and is associated with an increased incidence of iron deficiency anaemia (Cohen & Gibor 1980). Studies have shown that up to 10% of women will have objectively measurable excessive menstrual bleeding at any one time, but it is calculated that as many as 25% of women will complain of excessive menstrual bleeding at some time (Fraser 1985).

It has become increasingly evident that the objective measurement of a woman's menstrual blood loss is extremely important in studies of dysfunctional uterine bleeding. The amount of menstrual blood loss bears no relation to uterine weight or endometrial surface area, or to clinical parameters such as the duration of bleeding and numbers or total weight of sanitary wear used: the recognition of clots in the menstrual flow and the woman's perception of her menstrual loss are also major sources of error in diagnosing excessive menstrual bleeding (Chimbera et al 1980, Fraser et al 1984). In fact, only 40% of women attending gynaecology clinics complaining of excessive menstrual bleeding may have a mean menstrual blood loss greater than 80 ml per period (Fraser et al 1984, Carroll et al 1989).

There is evidence that the majority of women with dysfunctional uterine bleeding have regular ovulatory cycles (Cameron 1989), and circulating hormone levels of women with dysfunctional uterine bleeding are no different from those of women with normal menstrual loss (Haynes et al 1979). During the last decade, advances have been made in understanding the pathophysiology of dysfunctional uterine bleeding by examining local uterine factors that are thought to play a role in the control of blood loss from the uterus. The majority of studies have concentrated on endometrial vasculature, prostaglandins, the coagulation and fibrinolytic enzyme systems, platelets, and mast cells in relation to normal and excessive menstrual bleeding.

UTERINE VASCULATURE

Much of the present knowledge of the role of endometrial blood vessels in the physiological process of menstruation, and indeed many hypotheses on the pathogenesis of excessive menstrual bleeding, stem from the original studies of Markee (1940). In this seminal work, endometrium of rabbits was explanted into the anterior chamber of the eye of Rhesus monkeys; endometrial regression associated with a decline in ovarian steroid levels, the coiling of spiral arterioles, intense vasoconstriction prior to menstrual bleeding from the dilated spiral arterioles and a return to vasoconstriction of the vessels were all described in great detail. Markee estimated that 70–75% of bleeding arose from the spiral arterioles either through damaged vessels into the endometrial stroma or through ruptured arterioles directly into the uterine cavity.

More recently, quantitative studies of uterine vasculature, and in particular endometrial spiral arterioles, have been undertaken to investigate the relation between vascular density and the amount of menstrual blood

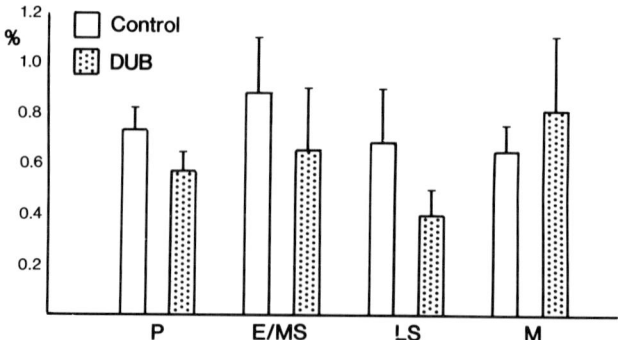

Fig. 10.1 Comparison of arterial density in the basal endometrium through the proliferative (P), early/mid-secretory (E/MS), late secretory (LS) and menstrual (M) phases of the cycle in women with normal menstrual blood loss (< 80 ml) and dysfunctional uterine (DUB) bleeding (DUB; > 80 ml). (Adapted from McKone et al 1991.)

loss. Although arterial density is greater in the myometrium adjacent to the endometrium than in basal endometrium (Rees et al 1984, Hourihan et al 1986) there is no variation in vessel density through the menstrual cycle in women with normal blood loss or dysfunctional uterine bleeding (Rees et al 1984a, McKone et al 1991). Increased numbers of thick-walled spiral arterioles have recently been identified in the functional endometrium of women with dysfunctional uterine bleeding (Robinson et al 1991). These vessels may represent remnant arterioles from incomplete menstrual shedding which have undergone further development in subsequent menstrual cycles. However, total arterial density in the endometrium of women with normal menstrual loss has been shown to be very similar to that in women with dysfunctional uterine bleeding (Fig. 10.1) Over the full range of possible menstrual blood loss, from a few millilitres to over a litre per cycle no correlation has been found between measured blood loss and arterial density in basal endometrium (Rees et al 1984a, McKone et al 1991). It would appear, therefore, that excessive menstrual bleeding in the absence of obvious pathology is not due to a proliferation in the number of arteries (though it may be due to other vascular abnormalities).

MORPHOLOGY OF MENSTRUAL HAEMOSTASIS

It is now well established that defective haemostasis occurs in the endometrial vasculature during normal menstruation, and it has been suggested that this is further compromised in patients with dysfunctional uterine bleeding (Sheppard 1984, 1990, Hourihan et al 1989). Vascular lesions, without haemostatic plugs, have been described in the endometrium just prior to the onset of menstruation (Christiaens et al 1980, Hourihan et al 1989), which probably coincide with the period of intensive vasoconstriction described by Markee (1940). During the first 20 h of menstrual bleeding, platelets and fibrin become involved in the haemostatic process with the formation of intravascular platelet plugs, although initially these do not occlude the vessel lumens (Christiaens et al 1980). A few hours later, complete occlusion of the vessels occurs, with a considerable amount of fibrin stabilizing the haemostatic platelet plug. Within 24 h these plugs have been shed with endometrial tissue; platelets and fibrin are consistently found in menstrual fluid (Fig. 10.2) during the first 48 h of menstrual bleeding (Christiaens et al 1981, Sheppard et al 1983a). Until the endometrial surface is completely re-epithelialized, vasoconstriction is probably more important and assures haemostasis.

Defects in this re-covering process, with and without accompanying haemostatic plugs, are more common and are present for a greater number of days in the endometrium of women with dysfunctional uterine bleeding than in women with normal menstruation (Hourihan et al 1989, Sheppard 1990). Whereas in normal menstruation haemostatic plugs usually remain intravascular, in dysfunctional uterine bleeding large haemostatic plugs

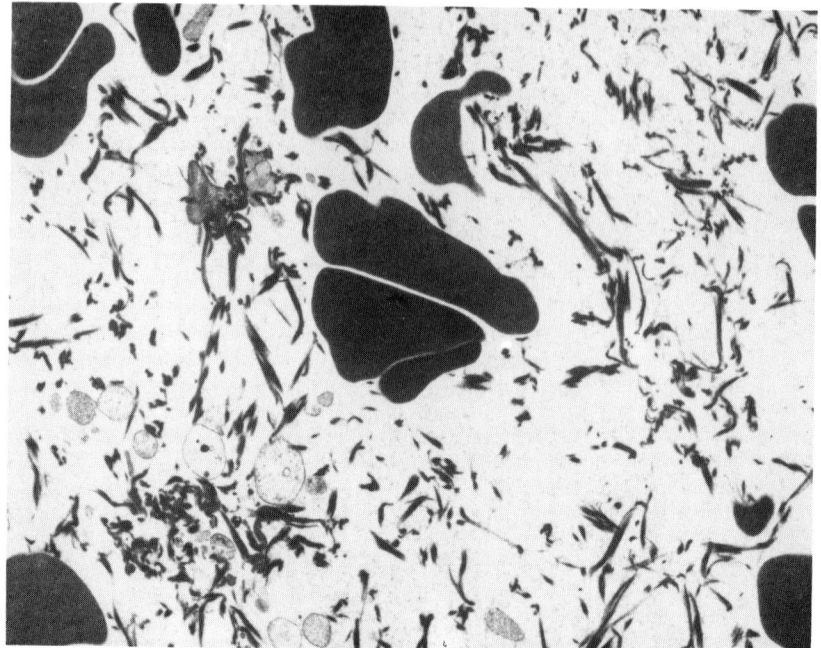

Fig. 10.2   Electron micrograph of part of a menstrual clot showing electron-dense fibrin fibres and platelets distributed between erythrocytes (× 6000).

have been observed protruding into the extravascular space of the endometrial stroma (van Eijkeren et al 1990). These plugs often consist of poorly interdigitated, granulated platelets with a very minor fibrin component (Fig. 10.3) and are probably less stable than those found in normal menstruation. In contrast to normal menstruation, re-canalized plugs with remnants of platelets and fibrin have also been described in endometrial blood vessels from women with dysfunctional uterine bleeding (van Eijkeren et al 1990). It is suggested that a diminished capacity of platelets to aggregate, coupled with reduced fibrin deposition, during the process of menstruation in women with dysfunctional uterine bleeding renders the haemostatic plugs more fragile, allowing blood to flow more freely past dislodged thrombi.

Platelets and fibrin play a vitally important part in haemostasis during the process of menstruation. Consumption of platelet aggregates in blood vessels of the functional endometrium during the haemostatic process of menstruation leads to only small numbers being found in menstrual discharge (De Merre et al 1967). Ultrastructural studies have shown that menstrual platelets are largely devoid of granules (Fig. 10.4), appear to have been exposed to an aggregating stimulus, and are probably spent (Sheppard et al 1983a). When challenged with aggregating stimuli such as adenosine diphosphate or collagen, the platelets fail to aggregate and produce little cyclo-oxygenase product from arachidonic acid (Rees et al 1984b). There is, however, no relation between platelet function and the degree of menstrual

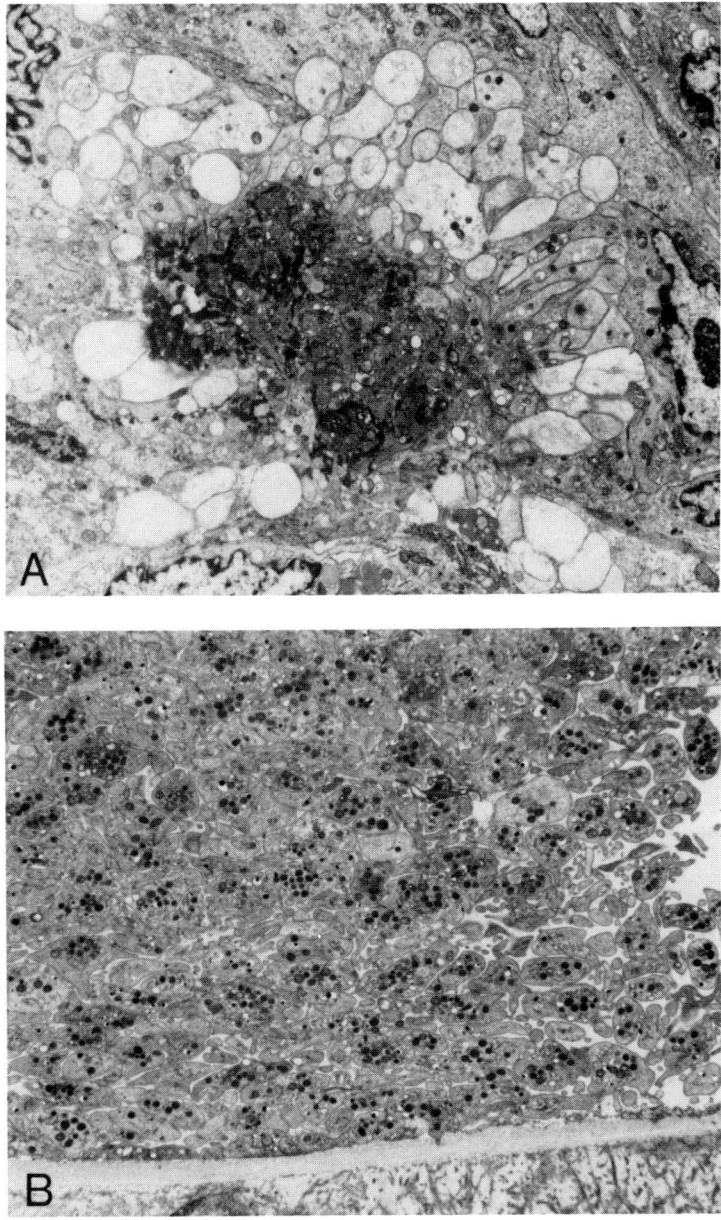

Fig. 10.3   Electron micrograph of part of a haemostatic plug in an endometrial blood vessel during menstruation in a woman with normal menstruation (**A**) and with dysfunctional uterine bleeding (**B**) (× 4500).

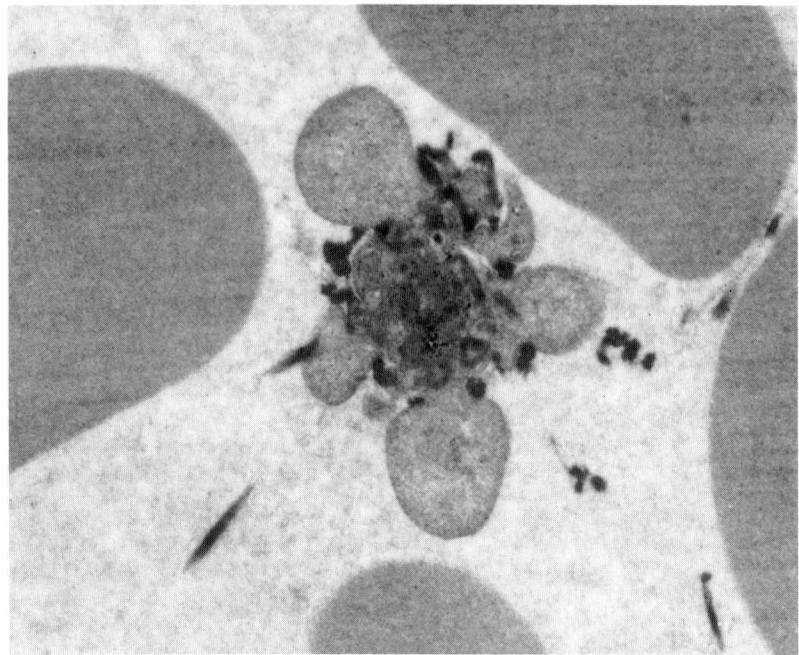

Fig. 10.4   Electron micrograph of a menstrual platelet which has undergone shape-change and granule-release during the process of aggregation and appears spent (× 15 000).

blood loss, suggesting that platelet abnormalities are unlikely to play an important role in the mechanism of dysfunctional uterine bleeding.

MENSTRUAL COAGULATION AND FIBRINOLYSIS

Activation of the coagulation and fibrinolytic enzyme systems occurs during menstruation. Blood coagulation factors are severely depleted in menstrual blood, indicating consumption of these components during menstruation (Hahn 1980). Compared with women with normal menstruation, no differences have been found in the coagulation factors in either menstrual fluid or peripheral blood plasma of women with dysfunctional uterine bleeding (Hahn et al 1976, Rees et al 1985).

Fibrinolytic activity results from the balance between plasminogen activators and their inhibitors. It was suggested many years ago that tissue activators of plasminogen may cause an increased local fibrinolysis that may interfere with haemostatic mechanisms (Astrup 1958), and it was further pointed out that the concentration of plasminogen activators in the endometrium might be of importance in the genesis of excessive menstrual bleeding (Albrechtsen 1956a). Early studies of plasminogen activator found high concentrations in both the uterus and menstrual fluid (Albrechtsen 1956a,b). It is generally accepted that menstrual blood contains no

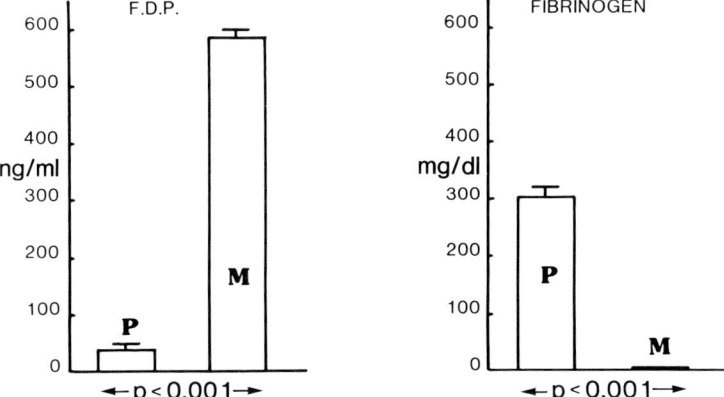

Fig. 10.5 A comparison of the levels of fibrinogen (right) and fibrin degradation products (left) in peripheral (P) and Menstrual (M) blood. Menstrual blood contains no fibrinogen but very high levels of fibrin degradation products.

fibrinogen but has high levels of fibrin degradation products (Fig. 10.5): this was thought to be the result of direct digestion of fibrinogen to breakdown products (Beller 1971). Subsequent morphological studies have, however, identified fibrin in menstrual clots from the uterine cavity and vagina of women with normal and dysfunctional uterine bleeding (Sheppard et al 1983a), and vigorous local fibrinolytic activity is now identified as a major mechanism in maintaining the fluidity of menstrual blood. A far higher level of tissue plasminogen activator antigen coupled with very low levels of

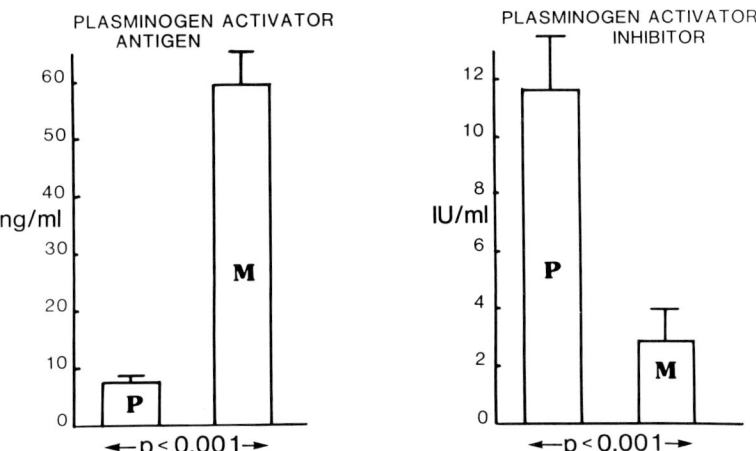

Fig. 10.6 A comparison of the levels of tissue plasminogen activator antigen and plasminogen activator inhibitor in menstrual (M) and peripheral (P) plasma. Menstrual plasma contains higher levels of antigen and lower levels of inhibitor than peripheral plasma.

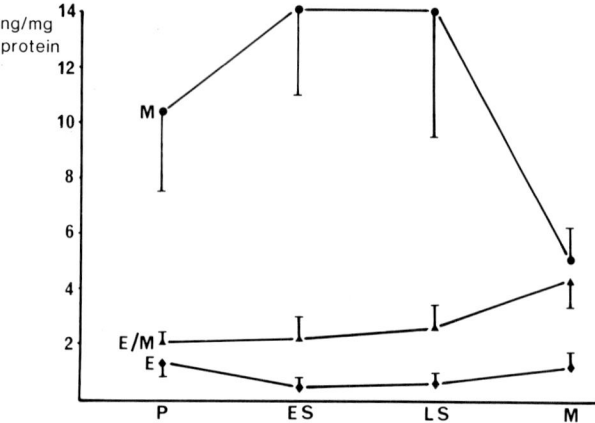

Fig. 10.7 Levels of tissue plasminogen activator (bars indicate S.D.s) in extracts of myometrium (M), the endometrial/myometrial border (E/M) and endometrium (E) taken at hysterectomy in the proliferative (P), early secretory (ES), late secretory (LS) and menstrual (M) phases of the cycle from women with normal menstrual cycles.

plasminogen activator inhibitor was found in menstrual fluid than in peripheral plasma (Fig. 10.6), a finding more noticeable in women with dysfunctional uterine bleeding (Sheppard et al 1990).

Evidence of the important role of increased local fibrinolytic activity in the pathogenesis of dysfunctional uterine bleeding is shown by the significantly higher levels of plasminogen activator in menstrual fluid of women with excessive menstrual loss (Bonnar et al 1983, Sheppard et al 1983b). This is further supported by treatment with antifibrinolytics, such as tranexamic acid (Nilsson & Rybo 1967, Bonnar et al 1980). Women with dysfunctional uterine bleeding have levels of tissue plasminogen activator in peripheral blood plasma similar to those of women with normal menstruation, suggesting that the higher levels in menstrual fluid are derived from the myometrium. Higher levels of tissue plasminogen activator are found in myometrium than in endometrium throughout the normal menstrual cycle (Fig. 10.7). The activity varies not only from region to region in the uterus (Shaw et al 1980) but also through the menstrual cycle; it increases considerably in the late secretory phase of the cycle (Rybo 1966, Shaw et al 1980, Hourihan et al 1990). Immunohistochemical staining of the uterine wall has shown that tissue plasminogen activator is predominantly localized in endothelial cells of small blood vessels of the myometrium throughout the cycle, and in capillaries and spiral arterioles of the endometrium in the late secretory/premenstrual phase of the cycle (Plate 10.1).

Increased endometrial fibrinolytic activity has been correlated with increased menstrual blood loss (Rybo 1966). Recently, significantly higher than normal levels of tissue plasminogen activator have been reported in late secretory phase endometrium extracts from women with dysfunctional

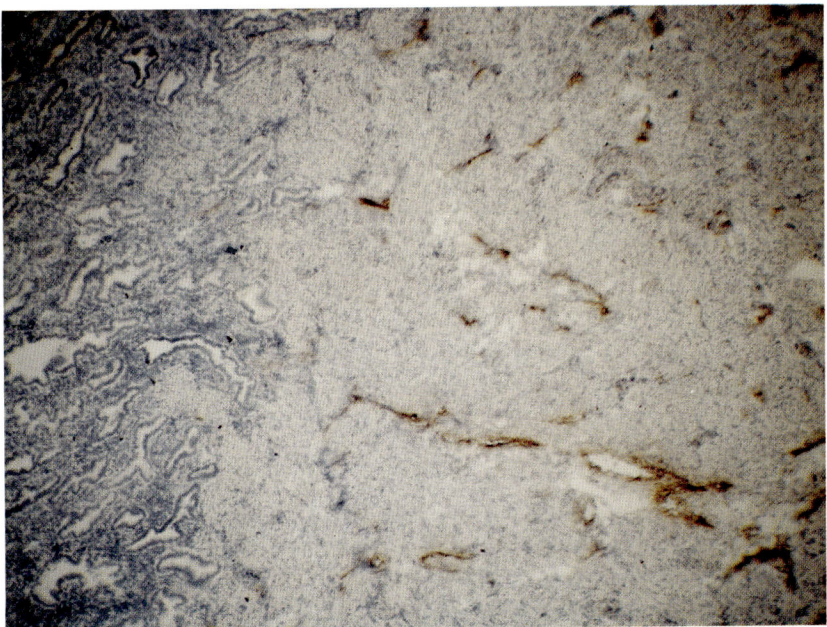

Plate 1a   Immunohistochemical localization of tissue plasminogen activator within blood vessels of the myometrium and endometrium in the late secretory phase of the menstrual cycle.

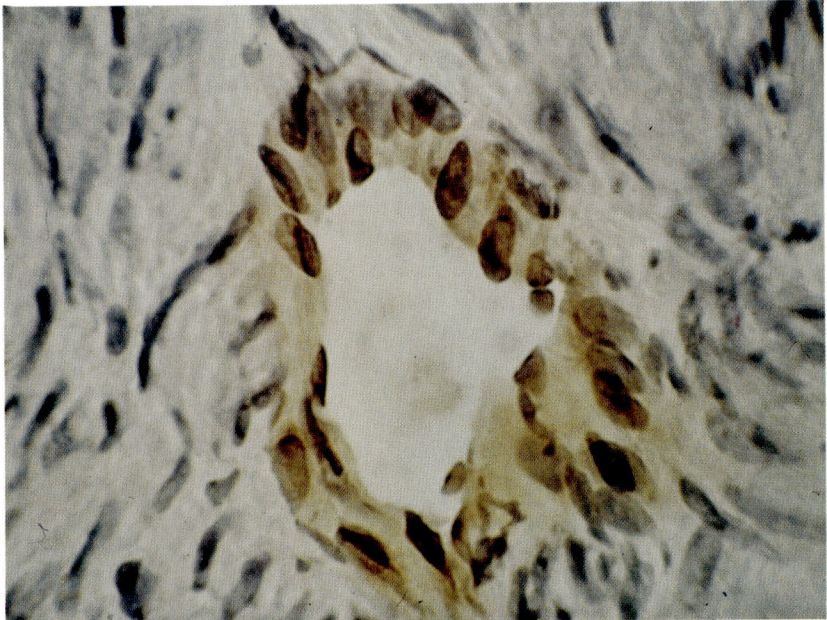

Plate 1b   Higher magnification of a capillary of the basal endometrium showing the tissue plasminogen activator localized in the endothelial cells lining the intima of the blood vessel.

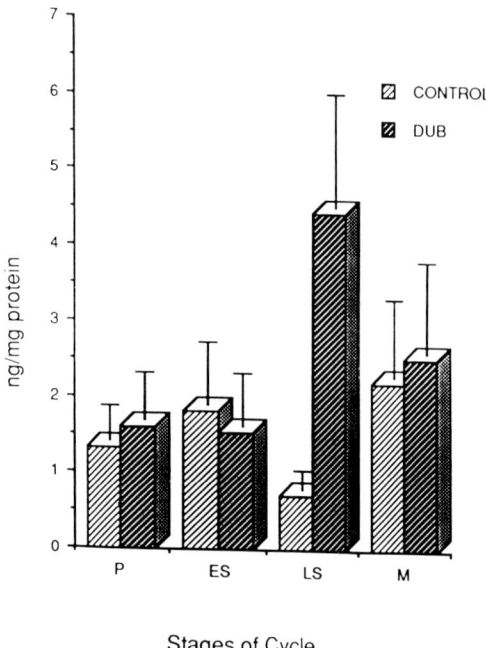

Stages of Cycle

Fig. 10.8   Tissue plasminogen activator antigen levels in extracts of endometrium from uteri removed at hysterectomy during the proliferative (P), early secretory (ES), late secretory (LS) and menstrual (M) phases of the cycle in women with normal menstrual blood loss (< 80 ml menstrual blood loss) and dysfunctional uterine bleeding (DUB; > 80 ml loss). (Adapted from Sheppard et al 1990.)

uterine bleeding (Fig. 10.8) (Sheppard et al 1990). In this study, a strong correlation was evident between the amount of menstrual blood loss and tissue plasminogen activator concentration in the late secretory phase of the cycle (Sheppard et al 1990), indicating that increased local release of fibrinolytic activator is a key factor in the aetiology of dysfunctional uterine bleeding.

PROSTAGLANDINS AND MENSTRUAL BLEEDING

Prostaglandins are intimately involved in haemostasis and individually have a variety of different effects on the haemostatic process. Prostaglandin E_2 (PGE_2) is a potent vasodilator, and prostaglandin $F_{2\alpha}$ ($PGF_{2\alpha}$) is a vasoconstrictor. Prostacyclin I_2 (PGI_2—usually measured as its stable metabolite 6-keto-$PGF_{1\alpha}$) is a vasodilator and inhibits platelet aggregation. Thromboxane A_2 (TXA_2) is a strong vasoconstrictor and stimulates platelet aggregation.

Prostaglandins have been implicated in the physiological process of menstruation since Pickles et al (1965) found high concentrations of PGE_2 and $PGF_{2\alpha}$ in endometrium and myometrium. The discovery that giving patients prostaglandin synthetase inhibitors, such as mefenamic acid, reduces menstrual blood loss suggests that excess uterine prostaglandin production is involved in the aetiology of dysfunctional uterine bleeding (Anderson et al 1976, Fraser et al 1983).

Prostaglandin production by the endometrium is influenced by changing levels of oestrogen and progesterone. The capacity of the endometrium to synthesize PGE_2 and $PGF_{2\alpha}$ increases greatly during the secretory phase of the menstrual cycle, reaching a maximum at the time of menstruation (Downie et al 1974). Although glandular epithelium has been shown to be the principal site of prostaglandin synthesis and degradation in the endometrium (Casey et al 1980, Rees et al 1982), no relation has been found between endometrial glandular density and the amount of menstrual blood loss (Rees et al 1984a, McKone et al 1991). Elevated levels of endometrial PGE_2 and $PGF_{2\alpha}$ throughout the menstrual cycle have, however, been described by Willman et al (1976) in women complaining of excessive menstrual loss. Other studies have shown that heavy menstrual blood loss is associated with an imbalance in endometrial synthesis of prostaglandins, with higher levels of PGE_2 and lower levels of $PGF_{2\alpha}$ (Smith et al 1981a). Endometrium from women with excessive menstrual bleeding has also been shown to have a greater capacity to synthesize 6-keto-$PGF_{1\alpha}$ than endometrium from women with normal menstrual loss (Smith et al 1981b, Makarainen & Ylikorkala 1986). Using a superfusion technique, Rees et al (1984a), found $PGF_{2\alpha}$ and 6-keto-$PGF_{1\alpha}$ to be the principal prostaglandins produced in the endometrium and myometrium, respectively. They were unable to find a correlation between the release of $PGF_{2\alpha}$, PGE_2 or 6-keto-

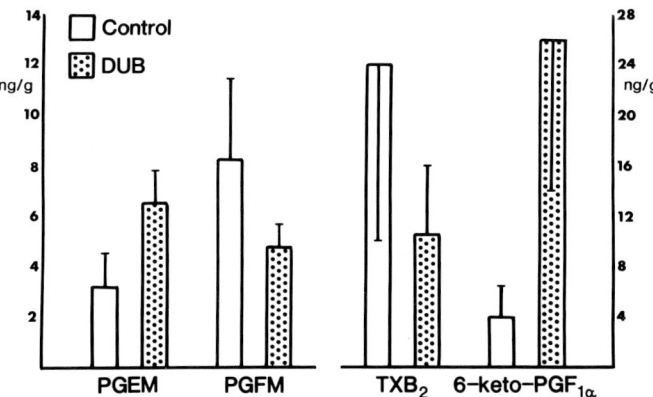

Fig. 10.9 Levels of the metabolites of prostaglandins PGE_2 (PGEM) and $PGF_{2\alpha}$ (PGFM) and of 6-keto-$PGF_{1\alpha}$ and thromboxane B_2 (TXB_2) in menstrual endometrium from women with normal menstrual blood loss and women with dysfunctional uterine bleeding (DUB). The vasodilators (PGEM and 6-keto-$PGF_{1\alpha}$) are higher and the vasoconstrictors lower (PGFM and TXB_2) in women with DUB than in women with normal menstrual blood loss. (Adapted from Sharma et al 1990a,b.)

$PGF_{1\alpha}$, or between the ratios of vasodilator to vasoconstrictor prostaglandins and menstrual blood loss, although during the first 2 days of menstruation, when the greatest menstrual flow occurs, a possible relation between menstrual blood loss and $PGF_{2\alpha}$, PGE_2 and $6\text{-keto-}PGF_{1\alpha}$ production in both endometrium and myometrium was observed. Recent studies have shown higher levels of $6\text{-keto-}PGF_{1\alpha}$ and the metabolite of PGE_2, and lower levels of thromboxane B_2 and the metabolite of $PGF_{2\alpha}$ (Fig. 10.9) in menstrual endometrium of women with dysfunctional uterine bleeding compared with normal menstrual blood loss (Sharma et al 1990a,b), supporting the suggestion that dysfunctional uterine bleeding is associated with a shift towards the production of higher levels of vasodilatory prostaglandins and away from prostaglandins that stimulate vasoconstriction and platelet aggregation. An interaction between prostaglandins produced by the myometrium and endometrium is probably a key factor in the control of the amount of blood loss during menstruation.

MAST CELLS IN THE UTERUS

Mast cells, which contain and release heparin and histamine, are irregularly distributed throughout the uterine endometrium and myometrium, often in close proximity to capillaries or small venules (Fig. 10.10). Characteristic cytoplasmic granules make the cells readily identifiable by light and electron microscopy (Sheppard & Bonnar 1979). Quantitative and qualitative

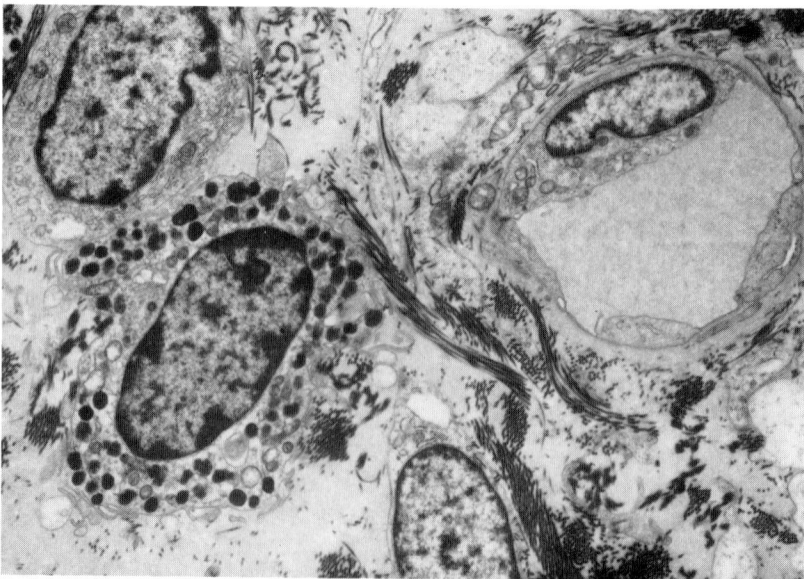

Fig. 10.10   An electron micrograph of a mast cell, with characteristic cytoplasmic granules, in close proximity to a blood vessel of the endometrial stroma of a women with dysfunctional uterine bleeding (× 3500).

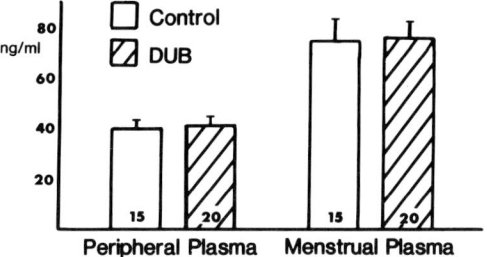

Fig. 10.11   A comparison of histamine levels (mean$^+$ S.E.M.) in peripheral and menstrual plasma in a group of women with normal menstruation and a group with dysfunctional uterine bleeding (DUB). Although the levels in menstrual plasma are significantly higher than in peripheral plasma (p < 0.01), no difference is seen between the levels in women with normal menstruation compared with dysfunctional uterine bleeding. (Adapted from Drudy, Sheppard and Bonnar 1991c.)

studies have shown that mast cells predominate in the myometrium, but in the endometrium undergo structural and numerical changes throughout the menstrual cycle: mast cell degranulation occurs principally during the premenstrual phase of the cycle (Drudy et al 1991a, b).

Heparin-like activity and histamine have been identified in menstrual fluid, which suggests that these metabolic products of mast cells may be involved in the mechanism of menstrual bleeding (Foley et al 1978, Drudy et al 1991c). The histamine released from mast cells may mediate contraction of endothelial cells, causing gaps to appear in the lining of blood vessels, with leakage of erythrocytes into the endometrial stroma: the heparin-like activity may be important in maintaining menstrual blood in a fluid state. Histamine has also recently been shown to stimulate the release of tissue plasminogen activator, plasminogen activator inhibitor and Factor VIII from cultured endothelial cells (Hanss & Collen 1987, Hamilton & Sims 1987).

A cyclical variation in heparin-like activity in the uterus has been postulated, and although Foley et al (1978) found higher levels of heparin-like activity in uterine fluid of women with excessive menstrual bleeding than women with normal menstrual blood loss, they found no correlation between this activity and the presence of mast cells in the endometrium or myometrium.

Histamine levels in the uterine wall also undergo cyclical variation, with the highest levels found in the late secretory/premenstrual phase of the cycle (Drudy et al 1991c). Significantly higher concentrations of histamine are also found in menstrual fluid during the first 48 h of menstrual bleeding than in peripheral blood (Fig. 10.11). Similar concentrations of histamine are, however, found in the uterine wall and in menstrual fluid from women with dysfunctional uterine bleeding and women with normal menstrual blood loss. Although histamine may therefore be involved in the physiological process of menstruation, it does not appear that increased levels play a part in the aetiology of dysfunctional uterine bleeding.

CONCLUSIONS

Data on the mechanisms that initiate and control menstrual bleeding are of paramount importance in our understanding of the pathogenesis of dysfunctional uterine bleeding. Recent studies suggest that most excessive uterine bleeding is due to local endometrial or myometrial dysfunction. The precise mechanism of dysfunctional uterine bleeding still remains unclear, but there is increasing evidence that impaired haemostasis, coupled with increased uterine fibrinolysis and an imbalance of prostaglandin production, are the major factors involved. It is essential that future studies are undertaken in this area, to increase our knowledge of the relation between factors controlling blood loss from the uterus, and hence to permit advances to be made in treatment to restore normal menstrual function.

REFERENCES

Albrechtsen O K 1956a The fibrinolytic activity of the human endometrium. Acta Endocrinologica 23: 207–218

Albrechtsen O K 1956b The fibrinolytic activity of the human tissue. British Journal of Haematology 3: 284–291

Anderson A B M, Haynes P J, Guillebaud J, Turnbull A C 1976 Reduction of menstrual blood loss by prostaglandin synthetase inhibitors. Lancet 1: 774–776

Astrup T 1958 The haemostatic balance. Thrombosis et Diathesis Haemorrhagica 2: 347–357

Beller F K 1971 Observations on the clotting of menstrual blood and clot formation. American Journal of Obstetrics and Gynecology 11: 535–546

Bonnar J, Guillebaud J, Kasonde J, Sheppard B L 1980 Clinical applications of fibrinolytic inhibition in gynaecology. Journal of Clinical Pathology 33(suppl 14): 55–59

Bonnar J, Sheppard B L, Dockeray C J 1983 The haemostatic system and dysfunctional uterine bleeding. Research and Clinical Forums 5: 27–36

Cameron I T 1989 Dysfunctional uterine bleeding. Baillière's Clinics in Obstetrics and Gynaecology 3: 315–326

Carroll E, Hennelly B, Sheppard B L, Bonnar J 1989 Menstrual blood loss in patients referred to the gynaecology out-patient clinic with excessive menstrual bleeding. Irish Journal of Medical Science 158: 129–132

Casey M L, Hemsell D L, MacDonald P C, Johnston J M 1980 NAD + dependent 15-hydroxy-prostaglandin dehydrogenase activity in human endometrium. Prostaglandins 19: 115–122

Chimbera T H, Anderson A B M, Turnbull A C 1980 Relation between measured menstrual blood loss and patient's subjective assessment of loss, duration of bleeding, number of sanitary towels used, uterine weight and endometrial surface. British Journal of Obstetrics and Gynaecology 87: 603–609

Christiaens G C M L, Sixma J J, Haspels A A 1980 Morphology of haemostasis in menstrual endometrium. British Journal of Obstetrics and Gynaecology 87: 425–430

Christiaens G C M L, Sixma J J, Haspels A A 1981 Fibrin and platelets in menstrual discharge before and after the insertion of an intra-uterine contraceptive device. American Journal of Obstetrics and Gynecology 140: 793–798

Cohen B J B, Gibor J 1980 Anemia and menstrual blood loss. Obstetric and Gynecological Survey 35: 597–602

Daly L, Sheppard B L, Carroll E, Hennelly B, Bonnar J 1990 Coagulation and fibrinolysis in menstrual and peripheral blood in dysfunctional uterine bleeding. Irish Journal of Medical Science 159: 24

De Merre L J, Moss J D, Pattison D S 1967 The haematologic study of menstrual discharge. Obstetrics and Gynecology 30: 830–833

Dockeray C J, Sheppard B L, Bonnar J 1987 The fibrinolytic enzyme system in normal menstruation and excessive uterine bleeding and the effect of tranexamic acid. European Journal of Obstetrics, Gynaecology and Reproductive Biology 24: 309–318

Downie J, Poyser N L, Wunderlich M 1974 Levels of prostaglandins in human endometrium during the normal menstrual cycle. Journal of Physiology 236: 465–472

Drudy L, Sheppard B L, Bonnar J 1991a Mast cells in the normal uterus and in dysfunctional uterine bleeding. European Journal of Obstetrics, Gynaecology and Reproductive Biology 39: 193–201

Drudy L, Sheppard B L, Bonnar 1991b The ultrastructure of mast cells in the uterus throughout the normal menstrual cycle and in the postmenopause. Journal of Anatomy 175: 51–63

Drudy L, Sheppard B L, Bonnar 1991c Histamine concentration in the normal human uterus and in dysfunctional uterine bleeding. Submitted for publication

Foley M E, Griffin B D, Zugel M et al 1978 Heparin-like activity in uterine fluid. British Medical Journal ii: 322–324

Fraser I S 1985 The 'dysfunctional' uterus: dysmenorrhoea and dysfunctional uterine bleeding. In: Shearman R P (ed) Clinical reproductive endocrinology. Churchill Livingstone, Edinburgh, p 579–598

Fraser I S, McCarron G, Markham R, Robinson M, Smyth E 1983 Long term treatment of menorrhagia with mefenamic acid. Obstetrics and Gynecology 61: 109–114

Fraser I S, McCarron G, Markham R 1984 A preliminary study of factors influencing perception of menstrual blood loss volume. American Journal of Obstetrics and Gynecology 149: 788–793

Hahn L 1980 Composition of menstrual blood. In: Diczfalusy E, Fraser I S, Webb F T G (eds) Endometrial bleeding and steroidal contraception. Pitman Press, Bath, p 107–131

Hahn L, Rybo G 1975 Fibrinogen–fibrin degradation products in menstrual blood from women with normal and excessive menstrual blood losses. Acta Obstetrica et Gynecologica Scandinavica 54: 1–16

Hahn L, Cederblad G, Rybo G, Pehrsson N G, Korsan-Bengtsen K 1976 Blood coagulation, fibrinolysis and plasma protein in women with normal and excessive menstrual blood loss. British Journal of Obstetrics and Gynaecology 83: 974–980

Hamilton K K, Sima P J 1987 Changes in cytosolic Ca^{2+} associated with von Willebrand factor release in human endothelial cells exposed to histamine. Study of microcarrier cell monolayers using the fluorescent probe indo-1. Journal of Clinical Investigation 79: 600–608

Hanss M, Collen D 1987 Secretion of tissue-type plasminogen activator and plasminogen activator inhibitor by cultured human endothelial cells: modulation by thrombin, endotoxin and histamine. Journal of Laboratory and Clinical Medicine 109: 97–104

Haynes P J, Anderson A B M, Turnbull A C 1979 Patterns of menstrual blood loss in menorrhagia. Research and Clinical Forums 1: 73–78

Hourihan H M, Sheppard B L, Bonnar J 1986 A morphometric study of the effect of oral norethisterone and levonorgestrel on endometrial blood vessels. Contraception 34: 603–612

Hourihan H M, Sheppard B L, Bonnar J 1989 The morphologic characteristics of menstrual haemostasis in patients with unexplained menorrhagia. International Journal of Gynecological Pathology 8: 221–229

Hourihan H M, Sheppard B L, Brosens I 1990 Endometrial haemostasis. In: D'Arcangues C, Fraser I S, Newton J R, Odlind V (eds) Contraception and mechanisms of endometrial bleeding. Cambridge University Press, Cambridge, p 95–116

McKone E, Sheppard B L, Bonnar 1991 Uterine histology and menstrual blood loss. Irish Journal of Medical Science (in press)

Makarainen L, Ylikorkola O 1986 Primary and myoma associated menorrhagia; role of prostaglandin and effect of ibuprofen. British Journal of Obstetrics and Gynaecology 93: 974–978

Markee J E 1940 Menstruation in intraocular endometrial transplants in the rhesus monkey. Contributions to Embryology. Carnegie Institution of Washington publication number 518 28: 219–308

Nilsson L, Rybo G 1967 Treatment of menorrhagia with an antifibrinolytic, tranexamic acid. A double blind investigation. Acta Obstetrica et Gynecologica Scandinavia 46: 572–580

Pickles V R, Hall W J, Poest F A, Smith G N 1965 Prostaglandins in endometrium and menstrual fluid from normal and dysmenorrhoea subjects. British Journal of Obstetrics and Gynaecology 72: 185–195

Rees M C P, Parry D M, Anderson A B M, Turnbull A C 1982 Immunohistochemical localization of cyclo oxygenase in the human uterus. Prostaglandins 23: 207–214

Rees M C P, Dunhill M S, Anderson A B M, Turnbull A C 1984a Quantitative uterine histology during the menstrual cycle to measured menstrual blood loss. British Journal of Obstetrics and Gynaecology 91: 662–666

Rees M C P, Demers L M, Anderson A B M, Turnbull A C 1984b A functional study of platelets in menstrual fluid. British Journal of Obstetrics and Gynaecology 91: 667–672

Rees M C P, Anderson A B M, Demers L M, Turnbull A C 1984c Endometrial and myometrial prostaglandin release during the menstrual cycle in relation to menstrual blood loss. Journal of Clinical Endocrinology and Metabolism 58: 813–818

Rees M C P, Cederholm-Williams S A, Turnbull A C 1985 Coagulation factors and fibrinolytic proteins in menstrual fluid collected from normal and menorrhagic women. British Journal of Obstetrics and Gynaecology 92: 1164–1168

Robinson I A, Sheppard B L, Gillen J E 1991 Increased complexity of endometrial spiral arterioles in dysfunctional uterine bleeding (in press)

Rybo G 1966 Plasminogen activators in the endometrium ii. Clinical aspects. Acta Obstetrica et Gynecologica Scandinavica 45: 97–118

Rybo G 1982 Variations in menstrual blood loss. Research and Clinical Forums 4: 81–92

Sharma S C, Sheppard B L, Bonnar J 1990a Relationship of menstrual blood loss with uterine 6-keto-PGF$_1$ and TXB$_2$ levels in women with normal and dysfunctional uterine bleeding. Irish Journal of Medical Science 159: 27

Sharma S C, Sheppard B L, Bonnar J 1990b Endometrial tissue levels of PGE$_2$ and PGF$_2$ metabolites in women with normal menstruation and dysfunctional uterine bleeding. Irish Journal of Medical Science 159: 152

Shaw S T, Macaulay L K, Tanaka M S, Hohman W R, Moyer D L, Sun N C 1980 Plasminogen activator in human uterine tissue—relationship to location of sampling and time of ovarian cycle. Biochemical Medicine 24: 170–178

Sheppard B L 1984 The pathology of dysfunctional uterine bleeding. Clinics in Obstetrics and Gynaecology 11: 227–236

Sheppard B L 1990 Coagulation and electron microscopy studies in menorrhagia. In: Shaw R W (ed) Advances in reproductive endocrinology. Dysfunctional uterine bleeding. Parthenon Publishing, Carnforth, Lancs, vol 2, p 25–42

Sheppard B L, Bonnar J 1979 Mast cells in the human uterus. In: Pepys J, Edwards A M (eds) The mast cell. Pitman Medical Press, Bath, p 142–148

Sheppard B L, Dockeray C J, Bonnar J 1983a An ultrastructural study of menstrual blood in normal menstruation and dysfunctional uterine bleeding. British Journal of Obstetrics and Gynaecology 90: 259–265

Sheppard B L, Dockeray C J, Sharma S C, Bonnar J 1983b In: Jespersen J, Kluft C, Korsgaard O (eds) Clinical aspects of fibrinolysis and thrombolysis. South Jutland University Press, Esbjerg, p 421–433

Sheppard B L, Stack M, Jordan M, Bonnar J 1990 Plasminogen activator in the human uterus in normal menstruation and dysfunctional uterine bleeding. Irish Journal of Medical Science 159: 151

Sheppard B L, Sharma S C, Bonnar J 1991 Haemostatic mechanisms of excessive menstrual bleeding. Journal of the Irish Colleges of Physicians and Surgeons (in press)

Smith S K, Abel M H, Kelly R W, Baird D T 1981a Prostaglandin synthesis in the endometrium of women with ovular dysfunctional uterine bleeding. British Journal of Obstetrics and Gynaecology 88: 434

Smith S K, Kelly R W, Abel M H, Baird D T 1981b A role for prostacyclin (PGI$_2$) in excessive menstrual bleeding. Lancet 1: 522

van Eijkeren M A, Christiaens G C M L, Genze J J, Haspels A A, Sixma J J 1990 Morphology of menstrual hemostasis in essential menorrhagia (in press)

Willman E A, Collins W P, Clayton S G 1976 Studies on the involvement of prostaglandins in uterine symptomatology and pathology. British Journal of Obstetrics and Gynaecology 83: 337

11. Endometrial hyperplasia

Alex Ferenczy   Christine Bergeron

INTRODUCTION

The morphological diagnosis of endometrial hyperplasias has been more of a nightmare than a pleasure in diagnostic gynaecological pathology and, for all practical purposes, only a handful of experts can claim to be able to diagnose endometrial hyperplasia with consistent accuracy. This difficulty in histological diagnosis is the fundamental reason for our fragmentary knowledge of the natural history of endometrial hyperplasias, particularly with respect to their pathogenic development, interrelationship and association with carcinoma of the endometrium (Welch & Scully 1977, Fox & Buckley 1982, Ferenczy 1988, Silverberg 1988). Because of lack of consensus as to the risk of carcinoma, the management of endometrial hyperplasias has not been standardized and has ranged from hormonal therapy to hysterectomy, depending on the concept a given institution has adopted.

Histologically, the endometrium is indeed a complex tissue system (Ferenczy 1987). In addition to being a target for sex steroids (Shyamala & Ferenczy 1981) and various peptides (i.e. epidermal growth factor, insulin-related growth factors, etc.; Murphy et al 1987, Reynolds et al 1990), it is very susceptible to artefacts due to delayed fixation or inappropriate tissue sampling. For example, poor fixation may lead to autolytic changes and hence poor cutting and staining, whereas poor handling of the tissue may result in compression artefacts. These alterations in turn may mimic hyperplasia or well-differentiated adenocarcinoma (Table 11.1). On the other hand, perfectly fixed and prepared material may contain glands with only subtle cytological changes yet extensively involving either the endometrial stroma or the myometrium. Inconsistent diagnostic terms have also contributed to the poor understanding of endometrial hyperplasia (Winkler et al 1984). Pathologists differ in their use of names and morphological criteria for diagnosing hyperplasias and their subsets (Bhagavan et al 1984); even those who use similar histological terms disagree on their respective clinical significance (Winkler et al 1984). On the other hand, many clinicians often feel obliged to remove the uterus irrespective of the presumed natural history of a given type of hyperplastic endometrium.

Table 11.1   Mimics of hyperplasia and neoplasia of the endometrium

---

Basalis endometrium
Lower uterine segment endometrium
Proliferative/early secretory endometrium with compression or cracking artefacts
Endometrial polyps
Menstrual phase endometrium
Metaplasia
   Tubal
   Ciliated
   Squamous
   Oncocytic

Inconsistency of histological diagnosis of endometrial hyperplasia has led to inappropriate interpretation of, and discrepancies in, clinical studies (Welch & Scully 1977, Ferenczy 1988, Silverberg 1988). For example, while Bechner et al (1985) found that only 21% of their 150 cases of endometrial carcinomas had coexistent hyperplasia, others reported a 100% coexistence rate (Bhagavan et al 1984). The same phenomenon is observed in prospective studies addressing the issue of the malignant potential of hyperplasias. This ranged, for 'adenomatous' hyperplasia, from 12 to 27% (Gusberg & Kaplan 1963), and for 'atypical' hyperplasia from 14% (Chamlian & Taylor 1970) to 100% (Wentz 1974).

The difficulty of diagnosing endometrial hyperplasias histologically has been compounded by lack of statistically meaningful long-term longitudinal studies on patients with endometrial hyperplasia without disturbing their biological behaviour. In most reports, patients with endometrial hyperplasia presented with symptoms of abnormal uterine bleeding for which a dilatation and curettage were performed to rule out carcinoma (Gusberg et al 1974). Endometrial curettage under general anaesthesia often removes the abnormal endometrium, providing not only diagnosis but treatment as well. In other instances, the most abnormal area may be missed by the first curettage but discovered later and interpreted as 'hyperplasia progressed to carcinoma'. Other pitfalls of earlier prospective studies included hysterectomy soon (1 week to 1 year) after the original diagnosis, the use of ionizing radiotherapy to control uterine bleeding (Hertig & Sommers 1949), exogenous oestrogenic therapy (Kurman et al 1985), small number of patients (Gusberg et al 1974), premenopausal women with polycystic ovary syndrome (Chamlian & Taylor 1970), and only two groups of investigators ever illustrated histologically the lesions they were following on a prospective basis (Sherman & Brown 1979, Kurman et al 1985).

Radiation has been proved to be carcinogenic to the endometrium, whilst patients with the polycystic ovary syndrome have a genetic background with metabolic aberrations and a predisposition for developing endometrial hyperplasia and carcinoma. Clearly, these patients are not comparable with postmenopausal women without a history of chronic anovulation and the polycystic ovary syndrome.

Despite the innumerable flaws in studies of a prospective, retrospective and coexistent nature, a concept has developed according to which most, if not all, endometrial carcinomas arise from pre-existing fields of hyperplasia (Hertig & Sommers 1949). As a result, hyperplasia has been considered to be a pre-cancerous condition, although carcinoma risk has been suspected to be related to the degree of atypia present in a given hyperplasia. For example, hyperplasia with cytological atypia was considered to be 'biologically closer' to carcinoma than its non-atypical variant. However, since hyperplasia without atypia presumably preceded atypia, both conditions were considered carcinoma precursor lesions and formed a biologic continuum. According to the continuum concept, simple exaggeration of the normal proliferative state (anovulatory endometrium) progresses gradually to a highly atypical form of hyperplasia, to carcinoma in situ and, at the end of the spectrum, to overt invasion (Hertig & Sommers, 1949, Kurman et al 1985, Silverberg 1988).

In recent years attempts have been made to classify histologically and clinically this spectrum of hyperplasia into more homogenous and relevant categories with respect to their diagnosis and management (Colgan et al 1983, Fox 1984, Ausems et al 1985, Kurman et al 1985, Ferenczy & Bergeron 1989). The results of these laboratory and clinical studies have challenged the continuum concept originally suggested by Cullen in 1900 (Cullen 1900). Indeed, it appears today that the risk of progression to endometrial carcinoma is neither uniform nor even gradually increasing in women with hyperplasia, rather it is concentrated in those women with hyperplasia in which there is significant cytological atypia. In this chapter, we review the evidence that supports the two-disease hyperplasia and neoplasia concept in favour of the hyperplasia to neoplasia continuum concept. It will be shown that the revised concept has important implications for both the pathologist and the clinician, making diagnostic and treatment decisions more accurate and, hopefully, reproducible.

LABORATORY EVIDENCE

Histologically endometrial proliferations devoid of cytological atypia contain a variety of architectural alterations of endometrial glands that range from simple to complex. The former is by far the most common form of hyperplasia, and its overall architecture deviates little from normal proliferative endometrium. The glands vary in size: many are voluminous, others are dilated, others are normal or even small (Figs 11.1A and 11.2B). The lining epithelium is usually formed of tall and columnar cells with regular nuclear pseudostratification (Fig. 11.2) or, in cystic dilated glands, flat cuboidal cells. The ratio of stroma to glands is within normal limits because the stroma is also hyperplastic, and usually hypercellular. The gland cells lack cytologic atypia; mitoses are numerous and normal and are present both in the epithelial and stromal cells. Unlike in normal, cyclical

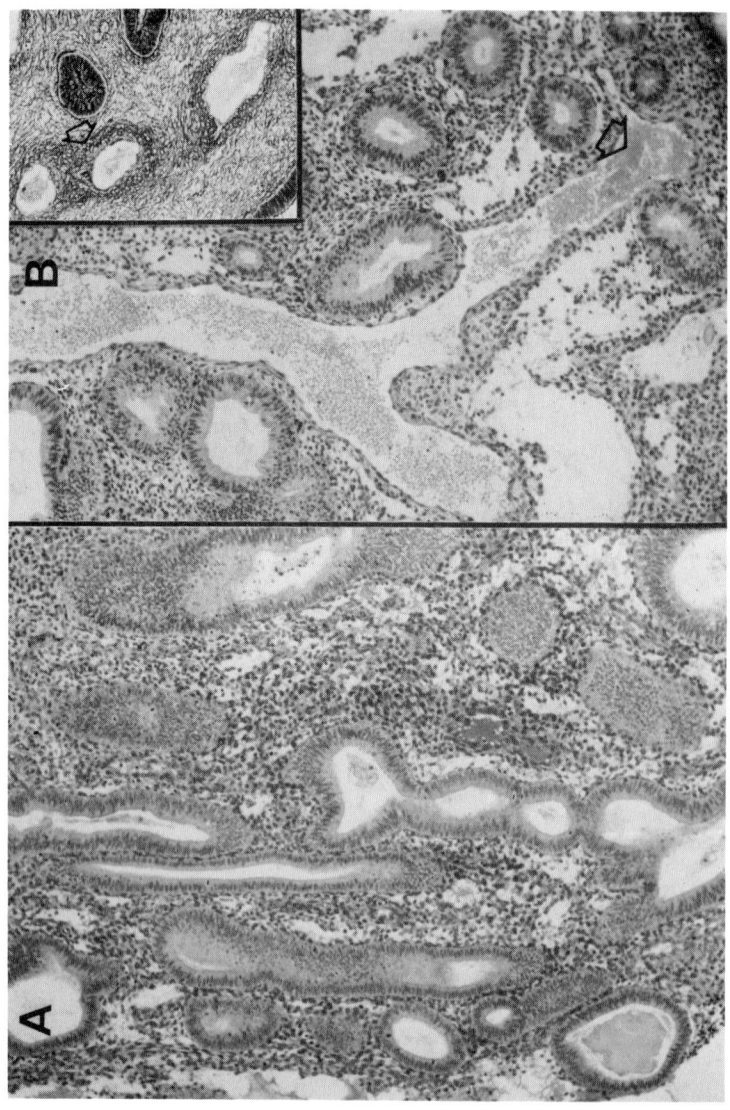

Fig. 11.1 Endometrial simple hyperplasia. **A** Voluminous glands supported by a compact stroma. The gland–stroma ratio is normal and architecturally, the glands deviate little from normal (H & E, × 100). **B** Dilated venous channel with early thrombus (arrow) (H & E, × 100). Inset: ectatic vessels with pericytic thickening (arrow) (Weigert elastic stain, × 100). (Reproduced with permission from Ferenczy 1982.)

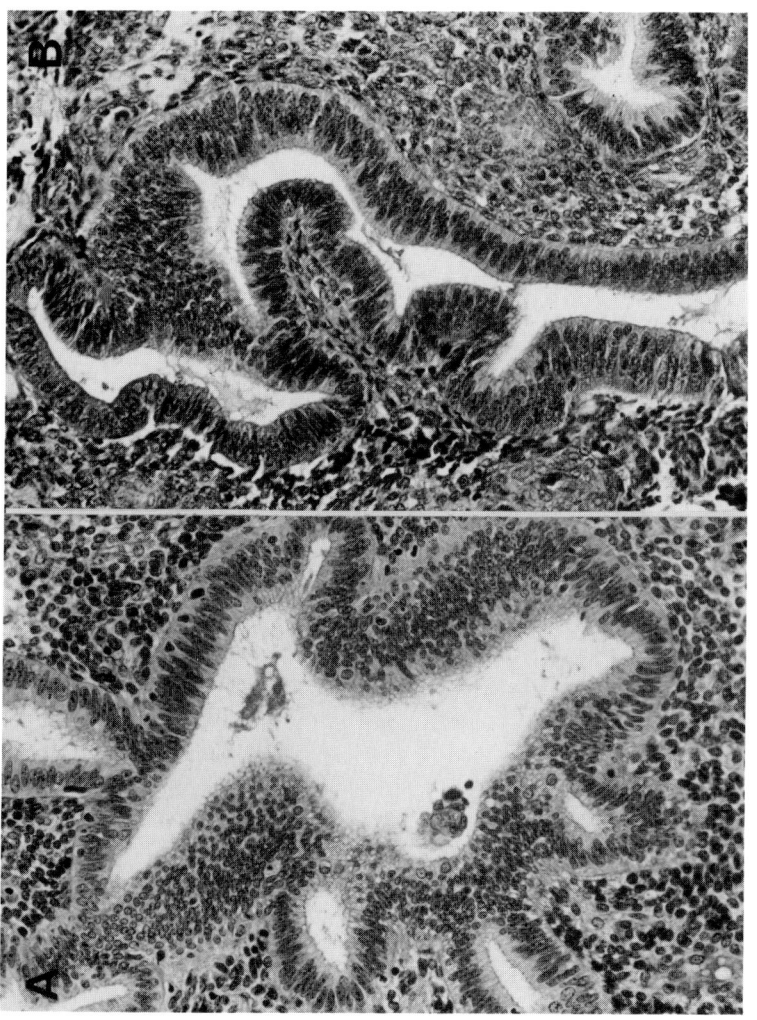

Fig. 11.2 Endometrial simple hyperplasia. **A** Hyperplastic gland with epithelial buddings into lumen and stroma. Note the pencil-shaped nuclei in surrounding compact stroma (H & E, × 380). **B** Voluminous gland lined by tall columnar cells in which nuclear pseudostratification is regular (H & E, × 300). (Reproduced with permission from Ferenczy 1982.)

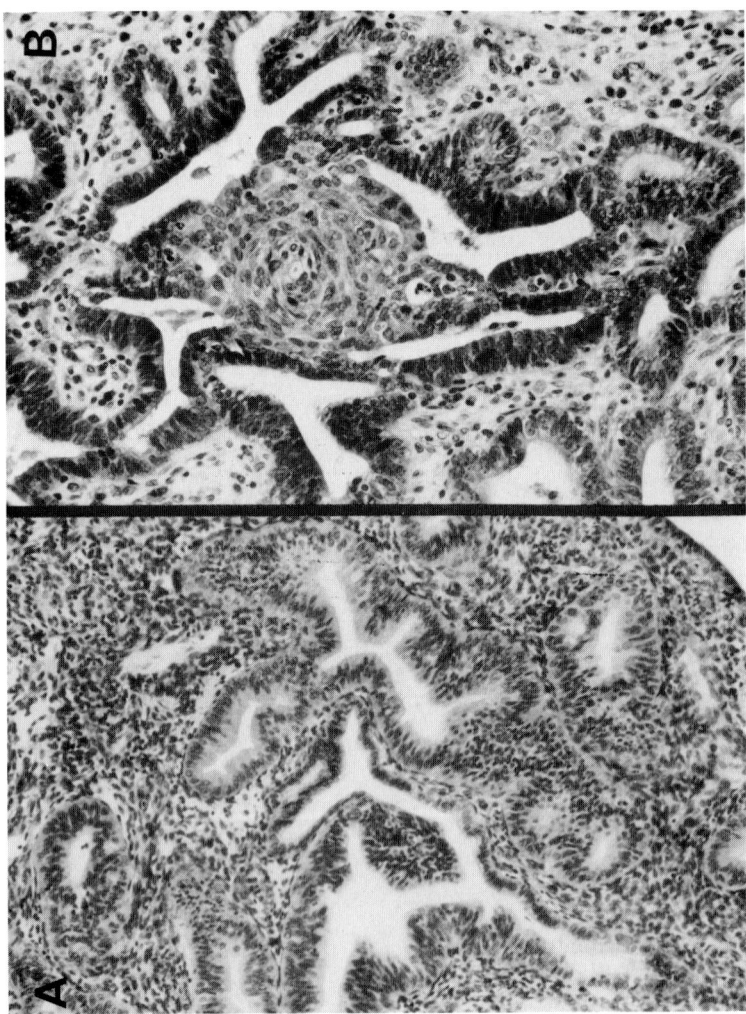

Fig. 11.3 Endometrial complex hyperplasia. **A** Glands are complex in their configuration and are in close relationship to each other. Epithelial buddings into the stroma and glandular lumen are frequent, as is Y-shaped gland pattern (H & E, × 100). **B** Hyperplastic glands devoid of cytological atypia are interconnected by squamous morule. This phenomenon should not be confused with adenocarcinoma with squamous differentiation (adenoacanthoma) (H & E, × 200). (Reproduced with permission from Ferenczy 1982.)

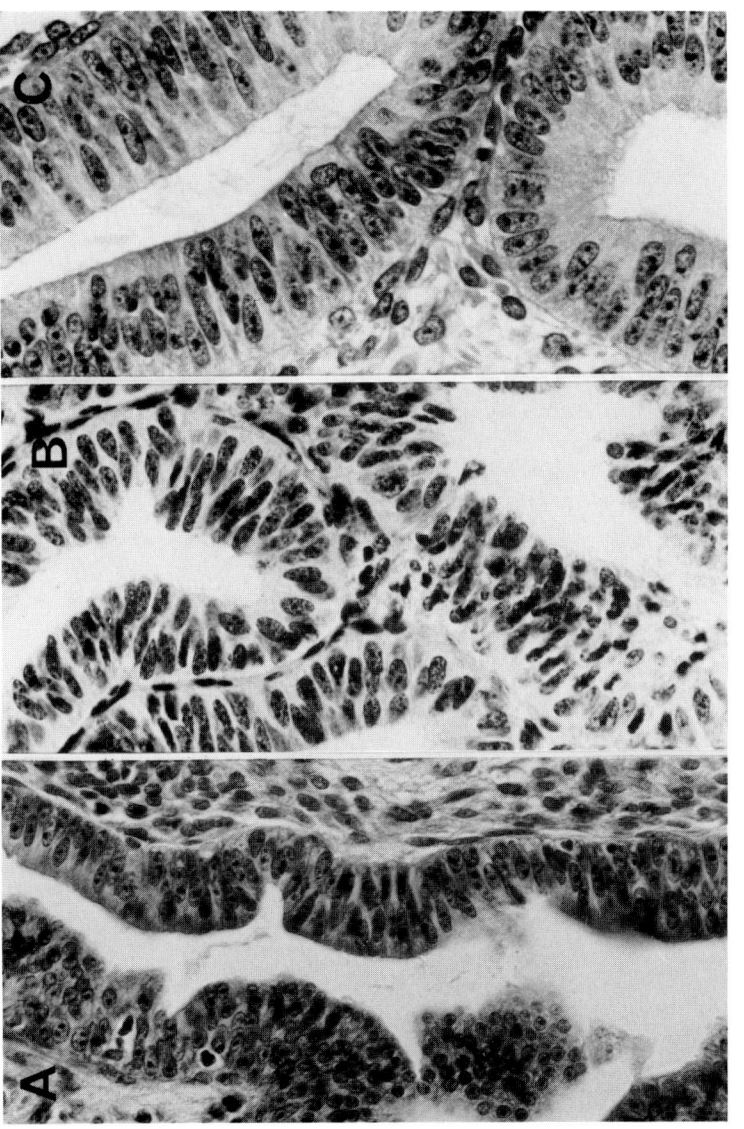

Fig. 11.4   Endometrial complex hyperplasia. **A** Detail of cytological presentations of gland lining cells. The commonest features of nuclear pseudostratification, regular nuclei, and enlarged nucleoli (H & E, × 400). **B** Tightly apposed glands with tall columnar cells and pencil-shaped nuclei arranged in a regular pseudostratified pattern (H & E, × 450). **C** Higher magnification of gland lining cells and their respective nuclei (H & E, × 550). (Reproduced with permission from Ferenczy 1982.)

proliferative endometrium, in this form of hyperplasia the stroma often contains numerous ectatic, often thrombosed vascular channels (Fig. 11.1B, inset). These lesions have traditionally been called anovulatory, persistent proliferative endometrium, cystic glandular hyperplasia or mild hyperplasia (Hertig & Sommers 1949, Beutler et al 1963, Vellios 1972, Gusberg et al 1974, Welch & Scully 1977, Tavassoli & Kraus 1978, Fox & Buckley 1982, Ferenczy 1983).

Most recently, the term simple hyperplasia was proposed by the International Society of Gynecologic Pathologists (Silverberg 1988), in its classification of endometrial hyperplasias into:

- Simple
- Complex
- Atypical.

The terms adenomatous hyperplasia, moderate hyperplasia, adenomatoid hyperplasia (Fox & Buckley 1982), cystic and adenomatous hyperplasia, slight atypical hyperplasia, glandular hyperplasia (Hertig & Sommers 1949, Beutler et al 1963, Welch & Scully 1977, Hendrickson & Kempson 1980, Ferenczy 1983) refer to voluminous glands with complex convolutions and epithelial buddings into the adjacent stroma (Fig. 11.3). The newly proposed term by ISGP to replace these names (representing a relatively rare form of endometrial hyperplasia), is *complex hyperplasia*. It is pertinent to point out that the epithelium of glands in complex hyperplasia, as in its simple counterpart, is composed tall columnar cells with regular pseudo-nuclear stratification devoid of atypia (Fig. 11.4). From a cytological point of view, the gland cells in both simple and complex hyperplasia are closely similar to those found in mid to late cyclical proliferative endometrium. In contrast to simple hyperplasia, the complex variant contains less stroma (Figs 11.3 and 11.4).

Simple and complex hyperplasias contrast with endometrial prolifer-ations in which glandular cells show nuclear enlargement, rounding, pleomorphism, loss of polarity, and clumped or coarse nuclear chromatin with macronucleoli (Fig. 11.5). The cytoplasm may be reduced or relatively abundant with a clear granular appearance and sometimes may be eosino-philic. These alterations in cytologic patterns are accompanied by glandular alterations as well, which include crowding of glands with 'back-to-back' pattern and intraluminal tufting without stromal support (Fig. 11.6A), which when fused together produce a cribriform or 'gland-in-gland' pattern (Fig. 11.6B). Intraluminal or intraepithelial inflammatory exudate as well as intraluminal epithelial or foam cells may be present (Fig. 11.6A). The stroma/gland ratio is usually low. While endometrial hyperplasia without cellular atypia tends to be diffuse, glands lined by atypical cells are always focal, although they may have a multifocal distribution in the endometrial mucosa. A plethora of names has been used for cytologically atypical endometrial lesions, including adenomatous hyperplasia (Winkler et al

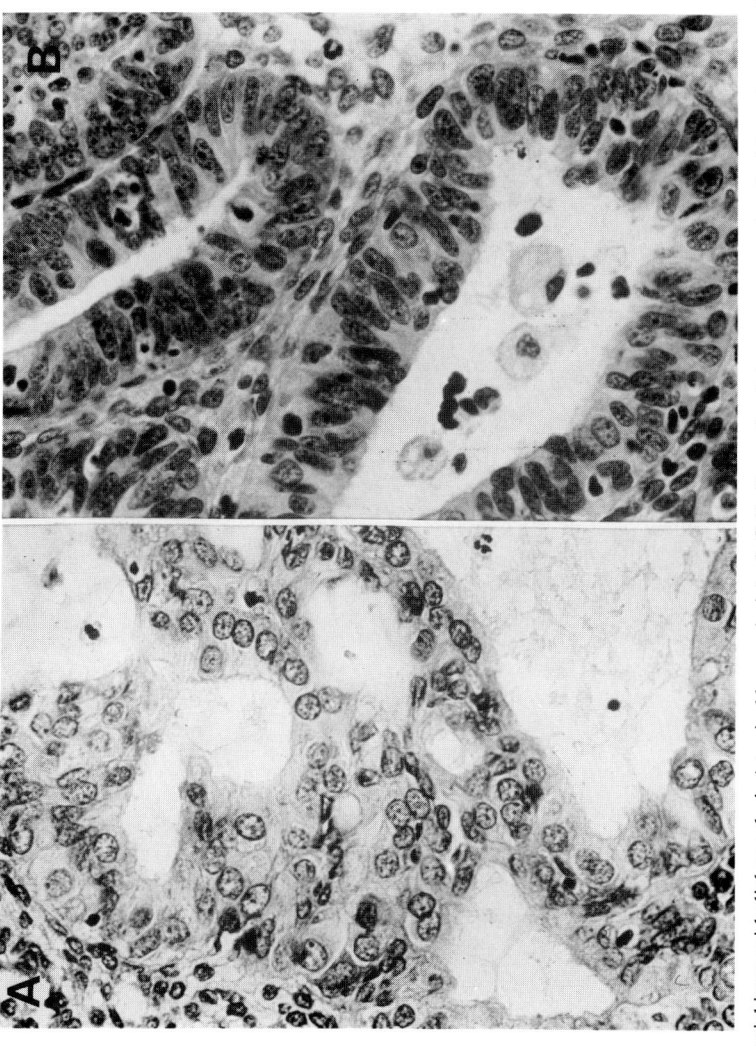

Fig. 11.5   Endometrial intraepithelial neoplasia (atypical hyperplasia).   **A** Cribriform glandular pattern associated with nuclear rounding, pleomorphism, loss of pseudostratification of nuclei in gland cells. The cytoplasm is pale, eosinophilic and abundant (H & E, × 850).   **B** There is significant cytologic atypia of gland lining cells. Nuclear pseudostratification is less regular than in hyperplasia without cytologic atypia and there is nuclear rounding, hyperchromasia with coarse chromatin, apoptosis, and the nucleoli are enlarged. Intraluminal foam cells are seen (H & E, × 800). (Reproduced with permission from Ferenczy 1982.)

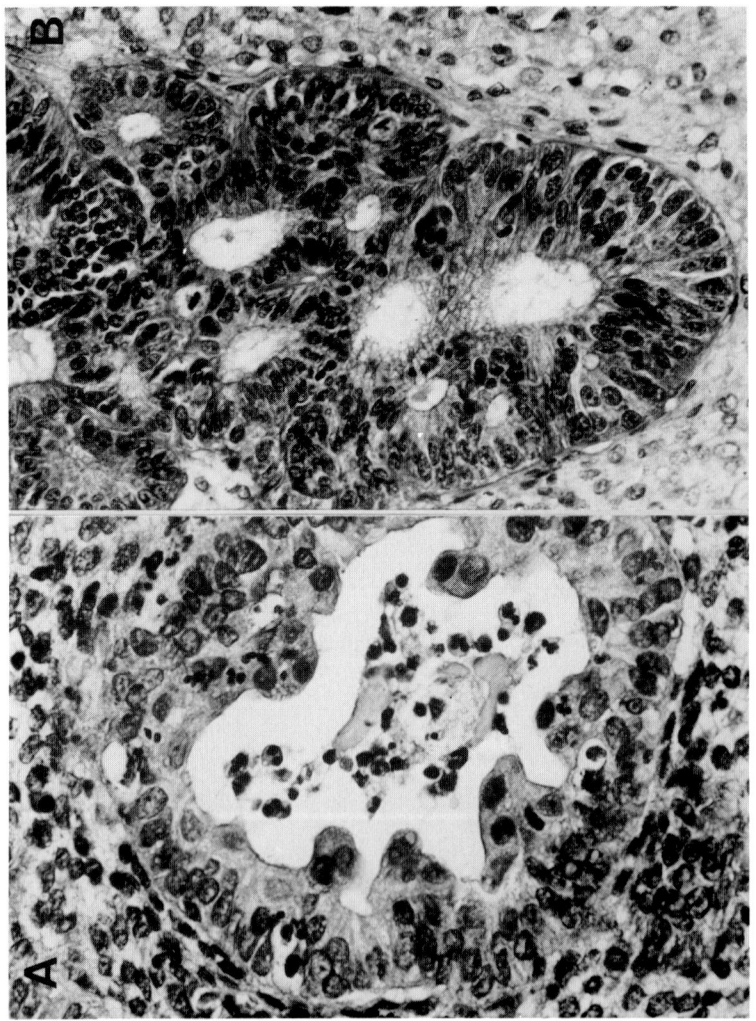

Fig. 11.6 Endometrial intraepithelial neoplasia (atypical hyperplasia). **A** Intraluminal papillary projections are associated with nuclear atypia and intraepithelial and intraluminal acute inflammatory exudate (H & E, × 800). **B** Cribriform glandular pattern associated with nuclear pleomorphism, hyperchromasia, macronucleoli and mitosis (H & E, × 350). (Reproduced with permission from Ferenczy 1982.)

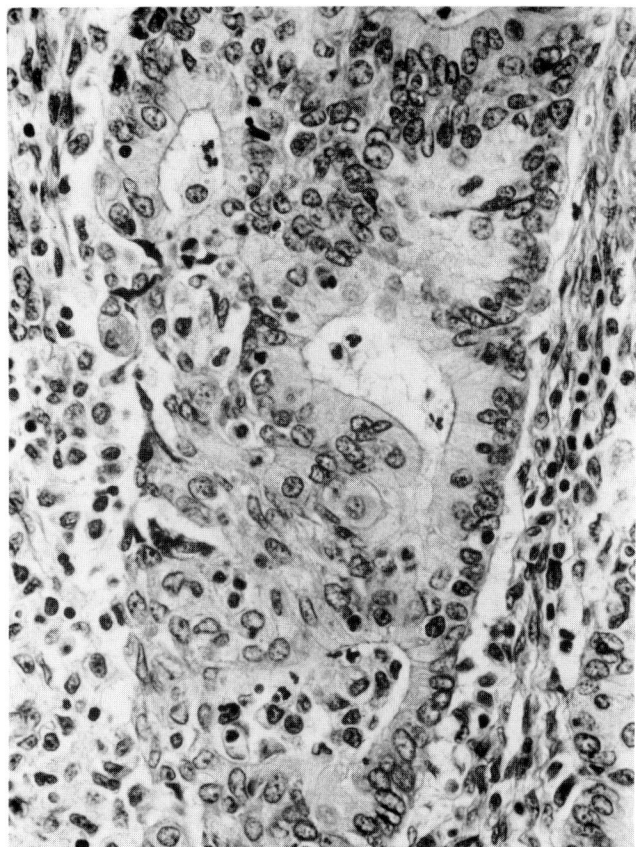

Fig. 11.7 Well-differentiated adenocarcinoma of the endometrium. Invasion of the stroma is evidenced by ragged outline of neoplastic gland cells (left) and an inflammatory stromal response (H & E, × 250). (Reproduced with permission from Ferenczy & Bergeron 1989.)

1984), atypical adenomatous hyperplasia, severe hyperplasia, glandular hyperplasia with cellular atypia, atypical complex hyperplasia, marked hyperplasia and carcinoma in situ (Hertig & Sommers 1949, Beutler et al 1963, Vellios 1974, Gusberg et al 1974, Welch & Scully 1977, Tavassoli & Kraus 1978, Fox & Buckley 1982, Ferenczy 1983, Kurman et al 1985). The International Society of Gynecologic Pathologists classified this rather infrequent lesion as atypical hyperplasia. The cytological pattern of atypical hyperplasia is closely similar to well-differentiated adenocarcinoma (Fig. 11.7).

Epithelial proliferations with cytological atypia that have become invasive represent adenocarcinoma, though it is often difficult to determine whether a carcinoma is genuinely invasive (Hendrickson et al 1983). In our opinion, carcinoma that invades the stroma (intraendometrial adenocarcinoma) (Fox & Buckley 1982) usually replaces large portions of pre-

Table 11.2   Morphological hallmarks of endometrial hyperplasia without (endometrial hyperplasia) and with cytological atypia (endometrial intraepithelial neoplasia)

	Endometrial hyperplasia	Endometrial intraepithelial neoplasia
Back to back glands	Rarely	Yes
Cribriform pattern, intraluminal epithelial projections	No	Yes
Regular nuclear pseudostratification of gland cells	Yes	No
Nuclear rounding, pleomorphism, hypochromasia, macronucleoli, intracellular–glandular inflammatory exudate	No	Yes

existing stroma; or the glands have ragged contours and extensive papillary pattern; or the glands are associated with a desmoplastic, inflammatory or necrotic reaction of the invaded stromal tissue; or combinations of these features may be present (Fig. 11.7) (Hendrickson & Kempson 1980, Kurman & Norris 1982, Silverberg 1988). These histological criteria delineate biologically significant lesions with a greater likelihood of metastasis than those in which invasion is absent. In our opinion, intraluminal epithelial bridging and acute inflammatory exudate within the gland cells or glandular lumens are features that may be seen in intraepithelial as well as intraendometrial/mucosal neoplasia (Fox & Buckley 1982) of the endometrium. As such they are not specific features of either of these entities. Table 11.2 details the morphological markers that are useful to distinguish hyperplasia without cytological atypia from its atypical counterpart.

Among the many experimental laboratory methods employed to give insight into the subclassification of endometrial hyperplasias, morphometry has provided the most consistent criteria for discriminating between histologically and clinically distinct lesions. Morphometry uses quantitative cytomorphology, which allows semi-objective assessment of a variety of morphological features and has increasingly been applied to diagnostic pathology (Baak et al 1988, Norris et al 1989) (see Ch. 2). Stereological features and nuclear parameters have been measured so that one lesion can be compared with another. The most consistent stereological discriminating parameters in the endometrium are the volume percentage of the epithelium and of the glands and the inner surface density of the glands (Baak et al 1988). The most consistent nuclear discriminating parameters are the mean and standard deviation of the longest nuclear axis, nuclear area and nuclear perimeter (Table 11.3) (Colgan et al 1983, Ausems et al 1985, Fu et al 1988, Baak et al 1988, Norris et al 1989). These parameters best express the degree of dispersion which on histology correspond to large and pleomorphic nuclei (Fig. 11.5). Hyperplasias without cytologic atypia contain morphometric discrimination parameters closer to normal than

Table 11.3 Biomorphological characteristics of endometrial hyperplasia without (endometrial hyperplasia) and with cytologic atypia (endometrial intraepithelial neoplasia)

	Endometrial hyperplasia	Endometrial intraepithelial neoplasia
Volume percentage epithelium	20	60
Standard deviation of nuclear area	10	15
Standard deviation of nuclear perimeter	3	4
DNA S-phase duration	Short	Prolonged
Potential doubling time	Short	Prolonged
Nuclear organizer region epithelial/ stromal ratio	1.5	2.5
Intracellular organelles	Uniform	Pleomorphic
Cell/nuclear membranes	Regular	Irregular
Cilia	Many	Few

invasive carcinoma, while those with cytological atypia tend to resemble carcinomas. In one study, 95% of 39 cases of hyperplasia were correctly correlated with the histological diagnosis (Norris et al 1989); in another (Colgan et al 1983), nuclear morphometry predicted progression of hyperplasia with cytological atypia to carcinoma with 80% accuracy, and in yet another, 8 of 42 (17%) cases progressed to carcinoma (Ausems et al 1985). It should be mentioned, however, that in the latter study, many cases with similar morphometric values failed to progress to invasion, whereas on occasion lesions without significant deviation from normal did so (Ausems et al 1985).

Other techniques used measured DNA content by Feulgen microspectrophotometry and flow cytometry. The results obtained, however, failed to distinguish endometrial proliferations with or without invasive potential (Feichter et al 1982, Iversen 1986, Lindahl et al 1987). Unlike nuclear aneuploidy found in pre-cancerous and cancerous conditions, most well-differentiated endometrial adenocarcinoma cells, as well as their precursors, contain diploid or near diploid nuclear DNA in all respects similar to that found in normal or hyperplastic gland cells (Feichter et al 1982, Iversen 1986, Lindahl et al 1987). The apparently 'normal' DNA content of invasive and non-invasive endometrial neoplasia is typical of sex-steroid target organs, including the breast (Trent 1985) and prostate (Stephenson et al 1987) and may correspond to subtle numerical (trisomy 1q or 10) rather than structural alterations of the chromosomes (Gibas & Rubin 1987). The clinical implication of diploid carcinomas lies in their favourable prognosis in comparison with those with aneuploid DNA values (Friedlander et al 1983). Histologically, nuclear diploidy produces normo- and often hypochromasia of nuclei on haematoxylin and eosin sections, making distinction between exuberant hyperplasia and early, well-differentiated adenocarcinoma difficult on the basis of the appearance of nuclear chromatin alone.

The available and pertinent laboratory data indicate that gland cells in hyperplasia with and without cytological atypia are different cell populations. The former is correlated with cytological alterations that are found in invasive carcinoma, whereas the latter is present in glandular structures which have simply increased in the amount or volume compared with normal, cyclical proliferative endometrium. It follows that if cytological atypia distinguishes carcinoma precursors (intraepithelial neoplasia) from non-precursors (hyperplasia) then lesions with and without atypia should be named differently to emphasize their different morphology and, as a corollary, different clinical behaviour. Lesions without atypia are best referred to as endometrial hyperplasia, and we prefer the unifying generic term endometrial intraepithelial neoplasia for lesions with significant cytological atypia. Thus we propose classification as follows:

- Endometrial hyperplasia
- Endometrial intraepithelial neoplasia
- Invasive carcinoma.

According to the intraepithelial concept in general, the term neoplasia is not synonymous with invasive carcinoma but corresponds to lesions that tend to persist rather than spontaneously regress, and in contrast to hyperplasia, if untreated, tend to recur after conservative treatment and may progress to carcinoma.

Most recently using the argyrophil method, nucleolar organizer regions have been evaluated in the nuclei of endometrial hyperplasia and carcinoma (Wilkinson et al 1990, Coumbe et al 1990). Nuclear organizer regions are loops of DNA which transcribe to ribosomal RNA and are increased in number in hyperplasia and neoplasia. In one study the highest epithelial nuclear organizer region counts were found in normal, cyclical proliferative endometrium and invasive carcinoma, correlating with the high mitotic activity observed in these endometria (Wilkinson et al 1990). In another work, however, focusing on the mean nuclear organizer region score (ratio), no significant difference was found between hyperplasia with and without architectural atypia, whereas the ratios observed in hyperplasia with atypia and invasive carcinoma were significantly different from hyperplasia without atypia (Table 11.3) (Coumbe et al 1990).

The DNA S-phase duration and potential doubling time of gland cells in hyperplasia without cytological atypia were similar to those of proliferative endometrium by in vitro autoradiography using the nuclear protein precursor tritiated thymidine (Ferenczy 1983). These kinetic characteristics were significantly longer in cytologically atypical lesions, including invasive carcinoma, than in hyperplasia without atypia. Prolongation of the DNA S-phase of the cell cycle and potential doubling time are characteristic cytokinetic features of both intraepithelial and invasive neoplasia at large. Unfortunately, autoradiography is not practical for routine diagnostic pathology for it requires fresh, unfixed specimens and requires short-term

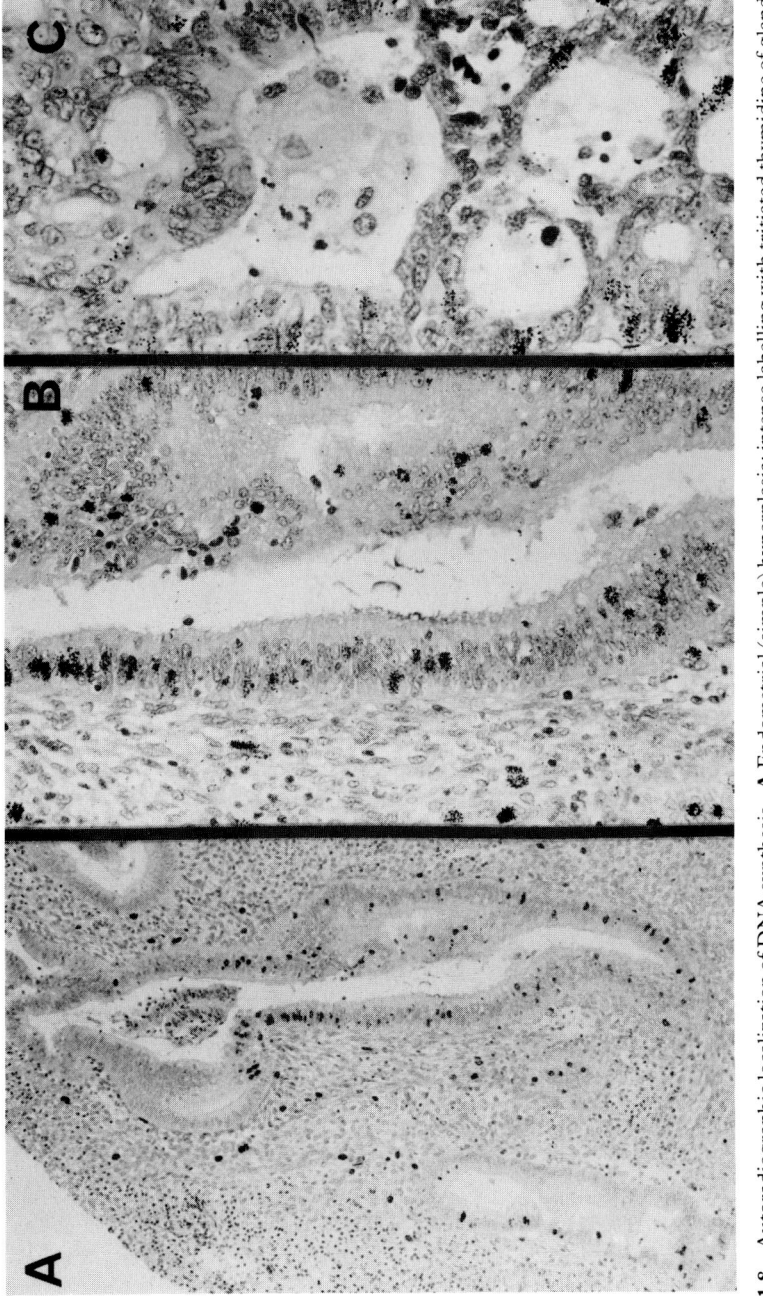

Fig. 11.8 Autoradiographic localization of DNA synthesis. **A** Endometrial (simple) hyperplasia: intense labelling with tritiated thymidine of gland lining cells and adjacent stromal fibroblasts (haematoxylin, × 80). **B** Detailed view of labelled gland and stromal cells (haematoxylin, × 250). **C** Endometrial intraepithelial neoplasia (atypical hyperplasia); nuclear labelling of gland cells is less conspicuous than in endometrial hyperplasia (haematoxylin, × 450). (Reproduced with permission from Ferenczy 1983.)

tissue cultures, radioactive isotopes and a dark-room for incubation of specimens (Fig. 11.8).

CLINICAL EVIDENCE

The only meaningful way to determine the biological behaviour of a presumed carcinoma precursor lesion would be to follow women with such lesions for a number of years and evaluate how many of them develop carcinoma. As suggested earlier, most prospective studies suffered from major pitfalls including inaccurate data analysis. Until 1980, only three prospective studies on postmenopausal women with hyperplasia of various degrees of morphological severity appeared with at least one year follow-up (Gusberg & Kaplan 1963, Wentz 1974, Sherman & Brown 1979, Silverberg 1988). In these studies, progression rates to carcinoma were significantly higher, at 57–100%, in women with hyperplasia with cytological atypia ('atypical hyperplasia, CIS'; Wentz 1974, Sherman & Brown 1979) than at 12–27%, in women with hyperplasia without atypia, ('adenomatous hyperplasia'; Gusberg & Kaplan 1963, Wentz 1974). Unfortunately, in only one of these three reports were the lesions illustrated.

Since 1985, two prospective studies of women with bleeding from hyperplasia have been published; follow-up was over 1.0–26.7 years. Ferenczy & Bergeron (1989) observed progression of hyperplasia to carcinoma in 33% of women with cytological atypia but in none of the women without cellular atypia; Kurman et al (1985), in contrast, observed progression to carcinoma in 37 and 4%, respectively. In the series of Kurman et al the exceptions to progression were two premenopausal women with polycystic ovary syndrome. In these women, endometrial hyperplasia without atypia 'progressed' to carcinoma. However, one of the two patients actually developed endometrial hyperplasia with cytological atypia before progressing to cancer; in the other patient, the slides were not available to review. Also, these women were suspected to be genetically and metabolically predisposed to developing carcinoma of the endometrium as a result of chronic anovulation (Fechner et al 1979). In a previous prospective study of women aged 35 years and younger with anovulation and cyto-logically atypical hyperplasia, a 14% progression rate to carcinoma was reported after follow-up over 14 years (Chamlian & Taylor 1970). Ad-mittedly, these women were strikingly different from their postmenopausal counterparts without a history of chronic anovulation with respect to their predisposition to endometrial carcinoma. Of great interest were the findings of prospective studies by Koss et al (1981, 1984). In their prospective studies, they found the same prevalence (9/1000) and incidence (9/1000) of hyperplasia and carcinoma in over 1000 asymptomatic, postmenopausal women followed for over 2 years. These observations are in great contrast to those reported for other carcinoma precursors in which invasive carcinomas are invariably less frequent than their pre-invasive variants (Koss et al

Table 11.4   Response, by morphology, to progestogenic therapy (data from Ferenczy & Gelfand 1989)

Cytological atypia	Complete response (%)
Yes	25
No	80

1981). Accordingly, the expected prevalence ratio is one carcinoma to nine precursors.

In addition to the progression rate differential in so-called hyperplasias with and without cytological atypia, their respective response to hormonal progestational therapy is also different (Wentz 1966, Eichner & Abellara 1971, Kurman et al 1985, Gal 1986, Ferenczy & Gelfand 1989). In a prospective study of postmenopausal women with histologically verified endometrial hyperplasia without atypia, secretory conversion and eventual atrophy have been observed in 80% of the 65 patients receiving progestogenic therapy (Table 11.4) (Ferenczy & Gelfand 1989). Others observed similar response rates to progestogens (Gal 1986, Kurman et al 1985). Most endometrial hyperplasias in patients who did not respond contained complex, glandular architecture (77%) compared with the responder group (13%) (Ferenczy & Gelfand 1989). Significantly, none of the 20% of 65 patients with persistent hyperplasia resistent to progestogen therapy progressed to carcinoma (see above; Ferenczy & Gelfand 1989).

In contrast to hyperplasia without atypia, the majority of women (15/20) with cytologically atypical lesions failed to respond to daily, relatively high doses of oral progestogenic therapy (Eichner & Abellara 1971, Kurman et al 1985, Ferenczy & Gelfand 1989). Even among those who initially responded to progestational agents, endometrial intraepithelial neoplasia tended to recur after therapy had been discontinued (Eichner & Abellara 1971, Ferenczy & Gelfand 1989).

The reason for progestogen-resistance of some hyperplasia and most endometrial intraepithelial neoplasia (Eichner & Abellara 1971, Gal 1986, Kurman et al 1985, Ferenczy & Gelfand 1989) is not clear. The major prerequisite for progestogen therapy is the presence of intranuclear progesterone receptors. Charcoal-coated binding assays (Shyamala & Ferenczy, 1981) and immunohistochemical studies (Bergeron et al 1988a) found high progesterone receptor concentrations in hyperplastic endometria (Fig. 11.9A), whereas in cytologically atypical lesions the levels were lower than in endometria (Fig. 11.9B) but above those found in invasive carcinoma. It is possible that progesterone receptors in cytologically atypical lesions are not functional, or that only a relatively small proportion of endometrial tissue contains high concentrations of progesterone receptors, or that progesterone receptors are concentrated in the stroma rather than the glandular epithelium. Indeed, progesterone receptors are predomi-

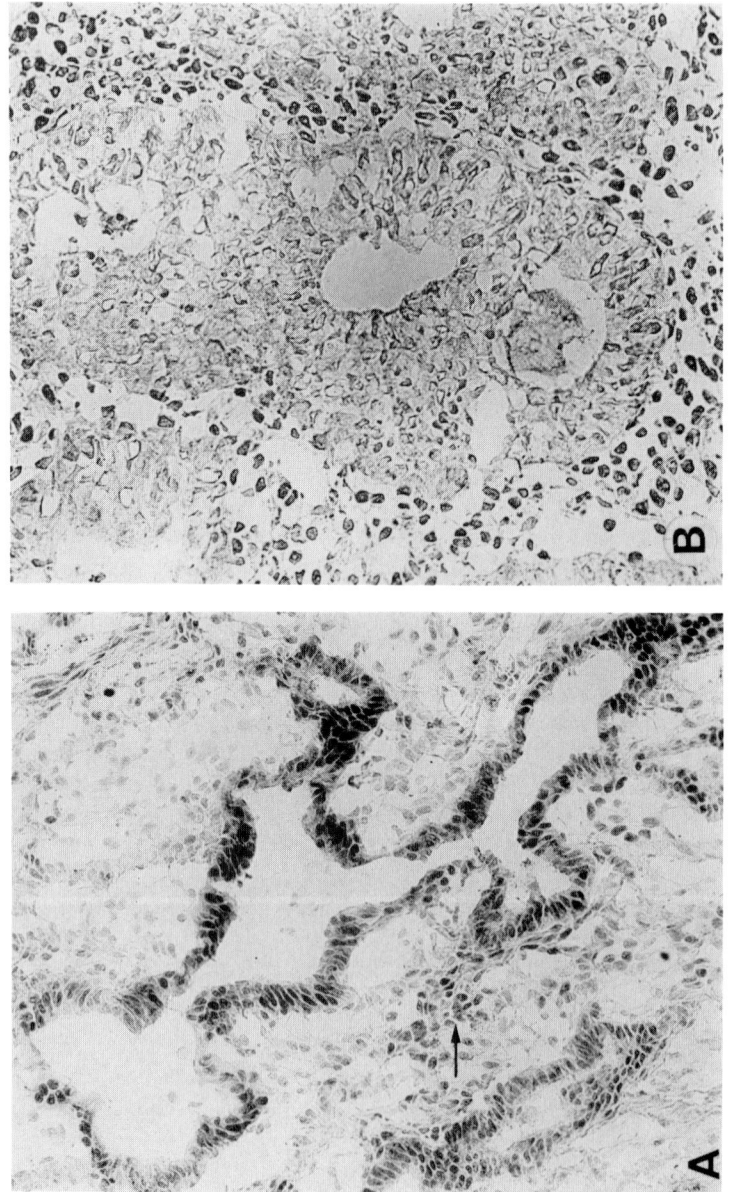

Fig. 11.9 Immunohistochemical localization of progesterone receptors. **A** Endometrial simple hyperplasia: intense nuclear staining reaction is observed in gland cells and stromal cells (arrow) (no counterstain, ×250). **B** Endometrial intraepithelial neoplasia (atypical hyperplasia): gland cells are devoid of staining reaction, whereas stromal cell nuclei stain strongly with antibody on progesterone receptor (no counterstain, ×450). (Reproduced with permission from Ferenczy & Bergeron 1989.)

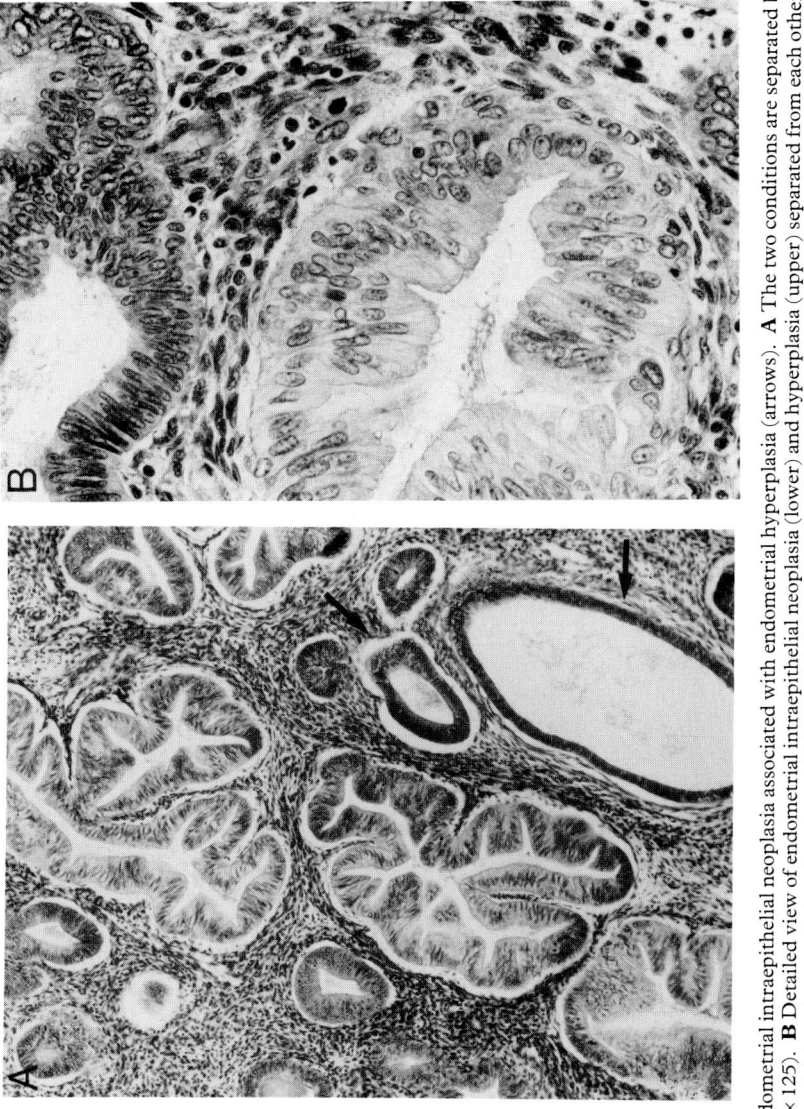

Fig. 11.10 Endometrial intraepithelial neoplasia associated with endometrial hyperplasia (arrows). **A** The two conditions are separated by intervening stroma (H & E, × 125). **B** Detailed view of endometrial intraepithelial neoplasia (lower) and hyperplasia (upper) separated from each other by fibrocellular stroma. The clear staining characteristics of endometrial intraepithelial neoplastic cells contrasts with the hyperchromatic but regularly arranged pencil-shaped nuclei of the adjacent hyperplasia (H & E, × 450). (Reproduced with permission from Ferenczy & Gelfand 1986.)

nantly found in the stroma of carcinoma precursors by immunohisto-chemistry (Bergeron et al 1988a), whereas in non-atypical hyperplastic endometrium, they are found both in the glands and the stroma (Fig. 11.9). Histologically, secretory differentiation in most glands with atypia and their supportive stroma is focal, partial and abortive, or only the stroma is decidualized, without secretory changes in the neighbouring endometrial glands of progestogen-resistant endometrial tissues.

RELATIONSHIP BETWEEN ENDOMETRIAL HYPERPLASIA AND NEOPLASIA

Coexistence of endometrial intraepithelial neoplasia and/or invasive carci-noma with hyperplasia in the same endometrium has been considered to be one of the most compelling pieces of evidence of a pathogenic continuum (Hertig & Sommers 1949, Beutler et al 1963, Gusberg & Kaplan 1963, Welch & Scully 1977, Tavassoli & Kraus 1978). However, this concept is not supported by either histological (Fig. 11.10) or immunohistochemical studies, in which virtually all cases of endometrial hyperplasia with coexistent intraepithelial or invasive neoplasia are distinct from each other and lack histological continuity (Bergeron et al 1988a,b). This is in contrast to the single-disease pathogenic concept according to which a direct histological interrelationship is demonstrable between invasive neoplasia and its non-invasive counterpart (Ferenczy & Winkler 1987, Dupont & Page 1985).

   The mechanism that operates in the development of both hyperplasia and endometrial interepithelial neoplasia/carcinoma in the same endometrium is not clear. In general, carcinogenesis requires initiation and promotion (potentiation) of cellular oncogenes in target cells. The initiator induces chromosomal alterations in the cells' nuclei which, if stimulated by a promoter, may develop into clinically overt cancer (Becker 1981). Initiators of human endometrial carcinogenesis other than ionizing radiation have not yet been identified (Lucas 1981, Satyaswaroop & Mortel 1981), but oestradiol and its receptors are considered potent promoters of endometrial proliferation (Clark et al 1985). Endometrial cells are heterogenous in their receptor content (Bergeron et al 1988a,b) and probably in their response to oncogenic stimulation and to sex-steroid promoters as well. The possibility is entertained that cells with the potential of 'cancer initiation' coexist with 'non-initiated' cells in the same endometrium in most women. The growth-promoting effect of oestradiol in the absence of (or failure to respond to) progestogenic growth inhibition may cause 'cancer-initiated' cells to develop into neoplasia, whilst their 'non-initiated' counterparts evolve into hyperplasia (Fig. 11.11). Such a phenomenon is particularly striking in didelphys uteri, in which one horn may show endometrial hyperplasia or atrophy and the other carcinoma (Eichner & Simak 1981). In tissue systems

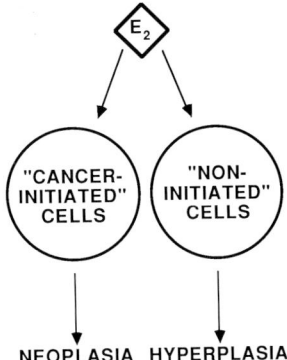

Fig. 11.11   Possible pathogenic mechanism of coexistent endometrial hyperplasia and neoplasia. Oestradiol (E_2), a potent growth promoter of endometrial epithelial cells, potentiates 'carcinoma-initiated' cells to develop into neoplasia, and 'non-initiated' cells to develop into hyperplasia. In such an endometrium, neoplasia coexists with hyperplasia. (Reproduced with permission from Ferenczy & Bergeron 1989.)

that are targets of steroid hormones, epithelial growth is dependent on mesenchymal support which in turn is influenced by sex-steroid hormones (Cunha et al 1983). Conversely, the epithelium controls the response of mesenchyme to these hormones by stimulating the function of appropriate receptors. The recently developed monoclonal antibodies to oestrogen receptor and progesterone receptor (King & Green 1984, Sullivan et al 1986) can trace sex-steroid receptors by immunohistochemistry and their relative distribution between the epithelium and the stroma can be evaluated as suggested earlier in this chapter. Both normal and hyperplastic endometria without cytological atypia display a high content of oestrogen receptor and progesterone receptor in the epithelium and the stroma on immunohistochemistry (Figs 11.9A and 11.12A) (Bergeron et al 1988a,b).

The results confirm the oestradiol-sensitivity of these tissues and suggest an intact oestrogen receptor mechanism. Their potential to respond to progesterone or progestogens is evidenced by their secretory differentiation on histology (Ferenczy & Gelfand 1989), high progesterone receptor concentrations, decrease in oestradiol-related ciliogenesis (Ferenczy & Richart 1974) and by the presence of oestradiol-induced growth factors in the stroma, including epidermal growth factor, β-transforming growth factor and insulin-like growth factor (Baird et al 1985, Murphy et al 1987). Although the presence of progesterone receptor in the stroma suggests the presence of functional oestrogen receptors and oestrogen sensitivity, progesterone receptor is only one measure of oestrogen action. The latter is better ascertained by measuring oestrogen-induced mitogenic action of the endometrial stroma. Presence of oestradiol induced growth factors in the stroma, including epidermal growth factor, β-transforming growth factor

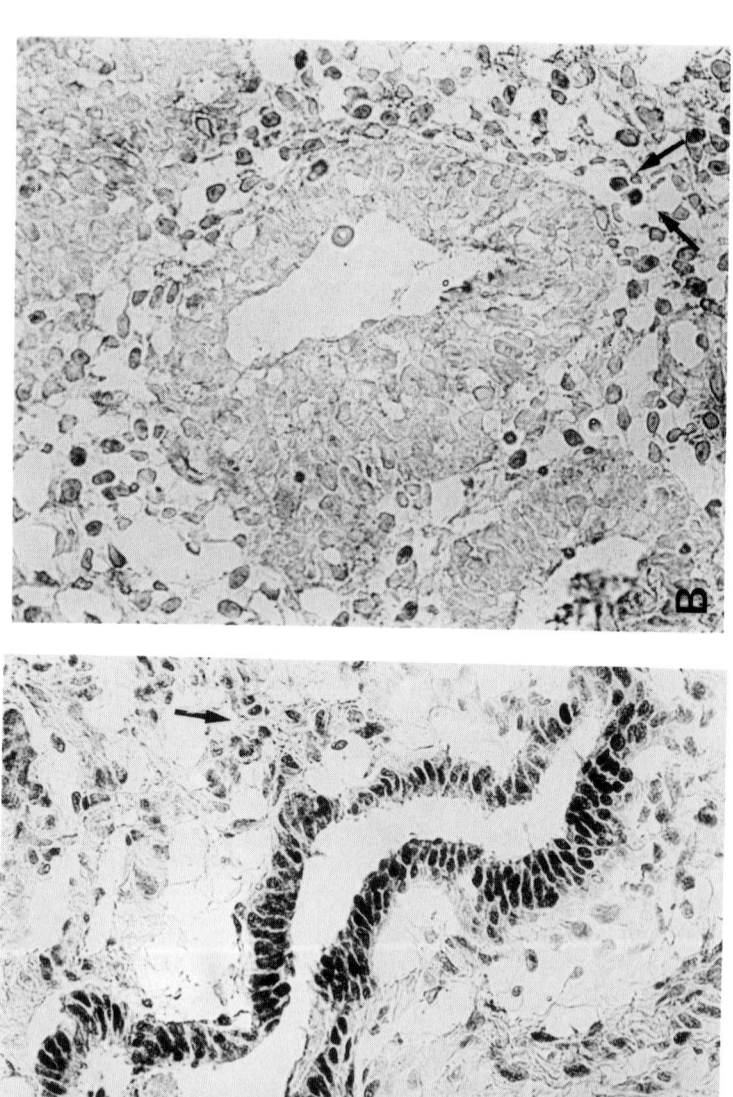

Fig. 11.12   Immunohistochemical localization of oestrogen receptors.   **A** Endometrial simple hyperplasia containing strong nuclear staining in both gland cells and stromal fibroblasts (arrow) (no counterstain, ×250).   **B** Endometrial intraepithelial neoplasia (atypical hyperplasia): gland cells are devoid of receptors in contrast to the strong nuclear staining reaction of stromal cells (arrows) (no counterstain, ×250). (Reproduced with permission from Ferenczy & Bergeron 1989.)

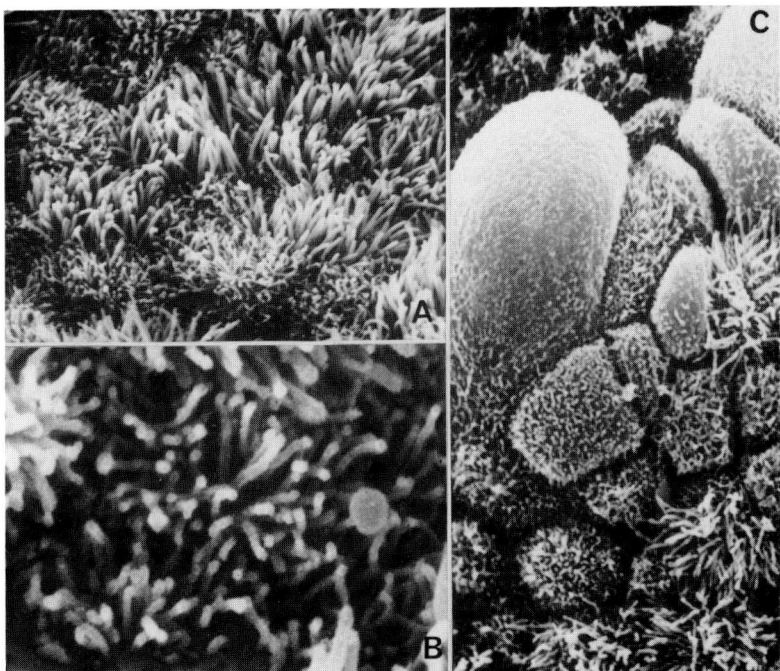

Fig. 11.13 Scanning electron microscopy of endometrial hyperplasia and intraepithelial neoplasia. **A** Endometrial simple hyperplasia: surface epithelial and gland cells contain numerous cilia (× 5600). **B** Non-ciliated cells have prominent surface microvilli (× 15 000). **C** Endometrial intraepithelial neoplasia (atypical hyperplasia): ciliated cells are fewer in number compared to hyperplastic endometrium, and non-ciliated cells have shorter surface microvilli. Cellular pleomorphism is evident (× 5000).

and insulin-like growth factor confirms that oestrogen receptors are functional (Baird et al 1985, Murphy et al 1987).

In contrast, endometria with cytologic atypia contain lower concentrations of oestrogen receptor and progesterone receptor in the epithelium (Figs 11.9B and 11.12B), and the levels are comparable to those of invasive carcinoma (Bergeron et al 1988a,b). Also, oestrogen-dependent ciliogenesis, microvilli and primary lysosomal activity are decreased and the nuclear membrane distended (Fig. 11.13). Interestingly, the oestrogen receptors and progesterone receptors in the stroma of cytologically atypical endometrial tissues, including invasive carcinoma, remain high. Whether oestrogen receptor and progesterone receptor play a role in mediating an oestradiol-dependent paracrine (extracellular) regulation of the epithelium as previously suggested remains to be determined.

That certain endometrial cancers are oestrogen-related is further substantiated by clinical observations. Typically, carcinomas that are associated with endometrial hyperplasia are seen in relatively young patients (less than 55 years old) with a hyperoestrogenic background, as evidenced by obesity and long-term oestrogen-only replacement therapy (Horwitz & Feinstein 1986). Typically also, these women have FIGO stage I, well-differentiated carcinomas with high oestrogen and progesterone receptor concentrations (Budwit-Novotny et al 1986, Bergeron et al 1988a,b). These carcinomas contrast with those discovered in elderly women whose meta-bolic background is consistent with hypo-oestrogenism as they tend to be under- rather than overweight and have never received oestrogen replace-ment therapy. Accordingly, there is atrophic rather than hyperplastic endometrium adjacent to poorly differentiated, progesterone receptor-poor carcinoma that has deep myometrial and vascular invasion (Budwit-Novotny et al 1986, Bergeron et al 1988a,b). These observations support the concept of two distinct pathogenic types of endometrial adenocarcinoma (Ober 1971, Boronow et al 1984, Deligdisch & Cohen 1985).

Recent reports have shown the effects of epidermal growth factor on the growth of endometrial cancer cell lines (Reynolds et al 1990) and the proliferative response of oestrogen-stimulated uterus associated with insulin-like growth factor I (Murphy et al 1987). The mitogenic activity of epidermal growth factor and insulin-like growth factor I is known to be mediated by receptors for these compounds. In the study by Berchuk et al (1989) and Reynolds et al (1990), epidermal growth factor receptors were found significantly less frequently in endometrial adenocarcinomas than in normal endometrium. The reason for this apparent loss of receptor by some tissues remains unclear and further studies are needed to clarify the factors that regulate expression of epidermal growth factor receptor in endometrial hyperplasia. In contrast, insulin-like growth factor I receptors were shown to be significantly 'up-regulated' in neoplastic endometrium (Talavera et al 1990). This suggests that progression of disease may be associated with insulin-like growth factor I stimulation. Whether there is a correlation between steroid receptors and insulin-like growth factor I receptor in endometrium remains to be determined. It is possible that the mitogenic activity of insulin-like growth factor I may also be influenced by oestrogen stimulation. Further studies are needed to understand this mechanism, but these observed differences in epidermal and insulin-like growth factor receptor expression in the endometrium may be involved in the deregulation of endometrial cell proliferation observed during its neoplastic growth.

THE TWO-DISEASE CONCEPT AND ITS CLINICAL IMPLICATIONS

The prerequisite for the appropriate management of diseases is their classification into reproducible subsets using clinically meaningful termin-ology (simple, complex, atypical; see p. 214). Based on the revised endo-metrial hyperplasia and neoplasia concept, it is proposed that hyperplasia is morphologically and clinically benign and has negligible, if any, carcinoma precursor potential (Ferenczy 1988). In contrast, endometrial intraepithelial neoplasia has morphological and clinical features similar to those of well-differentiated, invasive adenocarcinoma of the endometrium and is a significant precursor lesion. The single most important morphological feature distinguishing between hyperplasia and endometrial intraepithelial neoplasia is cellular atypia. It is hoped that the proposed classification (see p. 220) will lead to improved diagnostic accuracy and facilitate treatment decisions. Accordingly, the clinical response to the diagnosis of hyperplasia should consist of conservative, suppressive progestational therapy, whereas endometrial intraepithelial neoplasia is best managed by hysterectomy, provided the patient no longer desires to conceive and is not at significant surgical risk.

REFERENCES

Ausems E W M A, van der Kamp J-K, Baak J P A 1985 Nuclear morphometry in the determination of the prognosis of marked atypical endometrial hyperplasia. International Journal of Gynecological Pathology 4: 180–185

Baak J P A, Nauta J J P, Wisse-Bretelmans E C M, Bezemer P D 1988 Architectural and morphological features together are more important prognosticators in endometrial hyperplasias than nuclear morphological features alone. Journal of Pathology 154: 335–341

Baird A, Esch F, Mormede P et al 1985 Molecular characterization of fibroblast growth factor distribution and biological activities in various tissues. Recent Progress in Hormonal Research 42: 142–205

Bechner M E, Mori T, Silverberg S G 1985 Endometrial carcinoma: Nontumor factors in prognosis. International Journal of Gynecological Pathology 4: 131–145

Becker F F 1981 Recent concepts of initiation and promotion in carcinogenesis. American Journal of Pathology 105: 3–9

Berchuk A, Soisson A P, Olt G J et al 1989 Epidermal growth factor receptor expression in normal and malignant endometrium. American Journal of Obstetrics and Gynecology 161: 1247–1252

Bergeron C, Ferenczy A, Toft D O, Shyamala G 1988a Immunocytochemical study of progesterone receptors in hyperplastic and neoplastic endometrial tissues. Cancer Research 48: 6132–6136

Bergeron C, Ferenczy A, Shyamala G 1988b Distribution of estrogen receptors in various cell types of normal, hyperplastic and neoplastic endometrial tissues. Laboratory Investigation 58: 338–344

Beutler H K, Dockerty M B, Randall L M 1963 Precancerous lesions of the endometrium. American Journal of Obstetrics and Gynecology 86: 433–443

Bhagavan B S, Parmley T H, Rosenshein N B et al 1984 Comparison of estrogen-induced hyperplasia to endometrial carcinoma. Obstetrics and Gynecology 64: 12–15

Boronow R C, Morrow C P, Creasman W T 1984 Surgical staging in endometrial cancer: Clinical-pathological findings of a prospective study. Obstetrics and Gynecology 63: 825–832

Budwit-Novotny D A, McCarty K S, Cox E B et al 1986 Immunohistochemical analyses of estrogen receptor in endometrial adenocarcinoma using a monoclonal antibody. Cancer Research 46: 5419–5425

Chamlian D L, Taylor H B 1970 Endometrial hyperplasia in young women. Obstetrics and Gynecology 36: 659–666

Clark J H, Schrader W T, O'Malley B W 1985 Mechanisms of steroid hormone action. In: Wilson J D, Foster D W (eds) Textbook of endocrinology. W B Saunders, Philadelphia

Colgan T J, Norris H J, Foster W et al 1983 Predicting the outcome of endometrial hyperplasia by quantitative analysis of nuclear features using a linear discriminant function. International Journal of Gynecological Pathology 1: 347–352

Coumbe A, Mills B P, Brown L 1990 Nucleolar organizer regions in endometrial hyperplasia and neoplasia. Pathology Research and Practice 186: 254–259

Cullen T S 1900 Cancer of the uterus. Appelton, New York

Cunha G R, Chung L W K, Shannon J M et al 1983 Hormone-induced morphogenesis and growth: role of mesenchymal-epithelial interactions. Recent Progress in Hormonal Research 39: 559–598

Deligdisch L, Cohen C J 1985 Histologic correlates and virulence implications of endometrial carcinoma associated with adenomatous hyperplasia. Cancer 56: 1452–1455

Dupont W D, Page D L 1985 Risk factors for breast cancer in women with proliferative breast disease. New England Journal of Medicine 312: 146–151

Eichner E, Abellara M 1971 Endometrial hyperplasias treated by progestagens. Obstetrics and Gynecology 38: 739–741

Eichner E, Simak K A 1981 Uterus didelphys with adenocarcinoma in one horn and atypical endometrial hyperplasia in one other. Case report. American Journal of Obstetrics and Gynecology 139: 222–225

Fechner R E, Bossart M I, Spjut H J 1979 Ultrastructure of endometrial stromal foam cells. American Journal of Clinical Pathology 72: 628–633

Feichter G E, Hoffken H, Heep J et al 1982 DNA-flow-cytometric measurements on the normal, atrophic, hyperplastic, and neoplastic human endometrium. Virchows Archives (Pathological Anatomy and Histopathology) 398: 53–65

Ferenczy A 1977 Ultrastructural pathology of the uterus. In: Wynn R M (ed) Biology of the uterus. Plenum Press, New York, p 545–585

Ferenczy A 1982 The cytodynamics of endometrial hyperplasia and carcinoma I. Histology and ultrastructure. In: Fenoglio C M, Wolff M (eds) Progress in surgical pathology. Masson Publishing, New York, vol 4. p 95–113

Ferenczy A 1983 Cytodynamics of endometrial hyperplasia and neoplasia, part II: In vitro DNA histo-autoradiography. Human Pathology 14: 12–23

Ferenczy A 1987 Anatomy and histology of the uterine corpus. In: Kurman R (ed) Blaustein's pathology of the female genital tract, 3rd edn. Springer-Verlag, New York, p 257–291

Ferenczy A 1988 Endometrial hyperplasia and neoplasia: a two part disease concept. In: Berkowitz R C, Cohen C, Kale N G (eds) Contemporary issues in obstetrics and gynecology. Gynecology oncology. Churchill Livingstone, New York, vol 3 p 197–213

Ferenczy A, Bergeron C 1989 Endometrial hyperplasia and neoplasia. In: Wynn R M, Jollie W (eds) Biology of the uterus, 2nd edn, Plenum Publishing, New York, p 333–353

Ferenczy A, Gelfand M M 1986 Hyperplasia versus neoplasia: two tracts for the endometrium. Contemporary Obstetrics and Gynecology 28: 79–96

Ferenczy A, Gelfand M M 1989 The biologic significance of cytologic atypia in progestogen-treated endometrial hyperplasia. American Journal of Obstetrics and Gynecology 160: 126–131

Ferenczy A, Richart R M 1974 Female reproductive system: Dynamics of scan and transmission electron microscopy. John Wiley, New York

Ferenczy A, Winkler B 1987 Cervical intraepithelial neoplasia and condyloma. In: Kurman R (ed) Blaustein's pathology of the female genital tract, 3rd edn. Springer-Verlag, New York, p 177–217

Fox H 1984 The endometrial hyperplasias. Obstetrics and Gynecology Annual 13: 197–209

Fox H, Buckley C H 1982 The endometrial hyperplasias and their relationship to endometrial neoplasia. Histopathology 6: 493–590

Freidlander M L, Taylor I W, Russell P et al 1983 Ploidy as a prognostic factor in ovarian cancer. International Journal of Gynecologic Pathology 2: 55–63

Fu Y S, Ferenczy A, Huang I, Gelfand M M 1988 Digital imaging analysis of normal, hyperplastic and malignant endometrial cells in endometrial brushing samples. Analytical and Quantitative Cytology and Histology 10: 139–149

Gal D 1986 Hormonal therapy for lesions of the endometrium. Seminars in Oncology 13: 33–36

Gibas Z, Rubin S C 1987 Well-differentiated adenocarcinoma of endometrium with simple karyotypic changes: a case report. Cancer Genetics and Cytogenetics 25: 21–26

Gusberg S B, Kaplan A L 1963 Precursors of corpus cancer. IV. Adenomatous hyperplasia as stage 0 carcinoma of the endometrium. American Journal of Obstetrics and Gynecology 87: 662–678

Gusberg S B, Chen S J, Cohen C J 1974 Endometrial cancer: Factors influencing the choice of treatment. Gynecologic Oncology 2: 308–313

Hendrickson M R, Kempson R L 1980 Endometrial epithelial metaplasias: Proliferations frequently misdiagnosed as adenocarcinoma. Report of 89 cases and proposed classification. American Journal of Surgical Pathology 4: 525–542

Hendrickson M R, Ross J C, Kempson R L 1983 Toward the development of morphologic criteria for well-differentiated adenocarcinoma of the endometrium. American Journal of Surgical Pathology 7: 819–838

Hertig A T, Sommers S C 1949 Genesis of endometrial carcinoma. I. Study of prior biopsies. Cancer 2: 946–956

Horowitz R I, Feinstein A R 1986 Estrogens and endometrial cancer. Responses to arguments and current status of an epidemiologic controversy. American Journal of Medicine 81: 503–507

Iversen O E 1986 Flow cytometric deoxyribonucleic acid index: A prognostic factor in endometrial carcinoma. American Journal of Obstetrics and Gynecology 155: 770–776

King W J, Greene G L 1984 Monoclonal antibodies localize estrogen receptor in the nuclei of target cells. Nature 307: 745–747

Koss L G, Schreiber K, Oberlander S G et al 1981 Screening of asymptomatic women for endometrial cancer. Obstetrics and Gynecology 57: 681–691

Koss L G, Schreiber K, Oberlander S G et al 1984 Detection of endometrial carcinoma and hyperplasia in asymptomatic women. Obstetrics and Gynecology 64: 1–11

Kurman R J, Norris H J 1982 Evaluation of criteria for distinguishing atypical endometrial hyperplasia from well-differentiated carcinoma. Cancer 49: 2547–2559

Kurman R J, Kaminski P F, Norris H J 1985 The behavior of endometrial hyperplasia. A long-term study of untreated hyperplasia in 170 patients. Cancer 56: 403–412

Lindahl B, Alan P, Killander D et al 1987 Flow cytometric DNA analysis of normal and cancerous human endometrium and cytological-histopathological correlations. Anticancer Research 7: 781–790

Lucas W E 1981 Estrogen—a cause of gynecologic cancer? Cancer 48: 451–454

Murphy L J, Murphy L C, Friesen H G 1987 Estrogen induces insulin-like growth factor I expression in the rat uterus. Molecular Endocrinology 1: 445–450

Norris H J, Becker R L, Mikel U V 1989 A comparative morphometric and cytophotometric study of endometrial hyperplasia, atypical hyperplasia, and endometrial carcinoma. Human Pathology 20: 219–223

Ober W B 1971 Adenocarcinoma of the endometrium: a pathologist's view. In: Symposium on endometrial cancer. William Heinemann, London

Reynolds R K, Talavera F, Roberts J D et al 1990 Characterization of epidermal growth factor in benign and neoplastic human endometrium. Cancer (in press)

Satyaswaroop P G, Mortel R 1981 Endometrial carcinoma: An aberration of endometrial cell differentiation. American Journal of Obstetrics and Gynecology 140: 620–623

Sherman A I, Brown S 1979 The precursors of endometrial carcinoma. American Journal of Obstetrics and Gynecology. 135: 947–956

Shyamala G, Ferenczy A 1981 The effect of sodium molybdate on the cytoplasmic estrogen and progesterone receptors in human endometrial tissues. Diagnostic Gynecology and Obstetrics 3: 277–282

Silverberg S G 1988 Hyperplasia and carcinoma of the endometrium. Seminars in Diagnostic Pathology 5: 135–153

Sullivan W P, Beito R G, Proper J et al 1986 Preparation of monoclonal antibodies to the avian progesterone receptor. Endocrinology 119: 1549–1557

Stephenson R A, James B C, Gay H et al 1987 Flow cytometry of prostate cancer: Relationship of DNA content to survival. Cancer Research 47: 2504–2509

Talavera F, Reynolds R K, Roberts J A, Manon K M J 1990 Insulin-like growth factor I receptors in normal and neoplastic human endometrium. Cancer Research 50: 3019–3024

Tavassoli F, Kraus F T 1978 Endometrial lesions in uteri resected for atypical endometrial hyperplasia. American Journal of Clinical Pathology 70: 770–779

Trent J M 1985 Cytogenetic and molecular biologic alterations in human breast cancer: A review. Breast Cancer Research and Treatment 5: 221–229

Vellios F 1972 Endometrial hyperplasia, precursors of endometrial carcinoma. Pathology Annual 7: 201–229

Welch W R, Scully R E 1977 Precancerous lesions of the endometrium. Human Pathology 8: 503–512

Wentz W B 1966 Treatment of persistent endometrial hyperplasia with progestagen. American Journal of Obstetrics and Gynecology 96: 999–1004

Wentz S B 1974 Progestin therapy in endometrial hyperplasia. Gynecological Oncology 2: 362–368

Wilkinson N, Buckley C H, Chawner L, Fox H 1990 Nucleolar organizer regions in normal, hyperplastic, and neoplastic endometria. International Journal of Gynecological Pathology 9: 55–59

Winkler B, Alvarez S, Richart R M et al 1984 Pitfalls in the diagnosis of endometrial neoplasia. Obstetrics and Gynecology 64: 185

12. The diagnosis of molar disease

Sally A. Lane   Graham R. Taylor   Philip Quirke

INTRODUCTION

At first glance the diagnosis of molar pregnancy appears to be well defined, with clearly identified criteria on which to base clinical management. This is not the case, however, and many problems remain, especially at the borders of each diagnostic category. In this chapter we outline existing scientific knowledge of the biology of molar disease, discuss the available diagnostic techniques and their contribution to the reassessment of present views and, lastly, mention new molecular techniques that will help to answer many of the outstanding problems in this area.

BIOLOGY OF MOLAR DISEASE

Current knowledge of molar disease is derived mainly from the cytogenetic study of relatively limited amounts of clinical material. It has led to the division of this condition into several apparently distinct categories, namely complete hydatidiform mole, partial hydatidiform mole, and persistent trophoblastic disease (Vassilakos et al 1977, Szulman & Surti 1978a,b). Subsequently added to this classification were conditions such as placental site trophoblastic pseudotumour (Kurman et al 1976). The suggested methods of formation of molar pregnancy are shown in Figure 12.1 and described below.

Complete moles

Most complete moles have been shown to be diploid XX or XY and of paternal origin, arising by androgenesis, with the oocyte nucleus either absent or inactivated (Kajii & Ohama 1977, Wake et al 1978). This may be due to fertilization by a haploid sperm that duplicates without cytokinesis, a diploid sperm that has failed to undergo first or second meiotic division, or two haploid sperm synchronously (dispermy). The first two methods result in a diploid homozygous complete mole (46XX, as 46YY appears to be non-viable), and the third results in a diploid heterozygous complete mole (46XX or 46XY but not 46YY karyotype). Most complete moles appear to

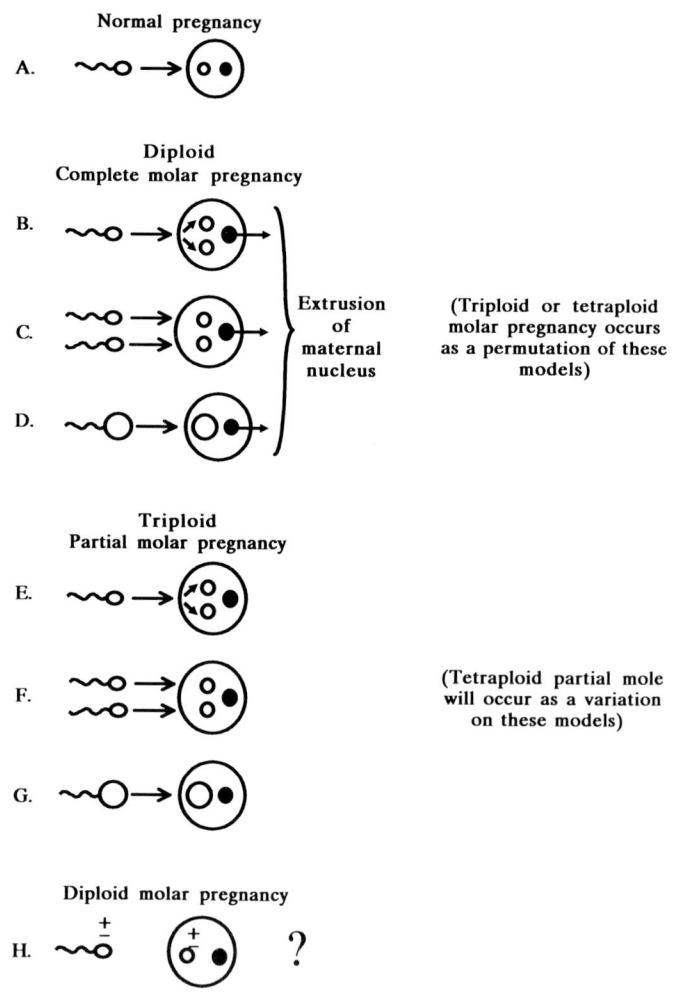

Fig. 12.1 Formation of molar pregnancy. **A** Normal sperm fertilizing an oocyte to give rise to a normal diploid conceptus. **B** Normal sperm fertilizing an oocyte with a subsequent abnormal meiosis. Extrusion of maternal DNA occurs. **C** Dispermic fertilization with extrusion of maternal DNA. **D** Fertilization by a diploid sperm with extrusion of maternal DNA. **E** Normal sperm fertilizing an oocyte with a subsequent abnormal meiosis giving rise to a triploid conceptus. **F** Dispermic fertilization giving rise to a triploid conceptus. **G** Diploid sperm giving rise to a triploid conceptus. **H** Theoretical model for a diploid molar pregnancy: gain or loss of genetic material concerned with placental development from the sperm; the duplicated material may be required for stimulation of placental development; the lost material would have to have a negative feedback effect on placental growth.

arise by the first method (Lawler et al 1979, Jacobs et al 1980) and it has been estimated that about 10% arise by dispermy (Patillo et al 1981, Ohama et al 1981). The cytoplasm of a complete mole is derived from the oocyte and so retains female mitochondrial DNA (Wallace et al 1982, Edwards et al 1984) as does the normal conceptus (Giles et al 1980). Thus a complete mole develops without the influence of the maternal nuclear contribution on fetoplacental development. Where the important areas controlling development are in the female genome is currently unknown. Rare cases of triploid (Vejerslev et al 1987b, Hemming et al 1988) and tetraploid complete moles (Jacobs et al 1978, Lage et al 1989) have been reported, and these are also thought to occur on the basis of a completely paternally-derived genome, with no maternal contribution.

Partial moles

Partial molar disease develops when there is a diploid fertilization of the oocyte with retention of the female haploid nucleus. This usually occurs on the basis of a dispermic fertilization of the oocyte (Jacobs et al 1982, Lawler et al 1982) but can occur only after fertilization by a single diploid sperm or a monospermic fertilization followed by an abnormal pronuclear division. Partial moles are therefore XXX or XXY and may be homozygous or heterozygous for the paternal contribution: the rare occurrence of XYY partial moles has also been described. The reason for the perturbation of the expected ratio of 1:2:1 of XXX:XXY:XYY is unclear. As far as we know, a single sperm fertilizing a digynic oocyte does not give rise to a partial mole (Jacobs et al 1982, Lawler et al 1982) but to a triploid pregnancy.

The existence of diploid (Szulman & Surti 1978a, Teng & Ballon 1984, Ohama et al 1986) and tetraploid (Surti et al 1986) partial moles has been reported. Little systematic study has appeared on this subject and thus controversy still exists in this area. The biological basis of the diploid partial mole is unknown but, if it truly exists, it might arise due to a paternal trisomy (Honore et al 1974, Vassilakos et al 1977) or a maternal chromosomal deletion, allowing an excess paternal influence on development. This area was reviewed in depth by Vejerslev et al (1987a). It has been suggested that tetraploid partial moles occur because of the presence of three paternal haploid genomes and only one maternal contribution (Sheppard et al 1982, Surti et al 1986), the excess of the paternal genomic material giving rise to the trophoblastic hyperplasia. No substantiated wholly maternally derived triploid partial mole has been reported (Vejerslev et al 1987a).

Persistent trophoblastic disease

Persistent trophoblastic disease is defined by a high serum β human chorionic gonadotrophin (β-hCG) concentration persisting for more than 4 weeks after a molar gestation or a progressively rising level any time after parturition or evacuation (Elston 1976). The WHO definition of gestational trophoblastic tumour (1983) includes this and histological evidence of choriocarcinoma, placental site trophoblastic tumour, or large or multiple metastases. Thus persistent trophoblastic disease may include all of these types of trophoblastic disease and little is known of the exact cause or biology of persistent trophoblastic disease. It follows 8–10% of cases of complete mole, but its occurrence cannot be predicted by current methods. Choriocarcinoma following complete mole has been assumed to arise from the paternally derived DNA of the complete mole. Azuma et al (1990) used restriction fragment length polymorphism analysis to show that this may not always be true: in two cases of choriocarcinoma following complete mole, one showed paternal restriction fragment length polymorphisms, and the other showed only maternal restriction fragment length polymorphisms. They conclude that the pathogenesis of choriocarcinoma can be variable.

The potential of a partial mole to progress to persistent trophoblastic disease is also unknown and, although most appear to resolve without treatment, persistent trophoblastic disease is still considered a significant risk, with reports of varying incidence (e.g. Vassilakos et al 1977, Szulman & Surti 1982, Ohama et al 1986, Lawler & Fisher 1987). Of recent reviews with a longer follow-up period, Bagshawe et al (1990) give an incidence of one case of persistent trophoblastic disease in 200 cases of partial mole (four of 857 registrations) compared with 1/12 after complete mole and 1/30 000 normal term births from the Charing Cross Hospital Registry. Rice et al (1990), from their referral base at the New England Trophoblastic Disease Center, reported 16/240 (6.6%) patients followed up for partial mole later developed persistent trophoblastic disease. Both groups were unable to determine criteria for identifying those patients who would progress to persistent trophoblastic disease although a higher than expected incidence has been ascribed to diploid partial moles by Teng & Ballon (1984). Further investigation by flow cytometry and molecular biological techniques of cases of persistent trophoblastic disease arising from partial mole would be valuable in determining whether such cases arise on the basis of histological misinterpretation or are truly partial moles. The current clinical practice is to follow all cases of molar disease, both complete mole and partial mole, by β-hCG assay, and in the UK these are registered centrally with the Royal College of Obstetricians and Gynaecologists.

Mouse experimental model

Since the discovery of the importance of the paternal contribution to molar pregnancy, experimental attempts have been made to reproduce this condition in mice by micromanipulation of the fertilization process. Two main sets of experiments have been performed. Firstly, the formation of diandric and digynic diploid conceptions (Surani & Barton 1983, Barton et al 1984), and, secondly, tripronucleate diandric and digynic triploid conceptions (Kaufman et al 1989).

Diandric conceptions produced trophoblastic hyperplasia with early loss of the embryo whereas digynic conceptions showed inhibition of trophoblastic development, although embryonic growth occurred to a greater degree than in the diandric cases. These and other experiments have led to the belief that maternal and paternal genomic contributions to the conception are involved unequally in placental and embryological development, with paternal genes being more concerned with the former and maternal genes with the latter. Such imprinting possibly arises by variable methylation of the male and female gametes when compared to autosomal DNA (McGrath & Solter 1984, Surani et al 1984, 1988). In the mouse, the most important paternal material appears to lie on chromosomes 6 and 8, whereas the maternal regions lie on 7 and 17 (Surani et al 1987, 1988).

Recent attempts to develop tripronucleate diandric and digynic triploid mouse conceptuses with retention of the oocyte nucleus failed to reproduce the human partial mole (Kaufman et al 1989). The diandric fetus was morphologically normal but underdeveloped, whereas the digynic fetus was consistently abnormal and underdeveloped. The placenta in each case appeared to develop normally. As it has not been possible to produce an experimental partial mole, further investigation of parental dosage in tetraploid moles has not yet been attempted. All of these experiments do, however, suggest that genomic imprinting in the male and female gonads during gametogenesis is important, and that much more of interest remains to be discovered.

CURRENT METHODS OF DIAGNOSIS

Clinical diagnosis

The diagnosis of molar pregnancy is often made by ultrasound, either as an incidental finding at an antenatal examination or as a result of the investigation of a large-for-dates uterus or abnormal bleeding per vaginam.

Curry et al (1975) identified patients at risk of persistent trophoblastic disease using clinical characteristics at the time of evacuation of the molar pregnancy. The best predictors were a uterus that was large-for-dates and bilateral enlarged cystic ovaries. When present, 57% of these patients progressed to persistent trophoblastic disease; this was later shown not to have sufficient predictive value to allow the use of prophylactic chemotherapy (Fasoli et al 1982, Kashimura et al 1986, Kim et al 1986). The follow-up of an established molar pregnancy and persistent trophoblastic disease is now most easily managed by radioimmunoassay of the concentration of β-hCG excreted by the trophoblastic element, measured in patients' serum or urine, and this is also useful for initial diagnosis and assessment of the bulk of trophoblastic disease. The recommendation of routine follow-up of all molar pregnancies has to some extent decreased the need for a precise histopathological diagnosis, but definitive tissue diagnosis may still be required, especially if invasive treatment methods are going to be employed.

Cytogenetic studies

Cytogenetic studies are usually performed on cultured chorionic villi, obtained at therapeutic removal or spontaneous abortion. Cells in mitosis are collected and chromosomes prepared for QM banding using Giemsa–trypsin and quinacrine staining. The latter method identifies variations in the banding patterns (heteromorphisms) and can determine the parental origin of specific chromosomes. These studies separated moles into the two major categories of complete mole and partial mole as discussed above, as well as establishing that there are rare cases of trisomy (Honore et al 1974, Vassilakos et al 1977, Lawler et al 1982) and tetraploidy in partial mole and complete mole (Surti et al 1986, Lage et al 1989) and a separate group of diploid partial moles (Vassilakos et al 1977, Szulman & Surti 1978a,b, Teng & Ballon 1984). The biological basis and frequency of these gestations remains to be established, as most published series are relatively small.

It has been reported that the chromosomal status of the mole may have prognostic implications: for example, heterozygous complete moles (XY, or XX where one X comes from each of two sperm) may have a higher incidence of persistent trophoblastic disease (Davis et al 1984, Kajii & Ohama 1984, Wake et al 1984, 1987), though this is contentious (Fisher & Lawler 1984, Lawler & Fisher 1987, Surti 1987).

Whilst cytogenetic analysis has proved valuable in the classification of these diseases, there are several drawbacks to the routine use of the method. Firstly, fresh material for these studies may be unavailable. Secondly, maternal tissue may be cultured in error and the interpretation of chromosomal patterns may be difficult, particularly in determining hetero-zygosity in XX complete moles. Lastly, some chorionic villi, although fresh, may not grow in culture. In these cases, alternative methods are required.

Histopathological diagnosis

Observer variation

Histopathological criteria for separating hydatidiform moles into the two groups of complete mole and partial mole have been identified by several authors (e.g. Szulman & Surti 1978a,b, Elston 1984), but problems still remain with inter- and intra-observer variation and limited sampling, particularly in the assessment of patchy hydropic change in otherwise normal placental tissue (Javey et al 1979, Messerli et al 1987, Hemmings et al, personal communication). In their frequently quoted paper, Javey et al (1979) reviewed sections from 256 patients on which their local histo-pathologists (University of Shiraz, Iran) had made a diagnosis of hydatidi-form mole and compared these initial diagnoses with those of Professor F. A. Langley of Manchester University (UK). It was found that there was a considerable difference of opinion amongst Shiraz pathologists over their diagnostic criteria and, on average, agreement between them and the visiting professor was obtained in only 55% of cases. They concluded that epidemiological studies, and in particular those conducted in several countries, should involve a panel of pathologists using strict histological definitions.

Hemming et al (unpublished observations) found a similar problem in their studies of flow cytometry and molar disease. They used kappa statistics to assess agreement above that expected by chance alone and found moderate to high values (good agreement) between observers for differentiating molar from non-molar placental tissue (kappa value of 0.77). There was, however, less agreement in separating partial moles and complete moles and a low level of agreement with the original diagnoses (kappa value of only 0.43).

Messerli et al (1987) studied the inter- and intra-pathologist variability in the diagnosis, using uniform diagnostic criteria, of 190 cases of trophoblastic disease. Initially all cases were reviewed blind by both pathologists and then a selected group was again reviewed blind by one of the pathologists. They found a lower level of agreement in diagnosing molar disease between the two pathologists (kappa value 0.53) than when the same pathologist reviewed the slides a second time (kappa value 0.87); greater variability was found for the diagnosis of partial mole (termed 'incomplete' in their definition), and about 70% agreement with the original diagnoses was obtained. All of these studies confirm that the histological diagnosis of molar pregnancy is subject to inter- and intra-observer variation and that supportive techniques are valuable in assisting a firm diagnosis.

Complete mole

A complete mole should be diagnosed only if there is gross vesicular change, this usually being evident as a 'bunch of grapes' macroscopically. Microscopically, the distended chorionic villi may show a lack of blood vessels and central degeneration resulting in 'cistern' formation. There is marked trophoblastic proliferation throughout the specimen, characteristically irregular all around the villi and also as extravillous trophoblast. Fetal parts are classically absent but, if present, the possibility of the coexistence of a twin pregnancy should be borne in mind.

Partial mole

A partial mole shows patchy vesicular change interspersed with normal villi. The vesicular villi more commonly show focal oedema with central 'cistern' formation than in complete mole and have an irregular 'geographical' outline. Cross-cutting of these may result in villous trophoblast 'inclusions'. Vessels with fetal red blood cells are usually present and fetal parts are also often found. Trophoblastic proliferation is generally less than in complete mole and more patchy.

Whilst it had been suggested, originally by Hertig (1937), that the potential for a subsequent choriocarcinoma to complicate a molar pregnancy is proportional to the degree of trophoblastic proliferation, this has not been confirmed by later authors (Elston & Bagshawe 1972, Curry et al 1975).

AgNORs

Nucleolar organizer regions are DNA loops that transcribe to RNA and are located in acrocentric chromosomes. They are associated with certain proteins—including RNA polymerase 1, C23 and B23, these being known as NOR-associated proteins—and are thought to be involved in RNA transcription. Since they stain with silver, they are also known as AgNORs.

Buys & Osinga (1984) showed that AgNORs were related to disulphide and sulphydryl groups on NOR-associated proteins, and suggested that these had functional significance in facilitating accessibility of the NOR loops. Other authors have suggested that carboxyl groups are also involved in the staining reaction (Olert et al 1979).

The technique used most commonly for the examination of AgNORs in tissues is an argyrophil staining method in one or three steps which can be used in paraffin-wax embedded tissues. The AgNORs appear as black dots in the nucleus, and measurements are usually made on 50–100 cells; there are thus the problems of sampling and tissue heterogeneity. There are also problems with inter- and intra-observer variation, the affinity of the nucleolus itself for silver (Tandler 1954), and with fixation (Griffiths et al 1989), but these have not been investigated in molar disease.

It is not known exactly whether AgNORs are a measure of cell proliferation or cellular ploidy. Suresh et al (1990) measured AgNOR counts in molar and hydropic pregnancies and found that such counts did correlate with the assumed ploidy status of complete moles, partial moles and hydropic abortions, in contrast to the more frequently reported association with proliferative activity in other tissues (Crocker et al 1988, Hall et al 1988, Derenzini et al 1989). Suresh et al (1990) conclude that, in the trophoblastic hyperplasia seen in molar pregnancies, AgNOR counts do reflect cellular ploidy. In this study, however, ploidy status had only been assumed to be typical and was not confirmed by flow cytometry. Crocker et al (1989) further showed that there was no relationship between numbers of NOR-bearing chromosomes in metaphase and interphase AgNOR counts from the same specimens, which suggests that ploidy is not directly related to interphase AgNOR numbers (at least, in non-Hodgkins lymphoma). These findings are not conclusive and at present the use of AgNORs cannot be recommended; further study of these and other types of nuclear morphological changes seems warranted.

Flow cytometry

For a variety of reasons cytogenetic measurements are frequently un-available on the majority of molar pregnancies. In most cases, therefore, the

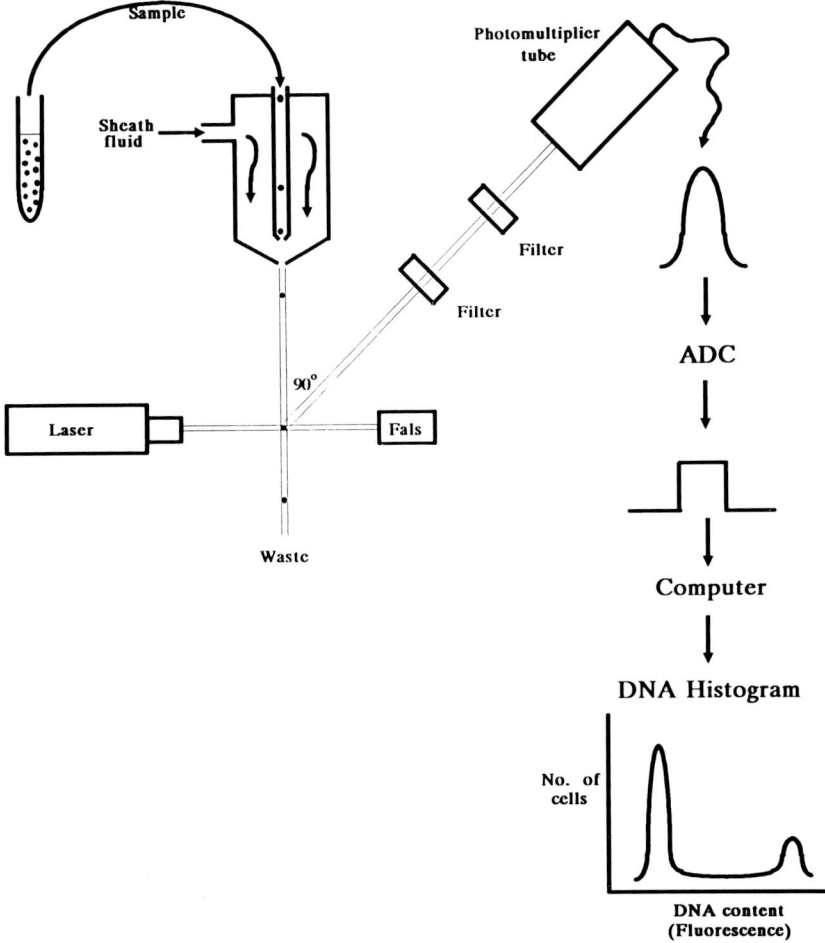

Fig. 12.2 Flow cytometry. Paraffin-wax sections are digested to give individual nuclei. These are suspended in fluid and injected into the flow cell of the flow cytometer under pressure. Sheath fluid controls the escape of the nuclei from the injection stylus. Individual cells are ejected from the nozzle of the flow cell and fall in a stream of fluid past the light source. Fluorescence from scattered light is collected at 90° and directly by the forward angle light scatter detector. The emitted fluorescence from the fluorochrome is collected at 90° and separated from the original light source by filters. The photomultiplier tube measures the amount of light and converts this into electricity which is subsequently changed into a digital signal for computer interpretation. A frequency distribution histogram is plotted of fluorescence (proportional to DNA content) against cell number to give a DNA histogram. Forward angle and 90° light scatter can also be measured for these cells to give information on the size and refractiveness of the particles.

diagnosis rests solely on the histopathological opinion and clinical data such as the ultrasound appearances and β-hCG levels. Partial moles are not infrequently diagnosed solely on histological grounds and thus other confirmatory evidence is lacking. In this situation, measurement of DNA content by flow cytometry is valuable since it can be performed on paraffin-wax embedded material (Hedley et al 1983, 1985).

Paraffin-wax embedded tissue extraction

Both normal maternal decidua and placental tissue must be present as analysis of paraffin blocks requires an internal standard, in this case decidua; external standards are unreliable owing to the variable loss of DNA from the tissue during fixation. Diploid decidua within the same block should lose the same proportion of DNA as the molar tissue, and thus the relative

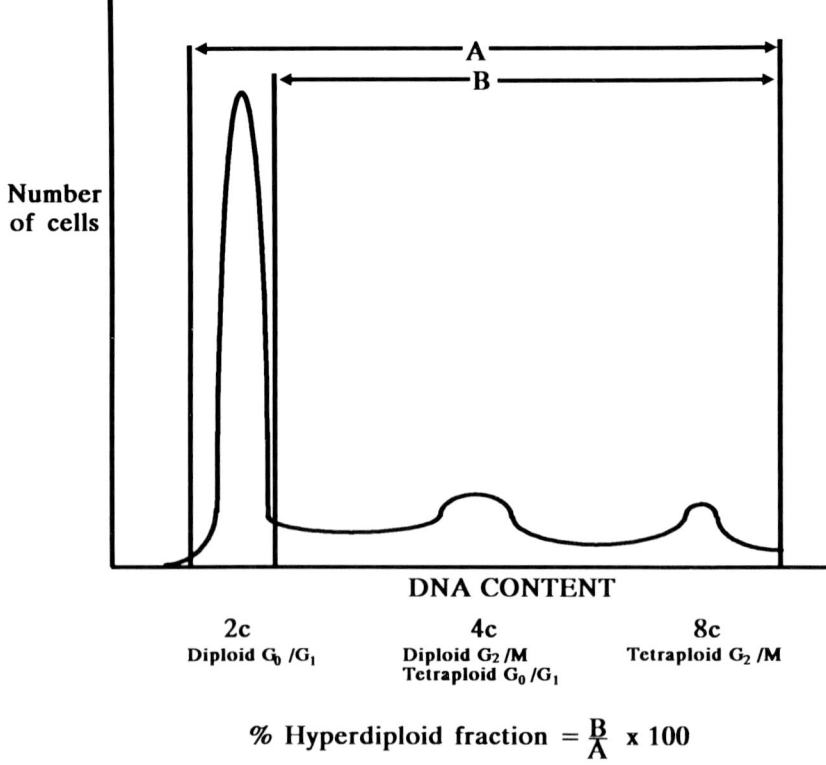

$$\% \text{ Hyperdiploid fraction} = \frac{B}{A} \times 100$$

Fig. 12.3 DNA histogram and the method of calculation of the hyperdiploid fraction. The total number of cells is measured (A) and then the number of cells greater than the first peak (G_0/G_1 peak) is quantitated (B). This value is then expressed as a percentage of the total number of cells and called the hyperdiploid fraction. The tetraploid G_0/G_1 and its octoploid G_2/M distort the results obtained by normal cell cycle analysis programmes.

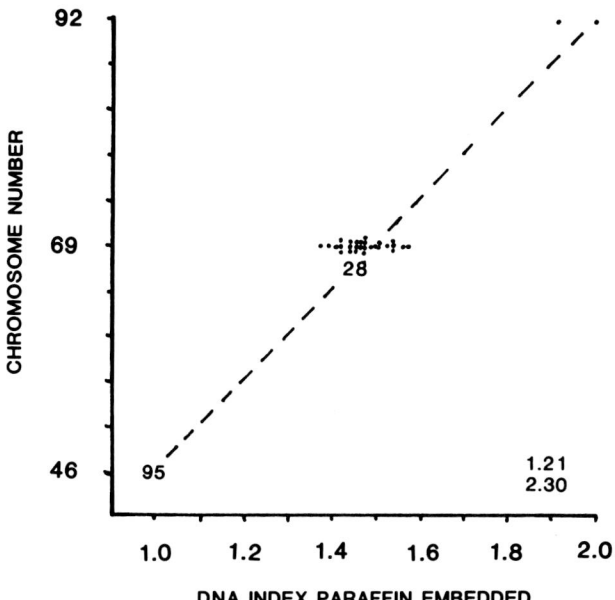

Fig. 12.4 Graph of the DNA index of 127 cases of normal placenta, partial mole and complete mole versus its theoretical chromosome number, (i.e. normal placental and complete mole, 46 chromosomes; partial mole, 69 chromosomes). The two tetraploid cases were presumed to have 92 chromosomes. Two aneuploid cases with DNA indices of 1.21 and 2.30 were also detected. There appears to be excellent correlation between the flow cytometry and the theoretical chromosome number.

difference between the diploid population and a triploid or tetraploid test population can be determined. For analysis the first peak is always assumed to be the diploid peak.

The technique

Sections, 40μm thick, are cut, dewaxed, rehydrated and digested by pepsin to yield nuclei. These are stained by a fluorescent dye such as propidium iodide or DAPI which binds stoichiometrically to DNA, then injected into a flow cell under pressure (Fig. 12.2). The individual cells pass through a light beam scattering the incident beam in all directions. Forward angle light scatter is proportional to cell size and 90° light scatter to the internal refractiveness of the cell. The DNA content of a cell is proportional to the amount of fluoresence emitted and is usually expressed as the DNA index. This is the ratio of the modal channel number of the G_0/G_1 phase of the first peak to the modal channel number of the G_0/G_1 phase cells in the second peak. In the case of molar pregnancy, maternal decidua, the internal control of diploid cells, forms the first peak. Thus diploid test cells have a DNA index of 1.0, triploid cells of 1.5, tetraploid cells of 2.0, etc. Indices that are not whole or half integers are usually regarded as DNA aneuploid, defined as the presence of an abnormal DNA stem line recognized by the appearance of at least two separate G_0/G_1 peaks on the DNA histogram (Hiddemann et al 1984).

Normal diploid placental tissue contains a small number of polyploid cells demonstrable by both cytogenetics (Makino et al 1963) and flow cytometry (Hemming et al 1987); tetraploid G_0/G_1 cells occupy the same position as diploid cells in G_2/M phase, which makes quantification of cell proliferation by standard computer programs inaccurate. We have developed another method for quantifying proliferation and polyploidy simultaneously by taking a simple estimate of the number of cells showing a DNA content greater than the diploid peak and expressing this fraction, the hyperdiploid fraction (Fig. 12.3), as a proportion of the total number of cells.

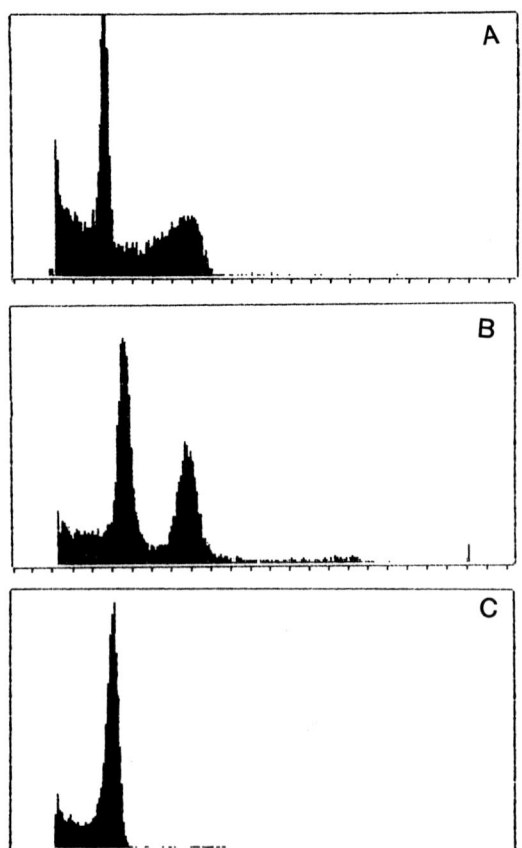

Fig. 12.5 DNA histograms obtained from paraffin embedded tissue of **A** diploid complete mole, **B** triploid partial mole and   **C** diploid partial mole.

Table 12.1   Flow cytometry data on ploidy in molar pregnancies

	Type of molar pregnancy			
DNA content	Partial mole[1]	Complete mole[1]	Persistent trophoblastic disease (complete mole)[2]	Persistent trophoblastic disease (partial mole)[2]
Diploid	10	46	41	0
Triploid	20	2	2	2
Tetraploid	1	0	0	0
DNA aneuploid	1	1	0	0
Total	32	49	43	2

[1]Hemming et al (1987).
[2]Hemming et al (1988).

Molar pregnancies

In molar pregnancies, flow cytometry is proving a more versatile method than cytogenetic studies for initial diagnosis and further study, DNA content being readily measured on fixed and paraffin wax embedded tissue. Like us, many authors have found no significant difference between the values of DNA in fresh and paraffin-wax embedded material (Fig. 12.4).

By flow cytometry, complete moles have been confirmed to be mainly diploid with high cell proliferation (Fig. 12.5A) and partial moles mainly triploid with a lower cell proliferation (Fig. 12.5B) (Fisher et al 1987, Hemming et al 1987, Lage et al 1988). A further minor group of cases with diploid histograms with a low cell proliferation have been categorized as possible diploid partial moles (Fig. 12.5C) (Davis et al 1987, Hemming et al 1987). Occasional cases of complete mole triploidy (Hemming et al 1987), complete mole and partial mole tetraploidy (Surti et al 1986, Hemming et al 1987, 1988, Lage et al 1989) and complete mole and partial mole DNA aneuploidy (Lawler et al 1982, Hemming et al 1987, Vejerslev et al 1987b) have been reported. Our data are summarized in Table 12.1.

The level of cell proliferation seen in complete moles was remarkably high (Hemming et al 1987, 1988), with complete mole histograms resembling measurements of in vitro cell cultures rather than solid tumours or hyperplastic lesions. This level was far in excess of that seen in first, second or third trimester placental tissue or triploid partial moles. The normal placentas showed a small degree of polyploidy. This polyploidy was increased in the complete moles, giving rise to a distinct tetraploid population in many cases (Fig. 12.6). By current definitions (Hiddemann et al 1984), these complete moles could be classified as DNA tetraploid by demonstrating a significant second population, but because of the natural inherent polyploidy of normal placenta (Makino et al 1963, Hemming et al 1987) we prefer to classify them as diploid. To do otherwise would require that placenta and other polyploid tissues such as bone marrow, liver and cardiac tissue should be categorized as DNA aneuploid according to standard definitions (Hiddemann et al 1984). Lage et al (1989) report a high level of tetraploid complete moles by flow cytometry and it is probable that these are identical to our diploid complete moles with a minor tetraploid population. Chromosomal studies do not usually demonstrate such natural polyploidy because it exists in only a small subpopulation. Occasionally a complete mole with a predominantly tetraploid population is seen and must be defined as a tetraploid complete mole. In the absence of a better definition, we categorize a molar pregnancy as DNA tetraploid if the tetraploid peak is greater than the diploid peak. The nature and importance of DNA aneuploid molar pregnancies remains to be established, but they have been reported previously (Hemming et al 1987). Until more data are available on such unusual pregnancies, the histopathological diagnosis remains the most important feature in these cases.

The high level of cell proliferation of complete moles does not predict the likelihood of progression to persistent trophoblastic disease (Hemming et al 1988): cases of persistent trophoblastic disease had identical flow cytometric histograms to complete moles and no differences were detectable. On the other hand, four of the cases of definite persistent trophoblastic disease were triploid, two with complete mole morphology and two with partial mole morphology but there were no tetraploid cases of persistent trophoblastic disease. Such cases with unusual ploidy suggest that flow cytometry and classical cytogenetics cannot absolutely predict the outcome of any given molar pregnancy without recourse to knowledge of the relative paternal and maternal contributions.

A further group of diploid pregnancies was detected that had the morphology of a partial mole with a low cell proliferation, and this group of cases represents a problem area. Such lesions may truly represent a group of diploid partial moles and, on expert histopathological review, all of our cases were confirmed to show the features of partial moles. Alternatively, these cases may have been labelled diploid because there was insufficient control material in the block and the single triploid peak was misinterpreted as diploid. All these cases were, however, re-run after further histological assessment to ensure that adequate maternal tissue was indeed present, and identical results were obtained. The diploid cases might also represent histologically misdiagnosed hydropic abortions or, finally, they might be true diploid partial moles arising on the basis of a trisomy rather than triploidy. Other workers have also described diploid partial moles by flow cytometry. Davis et al (1987) investigated 35 cases of partial mole using the criteria of Szulman & Surti (1978b). Six cases were triploid (17%) and 29 diploid (83%). Four cases were also karyotyped (two were triploid and two diploid). No complications occurred in the triploid group, but five of 25 diploid cases (20%) progressed to definite persistent trophoblastic disease. The diploid cases with progression differed from triploid and diploid cases without progression in having a greater frequency of presenting clinically as

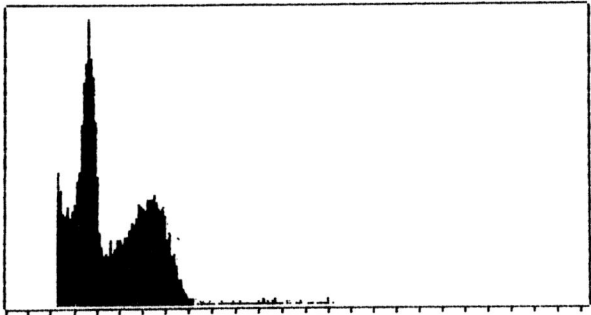

Fig. 12.6   DNA histogram of a diploid complete mole showing a substantial tetraploid population, raising difficulties as to the correct classification of the DNA status of this molar pregnancy. Since a variable number of tetraploid G_0/G_1 cells are frequently seen, this complete mole was classified as diploid.

a mole, a high β-hCG level (more than 20 000 mIU/ml), marked trophoblastic hyperplasia, and a low G_0/G_1 and high S phase fractions. They concluded that diploid molar pregnancies that had high cell proliferation were at increased risk of persistent trophoblastic disease. Their cases can, however, be explained in a different manner. The high proliferation diploid group could represent complete moles and not partial moles, with the low proliferation group being either diploid partial moles or, more likely, hydropic abortions. The very fact that 83% of their partial moles were diploid is very unusual and, taken in conjunction with the flow cytometry results, may actually represent a histological misdiagnosis.

A diploid partial mole was also reported from a series of 59 abortions of less than 15 weeks gestational age studied by flow cytometry (van Oven et al 1989). Four cases were classified as partial mole histologically and one of these had a diploid histogram. Six of 59 abortions gave triploid histograms, of which three were thought to be triploid pregnancies which were not partial moles. Likewise Lage et al (1988) found that two of seven partial moles studied by flow cytometry were diploid, but these were reclassified on histological review into a complete mole and a hydropic abortion. This situation is currently unresolved but requires further investigation, as Teng & Ballon (1984) have reported a greater potential for the development of persistent trophoblastic disease in diploid partial moles.

Martin et al (1989) claim to have isolated a high-risk group of DNA aneuploid molar pregnancies requiring treatment. They investigated 40 cases of histologically reviewed complete moles by flow cytometry. These were classified as diploid or DNA aneuploid, and an assessment of cell proliferation was performed. No attempt was made to identify triploid cases and any case with two stem lines was called DNA aneuploid. Thirteen of 40 cases were therefore 'DNA aneuploid'; three of the 13 did not require treatment and ten had persistent trophoblastic disease. Of the diploid cases,

IN SITU HYBRIDISATION

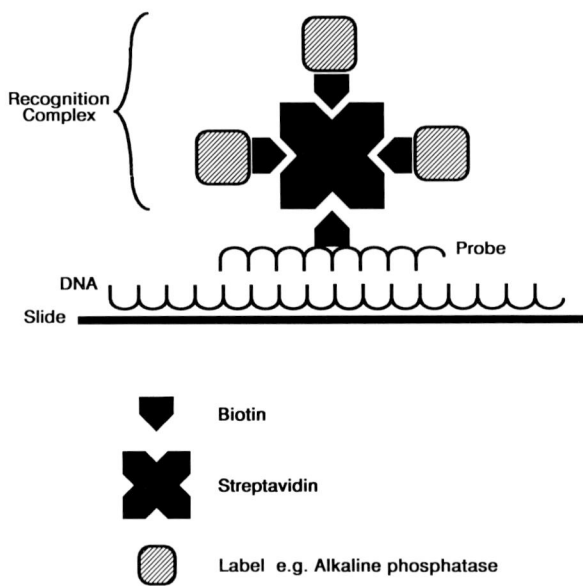

Recognition Complex

Probe

DNA

Slide

Biotin

Streptavidin

Label e.g. Alkaline phosphatase

Fig. 12.7   In situ hybridization. The DNA of a tissue section is exposed by proteolytic digestion and the DNA denatured into single strands by heating. A DNA probe or oligonucleotide probe, which has had biotin incorporated into it, is then hybridized with the slide. Subsequently streptavidin is applied, which binds to the biotin of any bound probe. This is followed by biotin labelled with a marker such as alkaline phosphatase, which generates a blue stain that can be recognized by light microscopy.

19 underwent spontaneous remission and eight were categorized as persistent trophoblastic disease, of which four showed metastatic disease. From our data and the literature, DNA aneuploidy and triploidy are rare in complete moles. The occurrence of 13/40 DNA aneuploid cases is therefore suspect, and the absence of metastatic disease in these cases also suggests that these data are highly unusual. Unless the demonstration of aneuploidy is supported by further studies, it cannot be used as a basis for clinical decision-making.

Whilst the definitions used in the flow cytometry of molar disease vary between workers, most generally agree that flow cytometric methods parallel cytogenetics and can be accurately performed on paraffin-wax embedded material. However, as stated above, a small number of cases do not fall into the two classical groups of diploid complete mole and triploid partial mole, and flow cytometry cannot be used to identify those patients who will progress to persistent trophoblastic disease. Other methods are still required, and newer molecular techniques may help in this assessment.

MOLECULAR TECHNOLOGY

In situ hybridization

In situ hybridization is a technique using nucleic acid probes to localize known DNA or RNA sequences in whole cells, tissue sections or chromosome preparations. The labelled probes associate with complimentary RNA or DNA target sequences to form a hybrid molecule which is then detected by its label (Fig. 12.7). With recent improvements in the creation of specific probes and in detection systems, particularly the development of non-radioactive methods with increased sensitivity, this technique is now becoming routine.

With respect to molar disease and the reported increased potential for persistent trophoblastic disease of heterozygous diploid complete mole (XX or XY), it would be possible to use a Y-chromosome probe to detect the XY complete moles, which should form approximately 50% of heterozygous complete moles. Dudding (unpublished observations) has investigated various methods of using the pH Y2.1 probe for the detection of the Y-chromosome by in situ hybridization and developed a non-isotopic method suitable for use in paraffin-wax embedded blocks. Using this on five cases of partial moles, he found two cases to be positive (Fig. 12.8) which is close to the expected frequency in partial mole. Owing to a shortage of material this technique was not assessed on a series of complete mole.

In situ hybridization appears currently to be of limited use in the

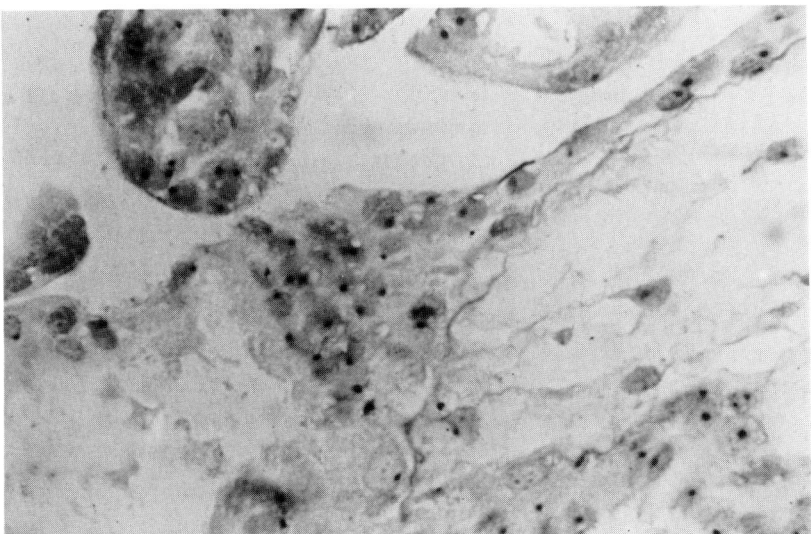

Fig. 12.8 Trophoblast from a partial mole showing one nuclear dot signifying the presence of a single Y chromosome as determined by in situ hybridization using a Y-chromosome probe, pH Y2.1. (Courtesy of Mr Nick Dudding.)

diagnosis of molar disease since it cannot reliably determine the relative genetic contribution from maternal and paternal sources.

DNA fingerprinting

Variations in gene products between individuals are usually not sufficiently great to identify maternal and paternal contributions. There appears, however, to be much greater variation in the non-transcribed DNA—simple tandem repetitive sequences of DNA ('minisatellites') found clustered in areas on the genome. Alterations in the number of such repeated sequences could arise owing to unequal exchanges during mitosis or meiosis, thus producing unique patterns of differing restriction fragment lengths for each individual. Jeffreys et al (1985) used Southern blots of human DNA with probes to known clusters of repetitive sequences and showed up to 50 polymorphic bands. They took DNA samples from 20 unrelated British Caucasians and showed that the minisatellite patterns on Southern blot analysis had few shared fragments and were highly specific for each individual. Using probability scores, even in cases of siblings (except identical twins), the likelihood of two people having the same DNA fingerprint was found to be not higher than 3×10^{-5}, and less if more than one probe was used. This test can be performed quickly and using only a drop of human blood. By comparison of the test material with maternal and paternal minisatellite fragments, biological parentage can be established. Such techniques have been applied to fresh molar material and have confirmed the androgenetic origin of complete moles (Saji et al 1989, Fisher et al 1989). Nobunaga et al (1990) and Takahashi et al (1990) report the use of DNA fingerprinting in the diagnosis of molar disease in fresh tissue. Furthermore, Takahashi et al (1990) corrected a histological diagnosis of partial mole to complete mole by DNA fingerprinting. However, these techniques cannot be easily applied to paraffin-wax embedded material because they require relatively large pieces of DNA for Southern blotting.

Polymerase chain reaction

PCR is now an established technique that can specifically amplify a given nucleic acid target sequence, thus avoiding the need for the sensitive detection system required by in situ hybridization. It uses two oligonucleotide primer sequences complementary to upstream sequences (5') and to the opposite strand downstream (3') of the target DNA (Fig. 12.9).

Extracted DNA, primers, the four individual deoxynucleotides and a DNA polymerase, usually Taq polymerase, are heated to 95°C to split the double-stranded DNA and then cooled to 55°C. At this temperature the primers hybridize upstream and downstream from the target DNA and a new complementary strand is synthesized onto both primers, catalysed by the Taq DNA polymerase at 72°C. The cycle of denaturation, hybridization and DNA synthesis is then repeated (usually 30 cycles), each time doubling

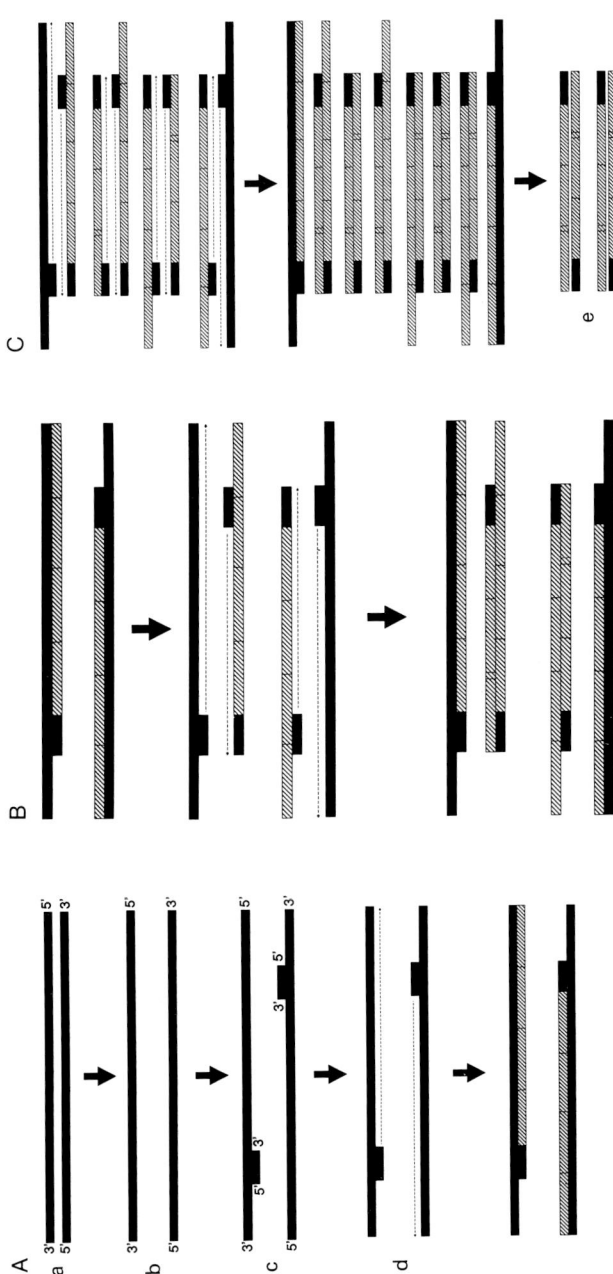

Fig. 12.9   The polymerase chain reaction.   **A** Template DNA (a) is heated to 90–95°C to separate the two strands (b). On cooling to 50–70°C the primers find their complementary sites and form a localized area of double-stranded DNA (c). On heating to 65–75°C the Taq polymerase synthesizes two new strands in each direction (d).   **B** A second round of identical temperature cycles break the four strands apart, allows the primers to bind on and creates four new strands.   **C** A third cycle leads to the production of a product of a restricted length as the primers begin to limit DNA synthesis in both directions. The final product is discrete fragments of the segment of interest (e).

the target DNA and leading to exponential amplification of this region. The amplified DNA becomes rapidly limited to the area between the primers, as shown in Figure 12.9.

There are similar benefits to this technique as for flow cytometry, in being able to use preserved and fixed tissue samples, although random strand breakage during fixation may limit the maximum size of DNA amplifiable (Shibata et al 1988, Jackson et al 1989a,b, 1990a,b). The technique is highly sensitive, and very small amounts of tissue can be used, even tissue removed from haematoxylin and eosin sections (Jackson et al 1989b).

There is a risk of false-positive results, and stringent anticontamination techniques must be performed with the inclusion of negative controls in each case. Ultraviolet light irradiation also helps to remove contamination (Sarkar & Sommer 1990).

Using this technique it is possible to amplify any human gene that has previously been sequenced. Since the region of the paternal DNA responsible for the fundamental defect causing molar pregnancy is unknown, only indirect evidence for the diagnosis can be obtained by polymerase chain reaction, by the determination of the relative parental contribution to the pregnancy. With the recent description of microsatellites, CA repeats and ALU polymorphisms, a paraffin-wax embedded tissue polymerase chain reaction-based test for molar disease is under development.

Microsatellites

Litt et al (1989) and Weber et al (1989) described polymorphisms in smaller repetitive sequences called microsatellites. These blocks of DNA, in the form $(CA)n$ or $(GT)n$ sequences repeated n times (where n is 10–60 or so), may number as many as 50 000–100 000 and have been found to be widely distributed through the human genome (Miesfeld et al 1981, Hamada et al 1982). The polymorphisms comprise alleles differing in length by units of two base pairs and so are not detectable by gel electrophoresis or Southern blotting, but after amplification by polymerase chain reaction they can be separated on a sequencing gel and a difference of only two base pairs can be detected as a polymorphism. The theory of the use of polymerase chain reaction amplifiable polymorphisms is outlined in Figure 12.10.

If maternal and paternal genomic DNA are both present in the test tissue, then a completely paternal origin can be excluded. If only paternal tissue is found, then a firm diagnosis of complete mole can be made. However, to be certain, the mother and father must be polymorphic at the locus chosen. This is easy to determine if paternal DNA is available from peripheral blood samples. If this is not the case (e.g. in referred material, if the father is unknown, or in retrospective investigations), then the situation becomes more difficult. In this context, a panel of highly polymorphic sequences must be used to rule out the presence of maternal DNA definitively. By comparing maternal and trophoblastic tissue CA repeats, it should be

Diagnosis of molar pregnancy by CA repeat

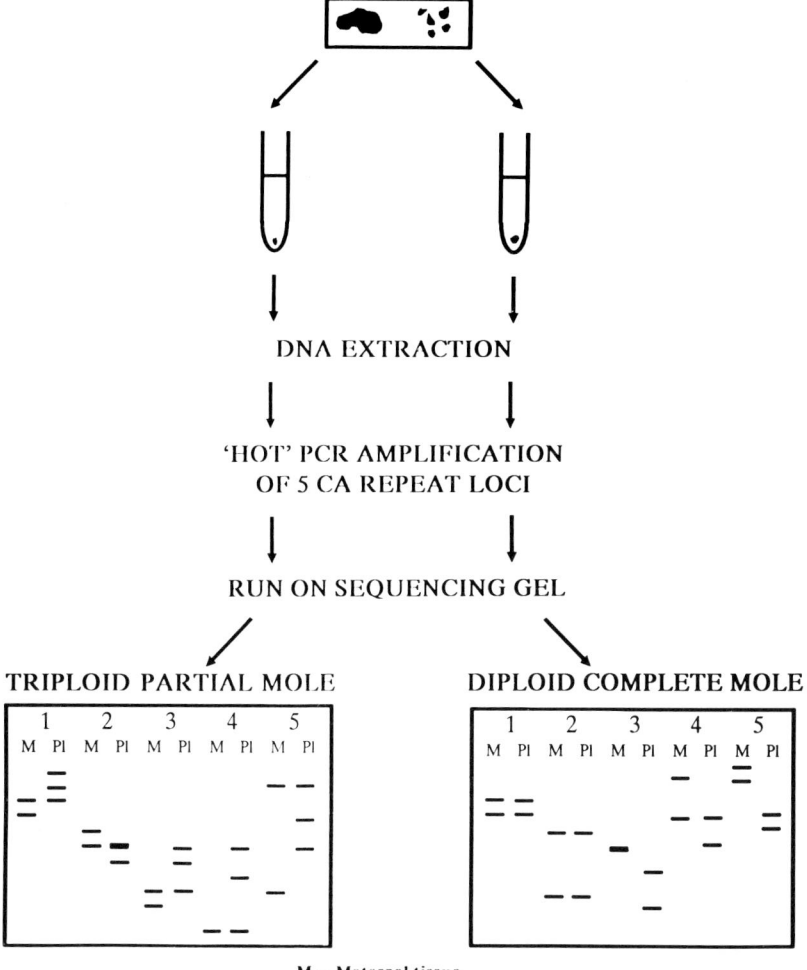

DNA EXTRACTION

'HOT' PCR AMPLIFICATION
OF 5 CA REPEAT LOCI

RUN ON SEQUENCING GEL

TRIPLOID PARTIAL MOLE   DIPLOID COMPLETE MOLE

M = Maternal tissue
Pl = Placental molar tissue

Fig. 12.10   The use of polymorphisms amplified by the polymerase chain reaction in the diagnosis of molar pregnancy. Endometrium and decidua from the mother are separated from placental molar villi on unstained glass sections by reference to haematoxylin and eosin slides cut before and after the test sample. The separated tissue is digested by proteinase K and DNA is extracted by phenol and chloroform. Five individual CA repeat polymerase chain reactions are performed on the DNA sample from decidua and also on the DNA from the placental or molar villi. These polymerase chain reactions contain radiolabelled primers. The amplified DNA is run on a sequencing gel to detect small variations in length caused by the variable number of CA repeats present on each allele. The sequencing gel is autoradiographed and one or two bands appear for each CA repeat for each sample. By comparison of the pattern produced, it is possible to determine whether any of the uniquely maternal CA repeat patterns are present in the placental or molar villous sample. If they are, then a maternal contribution is present and the gestation is not a complete mole. If only paternal CA repeats are present, then the gestation must be a complete mole. M, maternal tissue: Pl, placental molar tissue.

possible not only to diagnose the origin of such pregnancies, but also retrospectively to review problem cases such as triploid complete moles, tetraploidies, diploid partial moles and patients progressing to persistent trophoblastic disease, to determine their biological basis and to confirm or refute the established hypothesis that all complete moles contain only paternal nuclear DNA.

If it were possible reliably to separate pure trophoblast from the maternal circulation then it would be feasible to diagnose the pregnancy by CA repeats from the peripheral blood, as amplification of Y related sequences has already been performed for fetal sexing (Anon 1990, Lo et al 1990, Mueller et al 1990).

In conjunction with flow cytometry, polymerase chain reaction techniques should allow measurements of DNA content, cell proliferation and maternal/paternal genetic contributions. Such techniques will greatly aid in the diagnosis of molar pregnancy and should determine the genetic constitution of unusual cases. In addition, the techniques are rapid, sensitive and accurate, and can be performed on fresh or formalin-fixed, paraffin-wax embedded tissues at the time of receipt or retrospectively and provide a result within 24–48 h. Polymerase chain reaction diagnosis of molar pregnancy is in its early stages but shows much promise for the future.

CONCLUSIONS

There is a wide range of methods in use to study and define the diagnostic categories of molar disease. At present, diagnosis continues to rely heavily on clinical investigations, such as ultrasound and serum β-hCG levels, with histological assessment of molar tissue. However, intra-observer variation in the histological diagnosis remains a significant difficulty and, where available, newer methods such as flow cytometry or cytogenetics can enhance the accuracy of diagnosis. Whilst the biological basis of molar disease is relatively well established for diploid complete moles and triploid partial moles, there are exceptions to the rule. It is the investigation of these latter cases by a range of methods to ascertain their biological basis which will, we hope, lead to a more logical and complete classification of molar disease in terms of the parental origin.

In this respect, there are great hopes for newer molecular biological techniques that can be performed retrospectively on paraffin-wax embedded material. In the future, combinations of all these techniques may well prove more valuable than current methods, but too little work has been published to date to predict their exact role with confidence. The techniques may also assist in defining cases which progress to persistent trophoblastic disease as at present there are no available techniques to predict this accurately. The biological basis of the autonomous trophoblastic growth assumed to occur in this stage of the disease is also unknown.

Molar disease continues to provide a fascinating area for a greater understanding of the genes involved in placental and fetal growth and development.

REFERENCES

Anon 1990 Is it a boy? Lancet ii: 87–88
Azuma C, Saji F, Nobunaga T et al 1990 Studies on the pathogenesis of choriocarcinoma by analysis of restriction fragment length polymorphisms. Cancer Research 50: 488–491
Bagshawe K D, Lawler S D, Paradinas F J, Dent J, Brown P, Boxer G M 1990 Gestational trophoblastic tumours following initial diagnosis of partial hydatidiform mole. Lancet ii: 1074–1076
Barton S C, Surani M A H, Norris M L 1984 Role of paternal and maternal genomes in mouse development. Nature 311: 374–376
Buys C H C M, Osinga J 1984 Selective staining of the same set of nucleolar phosphoproteins by silver and Giemsa. A combined biochemical and cytochemical study on staining of NORs. Chromosoma 89: 387–396
Crocker J, Macartney J C, Smith P J 1988 Correlation between DNA flow cytometric and nucleolar organiser region data in non-Hodgkin's lymphomas. Journal of Pathology 154: 151–156
Crocker J, Janmohamed R M I, Armstrong S J, Hulten M, Leyland M J 1989 The relationship between numbers of interface NORs and NOR-bearing chromosomes in non-Hodgkin's lymphoma. Journal of Pathology 157: 166A
Curry S L, Hammond C B, Tyrey L, Creasman W T, Parker R T 1975 Hydatidiform mole diagnosis, management and follow-up of 347 patients. Obstetrics and Gynecology 45: 1–8
Davis J R, Surwit E A, Garay J P, Fortier K J 1984 Sex assignment in gestational trophoblastic neoplasia. American Journal of Obstetrics and Gynecology 148: 722–725
Davis J R, Kerrigan D P, Way D L, Weiner S A 1987 Partial hydatidiform moles: deoxyribonucleic acid content and course. American Journal of Obstetrics and Gynecology 157: 969–973
Derenzini M, Pession A, Farabegoli F, Trerè D, Badiali M, Dehan P 1989 Relationship between interphasic nucleolar organiser regions and growth rate in two neuroblastoma cell lines. American Journal of Pathology 134: 925–932
Edwards Y H, Jeremiah S J, McMillan S L, Povey S, Fisher R A, Lawler S D 1984 Complete hydatidiform moles combine maternal mitochondria with a paternal nuclear genome. Annals of Human Genetics 48: 119–127
Elston C W 1976 The histopathology of trophoblastic tumours. Journal of Clinical Pathology 29 (suppl 10): 111–131
Elston C W 1984 The pathology of trophoblastic disease: current status. Baillière's Clinics in Obstetrics and Gynaecology 2: 135–152
Elston C W, Bagshawe K D 1972 The value of histological grading in the management of hydatidiform mole. Journal of Obstetrics and Gynaecology of the British Commonwealth 79: 717–724
Fasoli M, Ratti E, Franceschi S, La Vecchia C, Pecorelli S, Mangioni C 1982 Management of gestational trophoblastic disease: results of a co-operative study. Obstetrics and Gynecology 60: 205–209
Fisher R A, Lawler S D 1984 Heterozygous complete hydatidiform moles: do they have a worse prognosis than homozygous complete moles? Lancet ii: 51
Fisher R A, Lawler S D, Ormerod M G, Imrie P R, Povey S 1987 Flow cytometry used to distinguish between complete and partial hydatidiform moles. Placenta 8: 249–256
Fisher R A, Povey S, Jeffreys A J, Martin C A, Patel I, Lawler S D 1989 Frequency of heterozygous complete hydatidiform moles, estimated by locus-specific minisatellite and Y chromosome-specific probes. Human Genetics 82: 259–263
Giles R E, Blanc H, Cann H M, Wallace D C 1980 Maternal inheritance of human mitochondrial DNA. Proceedings of the National Academy of Science USA 77: 6715–6719
Griffiths A P, Butler C W, Roberts P, Dixon M F, Quirke P 1989 Silver stained structures

(AgNORs), their dependence on tissue fixation and absence of prognostic relevance in rectal adenocarcinoma. Journal of Pathology 159: 121–127

Hall P A, Crocker J, Watts A, Stansfeld A G 1988 A comparison of nucleolar organizer region staining and Ki67 immunostaining in non-Hodgkin's lymphoma. Histopathology 12: 373–381

Hamada H, Petrino M G, Kakunaga T 1982 A novel repeated element with Z-DNA-forming potential is widely found in evolutionarily diverse eukaryotic genomes. Proceedings of the National Academy of Science USA 79: 6465–6469

Hedley D W, Friedlander M L, Taylor I W, Rugg C A, Musgrove E A 1983 Method for analysis of cellular DNA content of paraffin-embedded pathological material using flow cytometry. Journal of Histochemistry and Cytochemistry 31: 1333–1335

Hedley D W, Friedlander M L, Taylor I W 1985 Application of DNA flow cytometry to paraffin-embedded archival material for the study of aneuploidy and its clinical significance. Cytometry 6: 327–333

Hemming J D, Quirke P, Womack C, Wells M, Elston C W, Bird C C 1987 Diagnosis of molar pregnancy and persistent trophoblastic disease by flow cytometry. Journal of Clinical Pathology 40: 615–620

Hemming J D, Quirke P, Womack C, Wells M, Elston C W, Pennington G W 1988 Flow cytometry in persistent trophoblastic disease. Placenta 9: 615–621

Hemming J D, Wells, M, Womack C, Elston C W, Smeeton N C, Quirke P personal communication Interobserver variation in the histological diagnosis of hydatidiform mole

Hertig A T 1937 In: Discussion of paper by Phaneuf LE Hydatidiform mole and chorionepithelioma. New England Journal of Medicine 217: 775

Hiddemann W, Schumann J, Andreeff M et al 1984 Convention on nomenclature for DNA cytometry. Cytometry 5: 445–446

Honore L H, Dill F J, Poland B J 1974 The association of hydatidiform mole and trisomy 2. Obstetrics and Gynecology 43: 232–237

Jackson D P, Quirke P, Lewis F et al 1989a Detection of measles virus RNA in paraffin embedded tissue. Lancet i: 1391

Jackson D P, Bell S, Payne J et al 1989b Extraction and amplification of DNA from archival haematoxylin and eosin sections and cervical cytology Papanicolaou smears. Nucleic Acids Research 17: 10134

Jackson D P, Lewis F A, Taylor G R, Boylston A W, Quirke P 1990a Tissue extraction of DNA and RNA and analysis by the polymerase chain reaction. Journal of Clinical Pathology 43: 499–504

Jackson D P, Payne J, Bell S et al 1990b Extraction of DNA from exfoliative cytology specimens and its suitability for analysis by the polymerase chain reaction. Cytopathology 1: 87–96

Jacobs P A, Hassold T J, Matsuyama A M, Newlands I M 1978 Chromosome constitution of gestational trophoblastic disease. Lancet ii: 49

Jacobs P A, Wilson C M, Sprenkle J A, Rosenshein N B, Migeon B R 1980 Mechanism of origin of complete hydatidiform moles. Nature 286: 714–716

Jacobs P A, Szulman A E, Funkhouser J, Matsuura J, Wilson C C 1982 Human triploidy: relationship between parental origin of the additional haploid complement and development of partial hydatidiform mole. Annals of Human Genetics 46: 223–231

Javey H, Borazjani G, Behmard S, Langley F A 1979 Discrepancies in the histological diagnosis of hydatidiform mole. British Journal of Obstetrics and Gynaecology 86: 480–483

Jeffreys A J, Wilson V, Thein S L 1985 Individual-specific 'fingerprints' of human DNA. Nature 316: 76–79

Kajii T, Ohama K 1977 Androgenetic origin of hydatidiform mole. Nature 268: 633–634

Kajii T, Kurashige H, Ohama K, Uchino F 1984 XY and XX complete moles: clinical and morphological correlations. American Journal of Obstetrics and Gynecology 150: 57–64

Kashimura Y, Kashimura M, Sugimori H et al 1986 Prophylactic chemotherapy for hydatidiform mole: five to 15 years follow-up. Cancer 58: 624–629

Kaufman M H, Lee K K H, Speirs S 1989 Influence of diandric and digynic triploid genotypes on early mouse embryogenesis. Development 105: 137–145

Kim D S, Moon H, Kim K T, Moon Y J, Hwang Y Y 1986 Effects of prophylactic chemotherapy for persistent trophoblastic disease in patients with complete hydatidiform mole. Obstetrics and Gynecology 67: 690–694

Kurman R J, Scully R E, Norris H J 1976 Trophoblastic pseudotumor of the uterus. An exaggerated form of 'syncytial endometritis' simulating a malignant tumour. Cancer 38: 1214–1226

Lage J M, Driscoll S G, Yavner D L, Olivier A P, Mark S D, Weinberg D S 1988 Hydatidiform moles. Application of flow cytometry in diagnosis. American Journal of Clinical Pathology 89: 596–600

Lage J M, Weinberg D S, Yavner D L, Bieber F R 1989 The biology of tetraploid hydatidiform moles: histopathology, cytogenetics and flow cytometry. Human Pathology 20: 419–425

Lawler S D, Fisher R A 1986 Genetic aspects of gestational trophoblast tumours. In: Ichinoe K (ed) Trophoblastic diseases. Igaku-Shoin, Tokyo, p 22–33

Lawler S D, Fisher R A 1987 Genetic studies in hydatidiform mole with clinical correlations. Placenta 8: 77–88

Lawler S D, Pickthall V J, Fisher R A, Povey S, Wyn Evans M, Szulman A E 1979 Genetic studies of complete and partial hydatidiform moles. Lancet ii: 580

Lawler S D, Fisher R A, Pickthall V J, Povey S, Wyn Evans M 1982 Genetic studies on hydatidiform moles. I. The origin of partial moles. Cancer Genetics and Cytogenetics 5: 309–320

Litt M, Luty J A 1989 A hypervariable microsatellite revealed by in vitro amplification of a dinucleotide repeat within the cardiac muscle actin gene. American Journal of Human Genetics 44: 397–401

Lo Y-M D, Patel P, Sampietro M, Gillmer M D G, Fleming K A, Wainscoat J S 1990 Detection of single-copy fetal DNA sequence from maternal blood. Lancet 335: 1463–1464

Makino S, Sasaki M S, Fukushima T 1963 Preliminary notes on the chromosomes of human chorionic lesions. Proceedings of the Academy of Japan 39: 54–58

Martin D A, Sutton G P, Ulbright T M, Sledge G W, Stehman F B, Ehrlich C E 1989 DNA content as a prognostic index in gestational trophoblastic neoplasia. Gynecologic Oncology 34: 383–388

McGrath J, Solter D 1984 Completion of mouse embryogenesis requires both the maternal and paternal genomes. Cell 37: 179–183

Messerli M L, Parmley T, Woodruff J D, Lilienfeld A M, Bevilacqua L, Rosenshein N B 1987 Inter- and intra-pathologist variability in the diagnosis of gestational trophoblastic neoplasia. Obstetrics and Gynecology 69: 622–626

Miesfeld R, Krystal M, Arnheim N 1981 A member of a new repeated sequence family which is conserved throughout eukaryotic evolution is found between the human δ and β globin genes. Nucleic Acids Research 9: 5931–5947

Mueller U W, Hawes C S, Wright A E et al 1990 Isolation of fetal trophoblast cells from peripheral blood of pregnant women. Lancet ii: 197–200

Nobunaga T, Azuma C, Kimura T et al 1990 Differential diagnosis between complete mole and hydrophic abortus by deoxyribonucleic acid fingerprints. American Journal of Obstetrics and Gynecology 163: 634–638

Ohama K, Kajii T, Okamoto E et al 1981 Dispermic origin of XY hydatidiform moles. Nature 292: 551–552

Ohama K, Ueda K, Okamoto E, Takenaka M, Fujiwara A 1986 Cytogenetic and clinicopathologic studies of partial moles. Obstetrics and Gynecology 68: 259–262

Olert J, Sawatzki G, Kling H, Gebauer J 1979 Cytological and histochemical studies on the mechanism of the selective silver staining of nucleolus organizer regions (NORs). Histochemistry 60: 91–99

Patillo R A, Sasaki S, Katayama K P, Roesler M, Mattingly R F 1981 Genesis of 46XY hydatidiform mole. American Journal of Obstetrics and Gynecology 141: 104–106

Rice L W, Berkowitz R S, Lage J M, Goldstein D P, Bernstein M R 1990 Persistent gestational trophoblastic tumour after partial hydatidiform mole. Gynecologic Oncology 36: 358–362

Saji F, Tokugawa Y, Kimura T et al 1989 A new approach using DNA fingerprinting for the determination of androgenesis as a cause of hydatidiform mole. Placenta 10: 399–405

Sarkar G, Sommers S S 1990 Shedding light on PCR contamination. Nature 345: 27

Scully R E, Young R H 1981 Trophoblastic pseudotumor. A reappraisal. American Journal of Surgical Pathology 5: 75–76

Sheppard D M, Fisher R A, Lawler S D, Povey S 1982 Tetraploid conceptus with three paternal contributions. Human Genetics 62: 371–374

Shibata D K, Arnheim N, Martin W J 1988 Detection of human papilloma virus in paraffin embedded tissue using the polymerase chain reaction. Journal of Experimental Medicine 167: 225–230

Surani M A H, Barton S C 1983 Development of gynogenetic eggs in the mouse: implications for parthenogenetic embryos. Science 222: 1034–1036

Surani M A H, Barton S C, Norris M L 1984 Development of reconstituted mouse eggs suggests imprinting of the genome during gametogenesis. Nature 308: 548–550

Surani M A H, Barton S C, Norris M L 1987 Influence of parental chromosomes on spatial specificity in androgenetic-parthenogenetic chimaeras in the mouse. Nature 326: 395–397

Surani M A H, Reik W, Allen N D 1988 Transgenes as molecular probes for genomic imprinting. Trends in Genetics 4: 59–62

Suresh U R, Chawner L, Buckley C H, Fox H 1990 Do AgNOR counts reflect cellular ploidy or cellular proliferation? A study of trophoblastic tissue. Journal of Pathology 160: 213–215

Surti U 1987 Genetic concepts and techniques. In: Szulman A E, Buchsbaun H J (eds) Gestational trophoblastic diseases. Springer-Verlag, Berlin, pp 111–121

Surti U, Szulman A E, O'Brien S 1979 Complete (classic) hydatidiform mole with 46,XY karyotype of paternal origin. Human Genetics 51: 153–155

Surti U, Szulman A E, Wagner K, Leppert M, O'Brien S J 1986 Tetraploid partial hydatidiform moles: two cases with a triple paternal contribution and a 92,XXXY karyotype. Human Genetics 72: 15–21

Szulman A E, Surti U 1978a The syndromes of hydatidiform mole. I. Cytogenetic and morphologic correlations. American Journal of Obstetrics and Gynecology 131: 665–671

Szulman A E, Surti U 1978b The syndromes of hydatidiform mole. II. Morphologic evolution of the complete and partial mole. American Journal of Obstetrics and Gynecology 132: 20–27

Szulman A E, Surti U 1982 The clinicopathologic profile of the partial hydatidiform mole. Obstetrics and Gynecology 5: 597–602

Takahashi H, Kanazawa K, Ikarashi T, Sudo N, Tanaka K 1990 Discrepancy in the diagnosis of hydatidiform mole by macroscopic and microscopic findings and the deoxyribonucleic acid fingerprint method. American Journal of Obstetrics and Gynecology 163: 112–113

Tandler C J 1954 An argentaffin component of the nucleolus. Journal of Histochemistry and Cytochemistry 2: 165–166

Teng N N H, Ballon S C 1984 Partial hydatidiform mole with diploid karyotype: report of three cases. American Journal of Obstetrics and Gynecology 150: 961–964

van Oven M W, Schoots C J F, Oosterhuis J W, Keij J F, Dam-Meiring A, Huisjes H J 1989 The use of DNA flow cytometry in the diagnosis of triploidy in human abortions. Human Pathology 20: 238–242

Vassilakos P, Riotton G, Kajii T 1977 Hydatidiform mole: two entities. A morphological and cytogenetic study with some clinical considerations. American Journal of Obstetrics and Gynecology 127: 167–170

Vejerslev L O, Fisher R A, Surti U, Wake N 1987a Hydatidiform mole: cytogenetically unusual cases and their implications for the present classification. American Journal of Obstetrics and Gynecology 157: 180–184

Vejerslev L O, Larsen J K, Christensen I B J, Tommerup N 1987b DNA-aneuploidy in 46,XX hydatidiform moles. Cancer Genetics and Cytogenetics 27: 225–228

Wake N, Takagi N, Sasaki M 1978 Androgenesis as a cause of hydatidiform mole. Journal of the National Cancer Institute 60: 51–57

Wake N, Seki T, Fujita H et al 1984 Malignant potential of homozygous and heterozygous complete moles. Cancer Research 44: 1226–1230

Wake N, Fujino T, Hoshi S et al 1987 The propensity to malignancy of dispermic heterozygous moles. Placenta 8: 319–326

Wallace D C, Surti U, Adams C W, Szulman A E 1982 Complete moles have paternal chromosomes but maternal mitochondrial DNA. Human Genetics 61: 145–147

Weber J L, May P E 1989 Abundant class of human DNA polymorphisms which can be typed using the PCR. American Journal of Human Genetics 44: 388–396

WHO Scientific Group 1983 Gestational trophoblastic disease. WHO Technical Report Series 692, WHO, Geneva

13. Endocrine pathology of ovarian neoplasia

H. Fox

INTRODUCTION

The ovary is an endocrine organ and many ovarian neoplasms are associated with clinically overt endocrinological abnormalities. Most endocrinological syndromes due to ovarian neoplasia reflect overproduction of sex steroids but some, such as Cushing's syndrome or hyperthyroidism, pay eloquent tribute to the hormonal versatility of this complex organ.

Ovarian hormone synthesis is subordinate to pituitary gonadotrophins, which are themselves controlled by hypothalamic releasing factors. The ovary principally secretes oestrone, oestradiol and progesterone, but every steroid occurring as an intermediary along the synthetic pathway from pregnenolone to oestradiol, such as testosterone, androstenedione, dehydroepiandrosterone and 17-hydroxyprogesterone, is present in higher concentrations in ovarian venous blood than in the peripheral plasma.

Ovarian sex steroids are synthesized from cholesterol, which may be formed de novo from acetate or may be derived from the circulating plasma pool (Fig. 13.1). Cholesterol is first converted to pregnenolone and further steps in steroid synthesis are principally along one or other of two alternative pathways. One of these is the delta-4 pathway in which the first stage is conversion of pregnenolone to progesterone, a reaction dependent upon the enzymes 3-β-hydroxysteroid dehydrogenase and 5,4-isomerase; progesterone then undergoes 17-hydroxylation to yield 17-hydroxyprogesterone, and subsequent cleavage of the side chain produces androstenedione. The alternative, and probably predominant, delta-5 pathway involves conversion of pregnenolone to 17-hydroxypregnenolone and cleavage of the side-chain from this to yield dehydroepiandrosterone: this latter is converted to androstenedione by the hydroxysteroid and isomerase enzyme systems. Androstenedione is then aromatized directly to oestrone or converted to testosterone, which is then aromatized to oestradiol. Oestrone and oestradiol can undergo a reversible oxidation–reduction reaction.

The cellular sites of ovarian sex steroid synthesis are still not fully defined: there is no doubt that thecal cells can synthesize androstenedione, but it is uncertain whether thecal cells are capable of aromatization of this

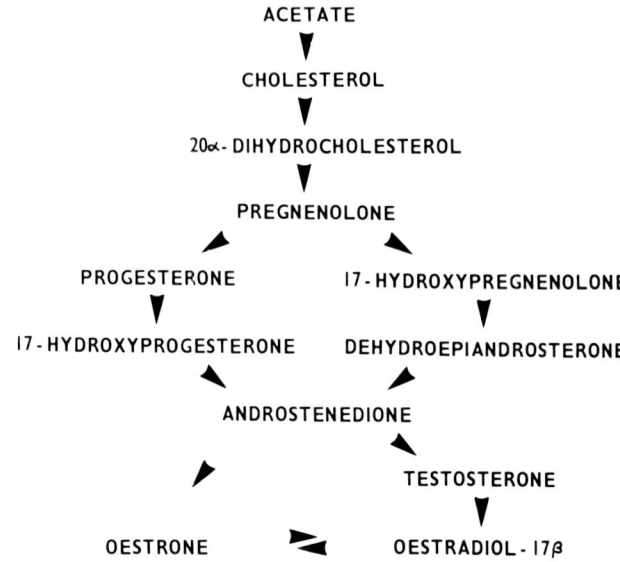

Fig. 13.1   Pathways of steroid biosynthesis in the ovary. The delta-4 pathway is on the left and the delta-5 pathway on the right. (Reproduced with permission from Fox & Langley 1976.)

androgen to oestrogens: one view is that thecally synthesized androstenedione is largely aromatized to oestrone by the body fat cells, only a small proportion, destined for intrafollicular secretion, being aromatized to oestrogens by the granulosa cells. An alternative concept is that all thecal-cell synthetized androstenedione is aromatized to oestrogens by the granulosa cells (Hillier 1981), these being the source of both intrafollicular and systemically secreted oestrogens.

The granulosa cells also secrete a number of non-steroidal substances, such as inhibin, oocyte maturation inhibitor, luteinization inhibitor, luteinization stimulator and follicle-regulatory factor (Ono et al 1986, Yen 1986, Ying 1988, McLachlan et al 1988), which control follicular development and function. The clinical significance of these regulators remains to be defined, but it has been suggested that both inhibin, which inhibits follicle-stimulating hormone secretion, and follicle-regulatory factor, which is involved in folliculogenesis, may serve as tumour markers in patients with granulosa cell tumours (Lappohn et al 1989, Rogers et al 1990).

ENDOCRINOLOGICAL SYNDROMES ASSOCIATED WITH OVARIAN NEOPLASMS

These fall into two broad groups:-

- Excess production of oestrogens and/or androgens
- Excess production of hormones other than sex steroids

Neoplasms associated with excess production of sex steroids

There are at least three possible mechanisms by which ovarian neoplasms may be associated with excess production of oestrogens or androgens:

- There may be direct synthesis and secretion of sex steroids by the neoplastic cells
- The tumour may be hormonally inert but associated with an endocrinologically active stroma
- The tumour may metabolize circulating hormones or substrates to oestrogens or androgens

It has to be borne in mind, when considering apparent sex hormone synthesis by an ovarian tumour, that hormones produced in the ovary may be metabolized in extraovarian sites and that the resulting clinical picture may be due to this extragonadally synthesized hormone rather than to the steroid originally produced by the ovarian neoplasm. Thus, for instance, a neoplasm secreting an androgen, such as androstenedione, may appear to be oestrogenic because of conversion of this substance to oestrone in the fat cells of the body.

A further consideration is that excess secretion of oestrogens in association with an ovarian neoplasm may be due to secretion by the tumour of gonadotrophins that stimulate oestrogen synthesis in the non-neoplastic ovarian tissue. This phenomenon is exemplified by the isosexual precocious pseudopuberty that may occur in young girls with a human chorionic gonadotrophin (hCG) secreting dysgerminoma or non-gestational ovarian choriocarcinoma.

Clinically detectable excess production of androgens will result in defeminization and virilization, whilst clinically apparent overproduction of oestrogens will lead to such symptoms as isosexual precocious pseudopuberty, menorrhagia or postmenopausal bleeding. It is often not realized that, during the reproductive years, hyperoestrogenism may manifest itself by amenorrhoea rather than excessive menstrual loss.

In the absence of hormone assays it is much easier to detect subclinical oestrogen excess than to recognize clinically covert androgen overproduction. There are no morphological 'markers' to allow for the recognition of an androgen effect and its differentiation from an oestrogen deficit: by contrast, the finding of proliferative activity in the endometrium many years after the menopause, of simple endometrial hyperplasia at any age and of vaginal cornification in the postmenopausal patient all permit an inappropriate oestrogen effect to be detected.

Direct synthesis and secretion of sex steroids by neoplastic cells

Virtually all the tumours that directly synthesize sex steroid hormones fall into either the sex cord–stromal or the steroid (lipid) cell categories. The steroid cell tumours have, until recently, been a poorly defined group and are afforded separate consideration in Chapter 14; they will not be discussed further in this chapter.

Granulosa cell tumours. The vast majority of granulosa cell tumours, whether of adult or juvenile type, are clinically oestrogenic (Fox & Langley 1976), not only being associated with symptoms such as isosexual precocious pseudopuberty, postmenopausal bleeding, menstrual abnormalities, painful enlargement of the breasts and, occasionally, an augumentation or a reactivation of the libido (the 'deuxième jeunesse' remarked upon by French authors) but also being associated with a high incidence of endometrial hyperplasia and, in about 5% of cases, with a well-differentiated endometrioid adenocarcinoma of the endometrium.

Despite, or possibly because of, the apparently clear-cut oestrogenic activity of granulosa cell tumours, there has been a striking paucity of endocrinological studies in women with such neoplasms. Those few patients who have been investigated have usually, though not invariably, had abnormally high levels of either plasma or urinary oestrogens that fell to normal after removal of the tumour (Jenner et al 1972, Target 1974, McCormack & Riddick 1976).

Granulosa cells, whether normal or neoplastic, appear to be devoid of the enzymes necessary for complete sex hormone synthesis (McKay et al 1949, Taki et al 1966) and generally lack the abundance of smooth endoplasmic reticulum and mitochondria with tubular cristae which characterize steroid-synthesizing cells (Klemi & Gronroos 1979, Genton 1980, Gaffney et al 1983). This does suggest, therefore, that oestrogen production by granulosa cell tumours is dependent upon preliminary synthesis of androgens by a thecal or stromal component. This view is compatible with studies showing that tissue slices or homogenates from granulosa cell tumours have an in vitro capacity to synthesize oestrogens from testosterone, androstenedione and dehydroepiandrosterone (Griffiths et al 1964, Besch et al 1966), for it is probable, indeed almost certain, that thecal or stromal cells were present in these preparations.

Immunocytochemical studies showed that oestradiol is present in the granulosa cell component of granulosa–theca cell tumours (Kurman et al 1979), but this does not disprove the concept that the final aromatization of androgenic precursors to oestrogens is the sole contribution of neoplastic granulosa cells to oestrogen synthesis, especially as some of the granulosa cells also stained positively for testosterone.

A small proportion of granulosa cell tumours appear to be androgenic rather than oestrogenic, several of these being associated with elevated plasma testosterone levels (Norris & Taylor 1969, Demopoulos & Bell 1983, Nakashima et al 1984, Dhont et al 1985). These virilizing granulosa cell tumours, though occasionally solid, have a particular tendency to be cystic, often macroscopically resembling a cystadenoma.

The mechanisms responsible for androgen synthesis by granulosa cell tumours are obscure. Tissue culture studies, however, have shown that whilst granulosa and thecal cells from normal follicles produce an excess of oestrogens over androgens, the reverse obtains for cells derived from atretic follicles (McNatty et al 1979). This has prompted the suggestion that the cells in virilizing granulosa cell tumours behave in a manner akin to those in an atretic follicle (Jarabak & Talerman 1983) which, it has to be assumed, lack or are deficient in aromatizing enzymes. An alternative explanation arises from an ultrastructural study of an androgenic granulosa cell neoplasm in which the morphological features regarded as characteristic of steroid-synthesizing cells were apparent only in non-neoplastic stromal cells that appeared to be showing Leydig, rather than thecal, cell differentiation (Demepoulos & Bell 1983).

Sex steroid synthesis is by the delta-4 pathway in at least some granulosa cell tumours (Dhont et al 1985). It is therefore not suprising that, very occasionally, neoplasms of this type have a predominantly progestational effect (Lomax et al 1977).

Thecomas. Thecal cell neoplasms are associated with a clinical picture identical to that encountered in granulosa cell tumours and thus usually appear to be oestrogenic. Thecal cells clearly have a capacity for steroid synthesis, and the ultrastructural appearances of the cells in a thecoma are typical of those of steroid-synthesizing cells (Salazar & Gonzalez-Angulo 1984). Oestradiol has been extracted, in considerable quantities, from a thecoma having an in vitro capacity to synthesize this oestrogen from androstenedione (Valette et al 1971), but the fact remains that non-neoplastic thecal cells are thought to be predominantly, if not solely, androgen-synthesizing. The paradox of the oestrogenic function of neoplastic thecal cells has not been resolved, though it is possible that their oestrogen effect is principally due to peripheral conversion of androstenedione to oestrone (Sasano et al 1989).

A number of virilizing thecal cell neoplasms have been described, but many of these appear to have been luteinized thecomas; these latter neoplasms contain groups of lutein cells and are androgenic in about 10% of cases (Zhang et al 1982). It is far from clear why a relatively small content of presumably androgenic lutein cells should produce a hormone effect that overshadows the oestrogenic activity of the thecoma, but it must be assumed that they are secreting a potent androgen that is not peripherally metabolized. Some androgenic thecomas contain Leydig cells, recognizable by their content of Reinke's crystals; these have been classed as stromal Leydig cell tumours (Zhang et al 1982), though it would be more logical to class them as Leydig cell-containing thecomas. There have, however, been a few reports of virilizing thecomas that apparently lacked a content of lutein or Leydig cells (Patton & Patton 1948, Nokes et al 1959); nothing is known about the metabolic capacities of such neoplasms, and there must always be a doubt as to whether more extensive sampling would have revealed a lutein cell component.

Sertoli–Leydig cell tumours. A high proportion of pure Sertoli cell tumours appear, clinically, to be oestrogenic, patients with these neoplasms commonly presenting with symptoms such as isosexual precocious pseudo-puberty or menorrhagia and having endometrial changes characteristic of oestrogenic stimulation (Fox & Langley 1976, Young & Scully 1984). One Sertoli cell tumour has been described which appeared to be secreting both oestrogens and progesterone (Tracy et al 1985), whilst a number of apparently androgenic Sertoli cell neoplasms have been reported (Fox & Langley 1976); most of these have been either poorly characterized or inadequately sampled, and it is highly probable that apparently androgenic Sertoli cell neoplasms are, in reality, incompletely sampled Sertoli–Leydig cell tumours.

Pure Leydig cell tumours fall conceptually within the category of Sertoli–Leydig cell tumours but are more conveniently classed as a form of steroid cell neoplasm: they are therefore discussed in Chapter 14.

Sertoli–Leydig cell tumours, which are probably Sertoli cell neoplasms with a reactive non-neoplastic stromal component that shows Leydig cell differentiation, are classically associated with clinical evidence of defemin-ization and virilization. In reality, only about one-third of patients with neoplasms of this type have symptoms and signs indicative of an androgen effect (Young & Scully 1985). Such patients usually first show defemin-ization, characterized by oligomenorrhoea, progressing to amenorrhoea, breast atrophy and loss of a normal female contour, followed by masculin-ization with acne, hirsutes, temporal hair recession, deepening of the voice and enlargement of the clitoris. Patients with such signs have an elevated plasma level of androgens, particularly androstenedione and testosterone (Mahesh et al 1970, Laatikainen et al 1972, Meldrum & Abraham 1979, Stegner & Lisboa 1984). In vitro studies have shown that Sertoli–Leydig cell tumour tissue is capable of synthesizing testosterone and a wide range of other androgens from pregnenolone and progesterone by both the delta-4 and delta-5 pathways (Kase & Conrad 1964, Younglai et al 1973, Stegner & Lisboa 1984, Nagamani et al 1989).

It is assumed, almost certainly correctly, that it is the Leydig cell component which is responsible for the androgenic activity of Sertoli–Leydig cell neoplasms. These cells have the typical fine structure associated with a steroid-synthesizing capacity (Kempson 1968, Fiz et al 1971, Murad et al 1973) and have been shown by immunocytochemistry to contain testosterone (Kurman et al 1978).

It has traditionally been thought that the incidence of clinical virilization increases progressively with decreasing degrees of differentiation of a Sertoli–Leydig cell tumour (Osborn & Yannone 1971), but in the largest reported series of neoplasms of this type no correlation could be shown between the incidence of clinical androgenic activity and the degree of differentiation of the tumour (Young & Scully 1985). A few Sertoli-Leydig cell tumours have appeared, on clinical grounds, to be oestrogenic (Detorres

1974, Genton & Schmid 1981, Young & Scully 1985, Dhont et al 1986): nothing is known about the metabolic characteristics of these unusual neoplasms.

Sclerosing stromal tumours. Between 10 and 25% of patients with ovarian tumours of this type have symptoms such as menorrhagia, or pathological findings such as endometrial hyperplasia, which suggest an oestrogenic effect (Gee & Russell 1979, Tang & Liu 1982). Two women with sclerosing stromal tumours had elevated preoperative levels of both oestrogens and androgens (Damjanov et al 1975, Yuen et al 1982), whilst a further two had raised levels only of androgens (Quinn et al 1981, Martinelli et al 1983). Enzymes typical of those involved in ovarian steroidogenesis, such as 17-β-hydroxysteroid dehydrogenase, have been detected in a sclerosing stromal tumour, and this neoplasm contained a population of cells with the ultrastructural features of steroid-synthesizing cells (Lam & Geittmann 1988). Whether the sclerosing stromal tumour is capable of full oestrogen synthesis or only of converting circulating oestrone to oestradiol remains uncertain.

Sex cord tumour with annular tubules. About 40% of patients with neoplasms of this type, unassociated with the Peutz–Jeghers syndrome, show clinical or pathological features suggestive of an oestrogenic effect (Crissman & Hart 1981, Ali 1981), though it is not yet fully clear whether such endocrinological activity is restricted to those tumours showing granulosa or Sertoli cell overgrowth. Oestrogen synthesis in these neoplasms appears to be via the delta-4 pathway (Crain 1986). Not entirely unexpectedly, two sex cord tumours with annular tubules have been described which were associated with a predominantly progestational effect (Czernobilsky et al 1985, Dolan et al 1986).

Sex cord tumours with annular tubules occurring in patients with the Peutz–Jeghers syndrome appear to be devoid of endocrinological activity. Ovarian tumours causing isosexual precocious pseudopuberty in young girls with the Peutz–Jeghers syndrome have been described, but these appear to have been of a unique nature, containing diffuse areas, cysts, tubules and papillae (Young et al 1983).

Epithelial tumours. In the vast majority of cases of apparently hormonally active epithelial tumours, the endocrine activity resides in the associated non-neoplastic stromal cells rather than in the neoplastic epithelial cells. There have, however, been a few genuine examples of virilizing or oestrogenic epithelial ovarian tumours which were not associated with stromal luteinization or hyperplasia, e.g. serous cystadenoma (Beauchamp et al 1989), and Brenner tumour (Kuhnel et al 1987, Lima et al 1989). The basis of this metabolic capacity of epithelial tumours is completely obscure, though it has been shown that tissue from an oestrogenic Brenner tumour was capable of in vitro aromatization of androgens to oestrogens (Kuhnel et al 1987).

Synthesis and secretion of sex steroids by tumours with an endocrinologically active stroma

The term 'tumours with functioning stroma' was introduced to describe ovarian neoplasms, either primary or metastatic, which fall outside the sex cord–stromal category but in which the stroma of the tumour contains steroid hormone-producing cells and the patient shows evidence of oestrogenic, androgenic or progestational effects (Morris & Scully 1958). The steroid hormone-secreting cells usually resemble luteinized thecal or stromal cells (Scully 1987) and are characteristically scattered in small nests or clumps throughout the tumour: in a minority of cases the luteinized cells form a peripheral shell around the neoplasm (Rutgers & Scully 1986). Occasionally the active stromal cells show Leydig cell differentiation and contain Reinkes crystals: such stromal Leydig cells may also be found either within or around the tumour (Hameed 1972, Sternberg & Roth 1973, Konishi et al 1986, Rutgers & Scully 1986). A final form of endocrinologically active stromal response to a tumour is seen in neoplasms lying adjacent to the ovarian hilum, which may show a hilar cell hyperplasia (Gardneau & Chabanne 1968, Derte & Foldes 1984, Rutgers & Scully 1986).

In all these various forms of endocrinologically active stromal response to an hormonally inert ovarian neoplasm, the active cells are rich in enzymes of steroidogenic type and, based on the few cases subjected to ultrastructural study, have the morphological characteristics of steroid-synthesizing cells (Scully 1987).

A functional stroma may be found in association with any type of epithelial or germ cell neoplasm but is noted most commonly in mucinous and endometrioid tumours: it is found infrequently in serous neoplasms. Functional stromas are also commonly seen in metastatic epithelial neoplasms of the ovary, most notably in Krukenberg's tumours; they are, however, rarely encountered in metastases from breast carcinomas. There is a particular association between germ cell neoplasms and a peripheral shell of luteinized stromal cells, this being seen most commonly with struma ovarii, ovarian carcinoid tumours and mature cystic teratomas.

Clinical virilization due to an epithelial or germ cell neoplasm with a functioning stroma is rare, occurring most commonly in, though not limited to, pregnant women with a Krukenberg's or primary mucinous tumour. It is extremely difficult to assess the possible oestrogenic effects of functional stromal cells in premenopausal women, but in those past the menopause there is a very high incidence of oestrogen effect, as determined either by plasma oestrogen assays, endometrial sampling or vaginal smears, in patients with epithelial ovarian tumours (Fox 1965, Fathalla 1968, Vesterinen et al 1978, Rome et al 1981, Heinonen et al 1982, Aiman et al 1986, Mahlck et al 1988). Clinical evidence of an oestrogen effect, as shown by postmenopausal bleeding from a hyperplastic or proliferative endometrium or, very uncommonly, swelling of the breasts, is by contrast relatively rare; it has been reported on occasion, however, in association with every type of primary epithelial tumour of the ovary, with metastatic epithelial neoplasms and, rather uncommonly, with germ cell tumours. It is usually assumed that any oestrogenic effect of a functional stroma is due to peripheral aromatization of androstenedione to oestrone, but it has been shown that cells derived from ovarian carcinomas are themselves capable of in vitro aromatization of testosterone to oestrogens (Thompson et al 1988).

A detailed correlation between clinical, endocrinological and morphological evidence of sex steroid secretion in association with epithelial or germ cell neoplasms and the presence of functionally active stromal cells has not been carried out. In general terms, however, there is a good, though far from absolute, correlation (Scully 1987).

The mechanisms responsible for the development of a functionally active stroma are far from clear though there has been no shortage of theories, amongst the more intellectually respectable of which are:

1. Stimulation of the stromal cells by hCG. This is almost certainly the cause of the virilizing stroma in tumours occurring in pregnancy; it probably also serves to explain the stromal luteinization found in association with syncytiotrophoblast-containing dysgerminomas. It is known that hCG is detectable by immunocytochemistry in many epithelial ovarian tumours (Mohabeer et al 1983), and it is possible that local hCG secretion by such neoplasms could induce stromal luteinization. Partial, though far from complete, support has been given to this hypothesis by the demonstration that hCG-synthesizing tumours are more commonly associated with stromal activation than are tumours lacking this synthetic capacity (Matias-Guiu & Prat 1990).

2. A mechanical hypothesis is that the stroma reacts to a tumour as it does to an expanding follicle, local pressure inducing the development of theca-like cells (Hughesdon 1958, Woodruff et al 1963). This hypothesis may well account for those slowly growing germ cell neoplasms with a peripheral rim of luteinized stromal cells, e.g. struma ovarii, but will not explain why a functionally active stroma should be more common in association with mucinous than serous tumours and in metastatic gastric than metastatic breast carcinomas.

3. The high levels of luteinizing hormone in many postmenopausal women with ovarian neoplasms could be responsible for the stromal luteinization (MacDonald et al 1976). This theory would not explain the by no means uncommon occurrence of stromal luteinization in epithelial and germ cell neoplasms occurring in premenopausal patients.

No all-embracing theory of the cause of stromal luteinization is therefore tenable, and it is probable that many different factors are involved, even in individual cases.

Production of sex steroids by tumour metabolism of circulating substrates

Sex steroid production as a result of tumour metabolism of circulating substrates probably only occurs in those neoplasms which contain trophoblastic tissue, i.e. choriocarcinoma and some cases of dysgerminoma. Trophoblastic tissue can metabolize circulating C19 steroids of adrenal origin, such as dehydroepiandrosterone sulphate, to oestrogens (Kirschner et al 1974). This may well account, in part at least, for the isosexual precocious pseudopuberty that occurs in some young girls with dysgerminoma (Zaloudek et al 1981) though, of course, hCG-induced stromal stimulation may also play a role in producing this symptom.

Neoplasms producing excess hormones other than sex steroids

Some ovarian tumours produce a predictable endocrinological syndrome, e.g. hyperthyroidism in association with a struma ovarii, whilst others show unpredictable, and apparently inexplicable, hormonal activity, e.g. aldosterone secretion by Sertoli cell neoplasms.

Predictable hormone synthesis

Struma ovarii. Biochemically proven hyperthyroidism develops in less than 5% of women with struma ovarii (Russell & Bannatyne 1989). A very high proportion of patients with struma ovarii and hyperthyroidism have an enlarged thyroid gland at the time of diagnosis or have a history of a previous partial thyroidectomy (Fox and Langley 1976) and this suggests that the ovarian thyroid tissue shares incidentally in a primary hyperthyroidism due to thyroid-stimulating immunoglobulins. Occasionally, however, the ovarian thyroid tissue is autonomous, probably because of adenomatous change, and causes hyperthyroidism whilst inhibiting the activity of the normally sited thyroid tissue (Perlmutter et al 1951).

Carcinoid tumours. Primary insular, but not trabecular, carcinoid tumours of the ovary are associated with the development of a typical carcinoid syndrome in one-third of cases (Qizilbash et al 1974, Robboy et al 1975). In contrast to intestinal carcinoid tumours, the carcinoid syndrome complicates ovarian neoplasms of this type in the absence of hepatic metastases; this is because serotonin, secreted by the ovarian tumour, enters directly into the systemic, rather than the portal, circulation and hence is not metabolized in the liver.

Rare, but not totally unexpected, hormonal effects of ovarian carcinoid tumours include the secretion of insulin, with resulting hypoglycaemic attacks (Margello et al 1988), and adrenocorticotrophic hormone production, with an accompanying Cushing's syndrome (Schlaghecke et al 1989).

Mucinous tumours. A few mucinous ovarian tumours, both benign and malignant, have been found to secrete considerable quantities of gastrin and have been responsible for the production of a Zollinger–Ellison syndrome (Cocco & Conway 1975, Bollen et al 1981, Morgan et al 1985, Primrose et al 1988, Maton et al 1989, de Broucker et al 1989, Garcia-Villanueva et al 1990). This is not altogether surprising, for a significant number of ovarian mucinous tumours are formed of gastric-type epithelium (Langley et al 1972).

Mature cystic teratoma. Instances of Cushing's syndrome (Axiotis et al 1987) and of hyperprolactinaemia (Palmer et al 1990), due respectively to a corticotroph cell adenoma and a prolactinoma developing in anterior pituitary tissue in a mature cystic teratoma, have been noted.

Unpredictable hormone synthesis

Examples of unexpected, and currently inexplicable, endocrinological activity by ovarian tumours include renin secretion, with resulting hypertension, by a Sertoli cell neoplasm (Korzets et al 1986), by a probable granulosa cell tumour (Tetu et al 1988) and by a leiomyosarcoma (Anderson et al 1989), and hyperaldosteronism associated with Sertoli–Leydig cell neoplasms (Ehrlich et al 1963, Todesco et al 1975) and a 'malignant sex cord stromal tumour' (Jackson et al 1986). In retrospect it appears possible that the hyperaldosteronism in these latter cases could have been due to tumour secretion of renin.

REFERENCES

Aiman J, Forney J P, Parker C R Jr 1986 Secretion of androgens and estrogens by normal and neoplastic ovaries in postmenopausal women. Obstetrics and Gynecology 68: 1
Ali F 1981 Sex cord tumor with annular tubules. Diagnostic Gynecology and Obstetrics 3: 137
Anderson P W, Macaulay L, Do Y S et al 1989 Extrarenal renin-secreting tumors: insight into hypertension and ovarian renin production. Medicine 68: 257
Axiotis C A, Lippes H A, Merino M G, de Lanerolle N C, Stewart A F, Kinder B 1987 Corticotroph cell pituitary adenoma within an ovarian teratoma: a new cause of Cushing's syndrome. American Journal of Surgical Pathology 11: 218
Beauchamp P J, Hughes R S, Schmidt W A 1989 Virilizing serous cystadenoma. Obstetrics and Gynecology 73: 513
Besch P G, Watson D J, Verys N, Hamwi G J, Barry R D, Barnett E B 1966 *In vitro* biosynthetic activity of endocrine tumors. VI. Malignant granulosa cell tumor. American Journal of Obstetrics and Gynecology 96: 466
Bollen E C, Lamers C B, Jansen J B, Larsson L I, Joosten H J 1981 Zollinger–Ellison syndrome due to a gastrin-producing ovarian cystadenocarcinoma. British Journal of Surgery 68: 776
Cocco A E, Conway S J 1975 Zollinger–Ellison syndrome associated with ovarian mucinous cystadenocarcinoma. New England Journal of Medicine 293: 485
Crain J C 1986 Ovarian sex cord tumor with annular tubules: steroid profile. Obstetrics and Gynecology 86: 75s
Crissman J D, Hart W R 1981 Ovarian sex cord tumors with annular tubules: an ultrastructural study of three cases. American Journal of Clinical Pathology 75: 11
Czernobilsky B, Gaedcke G, Dallenbach-Hellweg G 1985 Endometrioid differentiation in

ovarian sex cord tumor with annular tubules accompanied by gestational effect. Cancer 55: 738

Damjanov I, Drobnjak P, Grizelj V, Lomghino M 1975 Sclerosing stromal tumors of the ovary. Obstetrics and Gynecology 45: 675

de Broucker F, Caudron C, Sournia V, Adamsbaum C, Levesque M 1989 Syndrome de Zollinger–Ellison d'origine ovarienne: a propos d'un cas avec revue de la literature. Journal de Radiologie 70: 111

Demopoulos R I, Bell D A 1983 The fine structure of a virilizing human granulosa–theca cell tumor: observations on the nature of the hormone producing cell. Cancer 51: 1858

Derte Z, Foldes E 1984 Mucinous cystadenocarcinoma of the ovary with Leydig cell hyperplasia. Pathology Research and Practice 178: 400

Detorres E F 1974 Feminization in tumors of Sertoli–Leydig cells. Acta Cytologica 18: 187

Dhont M, Duvivier P, Vandekerckhove D 1985 A solid virilizing granulosa cell tumour. European Journal of Obstetrics, Gynaecology and Reproductive Biology 20: 253

Dhont M, Vandekerckhove F, Praet M, Vanluchen E, Vandekerckhove D 1986 A feminizing Sertoli–Leydig cell tumour in a postmenopausal woman: a case report. British Journal of Obstetrics and Gynaecology 95: 1171

Dolan J, Al-Timini A H, Richards S M et al 1986. Does ovarian sex cord tumour with annular tubules produce progesterone? Journal of Clinical Pathology 39: 29

Ehrlich E N, Dominguez O V, Samuels L T, Lynch D, Oberhelman H Jr, Warner N E 1963 Aldosteronism and precocious puberty due to an ovarian androblastoma (Sertoli cell tumor). Journal of Clinical Endocrinology 23: 358

Fathalla M F 1968 The role of the ovarian stroma in hormone production by ovarian tumours. Journal of Obstetrics and Gynaecology of the British Commonwealth 75: 78

Fiz G, Vital G I, Le Blanc M, Leng J, Vincendeau J, Leger H 1971 Etude d'un cas d'arrhenoblastome avec examen en ultrastructure. Bordeaux Medicin 4: 2145

Fox H 1965 Estrogenic activity of the serous cystadenoma of the ovary. Cancer 18: 401

Fox H, Langley F A 1976 Tumours of the ovary. Heinemann, London

Gaffney E F, Majmudar B, Hertzler G L, Zane R, Furlong B, Breding E 1983 Ovarian granulosa cell tumors: immunohistochemical localization of estradiol and ultrastructure, with functional correlations. Obstetrics and Gynecology 51: 311

Garcia-Villanueva M, Figuerola N B, Arbol L R et al 1990 Zollinger–Ellison syndrome due to a borderline mucinous cystadenoma of the ovary. Obstetrics and Gynecology 75: 549

Gardneau R, Chabanne F 1968 Dysembryome ovarien de type enteroide et bilio-hepatoide avec hyperplasie functionelle des cellules sympathicotropes de Berger: a propos d'une observation. Annales d'Anatomie Pathologique 13: 423

Gee D C, Russell P 1979 Sclerosing stromal tumours of the ovary. Histopathology 3: 367

Genton C Y 1980 Some observations on the fine structure of human granulosa cell tumours. Virchows Archiv A 387: 353

Genton C Y, Schmid J 1981 Ovarian Sertoli–Leydig cell tumor with hyperestrinism. Virchows Archiv 390: 243

Griffiths K, Grant J K, Symington T 1964 Steroid biosynthesis in vitro by granulosa-theca cell tissue. Journal of Endocrinology 30: 247

Hameed K 1972 Brenner tumor of the ovary with Leydig cell hyperplasia: a histological and ultrastructural study. Cancer 30: 945

Heinonen P K, Tuimala R, Pyykko O, Pystynen P 1982 Peripheral venous concentrations of oestrogens in postmenopausal women with ovarian cancer. British Journal of Obstetrics and Gynaecology 89: 84

Hillier S G 1981 Regulation of follicular oestrogen biosynthesis: a survey of current concepts. Journal of Endocrinology 89: 3

Hughesdon P E 1958 Thecal and allied reactions in epithelial ovarian tumours. Journal of Obstetrics and Gynaecology of the British Empire 65: 702

Jackson B, Valentine R, Wynn G 1986. Primary hyperaldosteronism due to malignant ovarian tumour. Australian and New Zealand Journal of Medicine 16: 69

Jarabak J, Talerman A 1983 Virilization due to a metastasizing granulosa cell tumor. International Journal of Gynecological Pathology 2: 316

Jenner M R, Kelch P R, Karlan S I, Grumbach M 1972 Hormonal changes in puberty. IV. Plasma estradiol, LH and FSH in prepubertal children, pubertal females and in precocious puberty, premature thelarche, hypogonadism and in a child with a feminizing ovarian tumor. Journal of Clinical Endocrinology and Metabolism 34: 521

Kase N, Conrad S H 1964 Steroid synthesis in abnormal ovaries. 1. Arrhenoblastoma. American Journal of Obstetrics and Gynecology 90: 1251

Kempson R L 1968 Ultrastructure of ovarian stromal cell tumors: Sertoli–Leydig cell tumor and lipid cell tumor. Archives of Pathology 86: 492

Klemi P J, Gronroos M 1979 An ultrastructural and clinical study of theca and granulosa cell tumors. International Journal of Gynaecology and Obstetrics 17: 219

Kirschner M A, Cohen F B, Jesperson P 1974 Estrogen production and its origin in men with gonadotropin-producing neoplasms. Journal of Clinical Endocrinology and Metabolism 30: 504

Konishi I, Fujii S, Ishikawa Y, Suzuki A, Okamura H, Mori T 1986 Ovarian fibroma with Leydig cell hyperplasia of the adjacent stroma: light and electron microscopic study. International Journal of Gynecological Pathology 5: 170

Korzets A, Nouriel H, Steiner Z et al 1986 A renin-producing ovarian Sertoli cell tumor. American Journal of Clinical Pathology 85: 242

Kuhnel R, Rao B R, Stolk J G, van Kessel H, Seldicnrijk C A, Willing A P 1987 Estrogen synthesizing rare malignant Brenner tumor of ovary with the presence of progesterone and androgen receptors in the absence of estrogen receptors. Gynecologic Oncology 26: 263

Kurman R J, Andrade G, Goebelsmann U, Taylor C R 1978 An immunohistological study of steroid localization in Sertoli–Leydig cell tumors of the ovary. Cancer 42: 1772

Kurman R J, Goebelsmann U, Taylor C R 1979 Steroid localization in granulosa–theca tumors of the ovary. Cancer 43: 2377

Laatikainen T, Pelkonen R, Vikho R 1972 Plasma steroids in two subjects with ovarian androgen producing tumours, androblastoma and gynandroblastoma. Journal of Clinical Endocrinology and Metabolism 34: 580

Lam R M Y, Geittmann P 1988 Sclerosing stromal tumor of the ovary: a light, electron microscopic and enzyme histochemical study. International Journal of Gynecological Pathology 7: 280

Langley F A, Cummins P A, Fox H 1972 An ultrastructural study of mucin secreting epithelia in ovarian neoplasms. Acta Pathologica et Microbiologica Scandinavia Section A 80 (Suppl 233): 76

Lappohn R E, Burger G H, Bouma J, Baugah M, Krans M, de Bruijn H W D 1989 Inhibin as a marker for granulosa cell tumors. New England Journal of Medicine 321: 790

Lima G R de, Lima O A de, Baracat E C, Vasserman J, Burnier M 1989 Virilizing Brenner tumor of the ovary: case report. Obstetrics and Gynecology 73: 895

Lomax C W, May H L, Panko W B, Thornton W N 1977 Progesterone production of an ovarian granulosa cell carcinoma. Obstetrics and Gynecology 50: 32s

McCormack T P, Riddick D H 1976 Hormonal function of a granulosa tumor. Obstetrics and Gynecology 48: 18s

MacDonald P C, Grodin J M, Edman C D, Vellios F, Siiteri P K 1976 Origin of estrogen in a postmenopausal woman with a nonendocrine tumor of the ovary and endometrial hyperplasia. Obstetrics and Gynecology 47: 644

McKay D G, Robinson D, Hertig A T 1949 Histochemical observations on granulosa cell tumors, thecomas and fibromas of the ovary. American Journal of Obstetrics and Gynecology 58: 625

McLachlan R I, Roberman D M, de Ketser D M, Burger H G 1988 Advances in the physiology of inhibin and inhibin-related peptides. Clinical Endocrinology 29: 77

McNatty K P, Makris A, DeGrazia C, Osathanondu R, Ryan K J 1979 The production of progesterone, androgens and estrogens by granulosa cells, thecal tissue and stromal tissue from human ovaries *in vitro*. Journal of Clinical Endocrinology and Metabolism 49: 687

Mahesh V B, McDonough P G, Deleo C A 1970 Endocrine studies in the arrhenoblastoma. American Journal of Obstetrics and Gynecology 107: 183

Mahlck C-G, Backstrom T, Kjellgren O 1988 Plasma level of estradiol in patients with ovarian malignant tumors. Gynecologic Oncology 30: 313

Margello S, Schwartz E, Horwith M, King M E, Gorden P, Alonso D R 1988 Ectopic insulin production by a primary ovarian carcinoid. Cancer 61: 800

Martinelli G, Govoni E, Pileri S, Grigioni F W, Doglioni C, Pelusi G 1983 Sclerosing stromal tumour of the ovary. Virchows Archiv 402: 155

Matias-Guiu X, Prat J 1990 Ovarian tumors with functioning stroma: an immunohistochemical study of 100 cases with human chorionic gonadotrophin monoclonal and polyclonal antibodies. Cancer 65: 2001

Maton P N, Mackem S N, Norton J A, Gardner J D, O'Dorisio T M, Jensen R T 1989 Ovarian carcinoma as a cause of Zollinger–Ellison syndrome: natural history, secretory products and response to provocative tests. Gastroenterology 77: 468

Meldrum A R, Abraham G E 1979 Peripheral and ovarian venous concentrations of various steroid hormones in virilizing ovarian tumors. Obstetrics and Gynecology 53: 36

Mohabeer J, Buckley C H, Fox H 1983 An immunohistochemical study of the incidence and significance of human chorionic gonadotrophin synthesis by epithelial ovarian neoplasms. Gynecologic Oncology 16: 78

Morgan D R, Wells M, MacDonald R C, Johnston D 1985 Zollinger–Ellison syndrome due to a gastrin secreting ovarian mucinous cystadenoma: case report. British Journal of Obstetrics and Gynaecology 92: 867

Morris J M, Scully R E 1958 Endocrine pathology of the ovary. Mosby, St. Louis

Murad T M, Mancini R, George J 1973 Ultrastructure of a virilizing ovarian Sertoli–Leydig cell tumor with familial incidence. Cancer 31: 1440

Nakashima N, Young R H, Scully R E 1984 Androgenic granulosa cell tumors of the ovary: a clinicopathologic analysis of 17 cases and review of the literature. Archives of Pathology and Laboratory Medicine 108: 786

Nagamani M, Stuart C A, Dinh T V 1989 Steroid biosynthesis in the Sertoli–Leydig cell tumor: effect of insulin and luteinizing hormone. American Journal of Obstetrics and Gynecology 161: 1738

Nokes J M, Claiborne H A, Reingold W N 1959 Thecoma with associated virilization. American Journal of Obstetrics and Gynecology 78: 722

Norris H J, Taylor H B 1969 Virilization associated with cystic granulosa tumors. Obstetrics and Gynecology 34: 629

Ono T, Campeau J D, Holmberg E A et al 1986 Biochemical and physiological characterization of follicle regulatory protein: a paracrine regulator of folliculogenesis. American Journal of Obstetrics and Gynecology 154: 709

Osborn R H, Yannone M E 1971 Plasma androgens in the normal and androgenic female: a review. Obstetrical and Gynecological Survey 26: 195

Palmer P E, Bogojavlemsky S, Bhan A K et al 1990 Prolactinoma in wall of ovarian dermoid cyst with hyperprolactinemia. Obstetrics and Gynecology 75: 540

Patton C L, Patton R J 1948 Ovarian thecoma: case report with contrasting symptomology. Illinois Medical Journal 94: 184

Perlmutter M, Mufson M, David M M 1951 Inhibition of a cervical thyroid gland by a functioning struma ovarii. Journal of Clinical Endocrinology 11: 621

Primrose J N, Maloney M, Wells M, Bulgim O, Johnston D 1988 Gastrin-producing ovarian mucinous cystadenoma:a cause of the Zollinger–Ellison syndrome. Surgery 104: 830

Qizilbash A H, Trebilcock R G, Patterson M C, Lamont K G 1974 Functioning primary carcinoid tumor of the ovary: a light and electron microscopic study with review of the literature. American Journal of Clinical Pathology 62: 629

Quinn M A, Oster A O, Fortune D, Hudson B 1981 Sclerosing stromal tumour of the ovary: case report with endocrine studies. British Journal of Obstetrics and Gynaecology 88: 555

Robboy S J, Norris H J, Scully R E 1975 Insular carcinoid primary in the ovary: a clinicopathologic analysis of 48 cases. Cancer 36: 404

Rogers K E, Marks J F, Ellefson M S et al 1990 Follicle regulating protein: a novel marker of granulosa cell cancer patients. Gynecologic Oncology 37: 381

Rome R M, Fortune D W, Quinn M A, Brown J B 1981 Functioning ovarian tumors in postmenopausal women. Obstetrics and Gynecology 57: 705

Russell P, Bannatyne P 1989 Surgical pathology of the ovaries. Churchill Livingstone, Edinburgh

Rutgers J L, Scully R E 1986 Functioning ovarian tumors with peripheral steroid cell proliferation: a report of twenty four cases. International Journal of Gynecological Pathology 5: 319

Salazar H, Gonzalez-Angulo A 1984 Ultrastructural diagnosis in gynaecological pathology. Clinics in Obstetrics and Gynaecology 11: 25

Sasano H, Okamoto M, Mason J I et al 1989 Immunohistochemical studies of steroidogenic enzymes (aromatase, 17α-hydroxylase and cholesterol side chain cleavage cytochromes P-450) in sex cord–stromal tumors of the ovary. Human Pathology 20: 452

Schlaghecke R, Kreuzpaintner G, Burrig K F, Juli E, Kley H K 1989 Cushing's syndrome due to ACTH-production of an ovarian carcinoid. Klinische Wochenschrift 67: 640

Scully R E 1987 Ovarian tumours with functioning stroma. In: Fox H (ed) Haines and Taylor: Obstetrical and gynaecological pathology, 3rd edn. Churchill Livingstone, Edinburgh, p 724

Stegner H E, Lisboa B P 1984 Steroid metabolism in androblastoma (Sertoli–Leydig cell tumor); a histopathological and biochemical study. International Journal of Gynecological Pathology 2: 410

Sternberg W H, Roth L M 1973 Ovarian stromal tumors containing Leydig cells. 1. Stromal–Leydig cell tumor and non-neoplastic transformation of ovarian stroma to Leydig cells. Cancer 32: 940

Taki I, Hamanaka M, Mori M 1966 Histochemical observations of enzymatic patterns in human ovaries. American Journal of Obstetrics and Gynecology 96: 386

Tang M, Liu T 1982 Ovarian sclerosing stromal tumors: clinicopathologic study of 10 cases. Chinese Medical Journal 95: 186

Target C S 1974 Estrogen excretion in a case of theca–granulosa cell tumor. American Journal of Obstetrics and Gynecology 119: 859

Tetu B, Leber M, Camilleri J-P 1988 Renin-producing ovarian tumor: a case report with immunohistological and electron-microscopic study. American Journal of Surgical Pathology 12: 634

Thompson M A, Adelson M P, Kaufman L M, Marshall L D, Cable D M 1988 Aromatization of testerone by epithelial cells cultured from patients with ovarian carcinoma. Cancer Research 48: 6491

Todesco S, Terribile E, Borsatti A, Mantero F 1975 Primary aldosteronism due to a malignant ovarian tumor. Journal of Clinical Endocrinology and Metabolism 41: 809

Valette C, Laymarie P, Castagnier M, Chamilian A 1971 Un cas de thecome de l'ovaire: hormonologie structure fine, histochimie, incubation. Annales d'Endocrinologie 52: 608

Vesterinen E, Purola E, Wahlstrom T 1978 Oestrogenic activity associated with ovarian cystadenomas after the menopause. Annales Chirurgiae at Gynaecologiae 67: 109

Woodruff J D, Williams T J, Goldberg B 1963 Hormone activity of the common ovarian neoplasms. American Journal of Obstetrics and Gynecology 87: 697

Yen S C 1986 The normal menstrual cycle. In: Yen S C, Jaffe R B (eds) Reproductive endocrinology, 2nd edn. W B Saunders, Philadelphia, p 200

Ying S Y 1988 Inhibins, activins and follistatins: gonadal proteins regulating the action of follicle stimulating hormone. Endocrinology Reviews 9: 267

Young R H, Scully R E 1984 Ovarian sex cord–stromal tumours: recent advances and current status. Clinics in Obstetrics and Gynecology 11: 93

Young R H, Scully R E 1985 Sertoli–Leydig cell tumors: a clinicopathologic analysis of 207 cases. American Journal of Surgical Pathology 9: 543

Young R H, Dickersin G R, Scully R E 1983 A distinctive ovarian sex cord–stromal tumor causing sexual precocity in the Peutz–Jeghers syndrome. American Journal of Surgical Pathology 7: 223

Younglai E V, Richmond H, Atyeo R, Johnson F L 1973 Arrhenoblastoma: in vivo and in vitro studies. American Journal of Obstetrics and Gynecology 116: 401

Yuen B H, Robertson I, Clement P B, Mincey E K 1982 Sclerosing stromal tumor of the ovary. Obstetrics and Gynecology 60: 252

Zaloudek C J, Tavassoli F, Norris H J 1981 Dysgerminoma with syncytiotrophoblastic giant cells: a histologically and clinically distinctive subtype of dysgerminoma. American Journal of Surgical Pathology 5: 361

Zhang J, Young R H, Arseneau J, Scully R E 1982 Ovarian stromal tumors containing lutein or Leydig cells (luteinized thecomas and stromal Leydig cell tumors): a clinicopathological analysis of fifty cases. International Journal of Gynecological Pathology 1: 270

14. Steroid cell tumours of the ovary

Robert H. Young   Robert E. Scully

INTRODUCTION

The terms 'adrenal rest tumour', 'adrenal-like tumour', 'masculinovo-blastoma', 'lipoid cell tumour', and 'lipid cell tumour' have been applied for many years to ovarian neoplasms composed entirely, or almost entirely, of cells resembling typical steroid-hormone secreting cells, that is lutein cells, Leydig cells, and adrenocortical cells. The first three terms have been largely discarded, and, as up to 25% of these tumours contain no stainable fat, the last two designations are often inaccurate. The term 'steroid cell tumour' has been proposed (Scully 1979) as more appropriate and has now been accepted by the World Health Organization group classifying ovarian tumours. This designation reflects both the morphological features of the neoplastic cells and their propensity to secrete steroid hormones.

Steroid cell tumours account for 0.1% of all ovarian neoplasms, and are derived in almost all cases from ovarian stromal cells or their luteinized derivatives, or from Leydig cells of hilar or stromal origin. An origin from cells of adrenocortical rests is unlikely, as adrenocortical rests have been described in the fetal ovary only once (Symmonds & Driscoll 1973) and have not been identified in the postnatal ovary. Even in cases in which raised serum cortisol concentrations or Cushing's syndrome, or both, have been associated with a steroid cell tumour, the intraovarian location of the tumours in such cases and their similarity to other steroid cell tumours without hypercortisolaemia favour the interpretation that the adrenal type hormones were secreted ectopically by gonadal steroid cells rather than adrenocortical rest cells. Adrenocortical rests have been found, however, in up to 27% of hysterectomy specimens in the broad ligament and are occasionally located in the ovarian hilus (Falls 1955), and it is possible that steroid cell tumours in these locations may have arisen in such rests.

Steroid cell tumours have been subclassified as stromal luteoma, Leydig cell tumour (hilus cell tumour and Leydig cell tumour, non-hilar type), and steroid cell tumour not otherwise specified (NOS) on the basis of knowledge or lack of knowledge of their cell of origin. The major clinical and pathological features of these neoplasms are compared in Table 14.1. Tumours composed of steroid cells arising from a background of spindle-

Table 14.1 Clinical and pathological features of steroid cell tumours (from Paraskevas & Scully 1989)

	Stromal luteoma	Hilus cell tumour		Steroid cell tumour NOS
		Reinke crystal positive	Reinke crystal negative	
Number of cases	25	12	9	63
Age range[1] (years)	28–74 (58)	32–75 (57)	34–82 (61)	2–80 (43)
Virilization or hirsutism (%)	12	83	33	52
Oestrogenic manifestations (%)	60	0	44	8
Duration of androgenic manifestations (years)	1.5–5	2–20	1–24	0.5–30
No endocrine abnormality (%)	20	17	23	27
Cushing's syndrome (%)	0	0	0	6
Mean diameter (CM)	1.3	2.4	1.8	8.4
Associated stromal hyperthecosis (%)	92	42	67	23
Associated endometrial hyperplasia or carcinoma (%)	88	8	33	24

[1]Means are given in parentheses.
NOS = not otherwise specified.

shaped cells, such as luteinized thecomas and stromal Leydig cell tumours (Zhang et al 1982), although closely related to steroid cell tumours, are not discussed in this chapter.

STROMAL LUTEOMA

The stromal luteoma (Scully 1964, Hayes & Scully 1987a) accounts for about 25% of steroid cell tumours. It is characterized by a location in the ovarian stroma and an absence of crystals of Reinke, the distinctive inclusions of Leydig cells. These neoplasms are by definition small because large steroid cell tumours are no longer confined to the ovarian stroma and must be designated steroid cell tumour NOS in the absence of crystals of Reinke. In view of its topography, the stromal luteoma must arise from luteinized stromal cells or their precursors, the spindle cells of the ovarian stroma. The presence of luteinized stromal cells (stromal hyperthecosis) elsewhere in the same or contralateral ovary in 90% of the cases supports a stromal origin (Hayes & Scully 1987a), as does the rare occurrence of a lesion intermediate between stromal hyperthecosis and stromal luteoma, namely nodular hyperthecosis. This is characterized by multiple nests of stromal lutein cells that are large enough to be visible on very careful gross examination, but do not form a single tumour mass.

Eighty per cent of stromal luteomas occur in postmenopausal women (Table 14.1) (Hayes & Scully 1987a). The initial symptom in 60% of cases is abnormal vaginal bleeding probably related to associated hyperoestrinism, although whether the tumour secretes oestrogen directly or an androgen that is converted peripherally to an oestrogen is unknown. As the tumour is not palpable, it is usually implicated as the probable cause of the bleeding only when it is identified as an incidental finding in a hysterectomy and bilateral salpingo-oophorectomy specimen. Androgenic manifestations are present in only 12% of cases. This profile of hormonal function is the converse of that associated with other categories of steroid cell tumour, which are usually androgenic and only occasionally oestrogenic. Associated stromal hyperthecosis may contribute to the clinical picture in some cases, particularly those in which there is a very long history of hormonal disturbance. At least one case of stromal luteoma has been associated with the insulin resistance/acanthosis nigricans/hyperandrogenism syndrome (Givens et al 1974), in which the ovaries are polycystic with stromal hyperthecosis (Dunaif et al 1985). All of the reported tumours have been benign, as expected in view of their small size and bland cytological features.

Stromal luteomas are almost always under 3 cm in diameter and, with rare exceptions, are unilateral. They are well circumscribed, solid, and usually grey-white or yellow, but one-third have red or brown areas (Fig. 14.1). Microscopic examination reveals an unencapsulated, rounded nodule (Fig. 14.2). composed of polyhedral cells arranged diffusely or in small nests (Fig. 14.3) and less commonly cords of cells which are more or less completely surrounded by ovarian stroma. Degenerative changes occur in

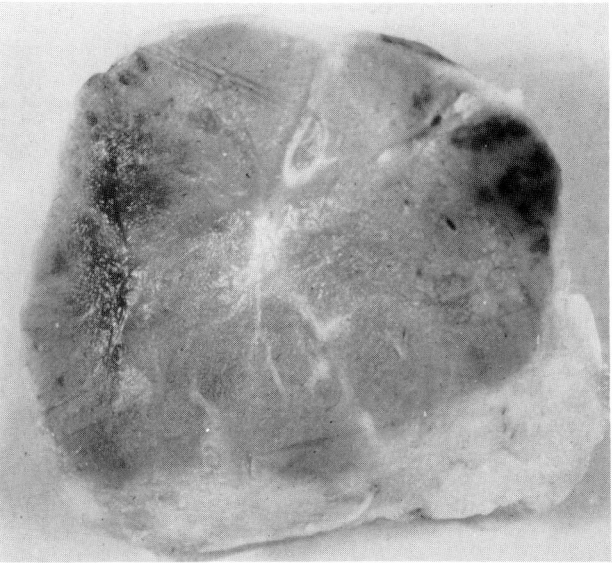

Fig. 14.1 Stromal luteoma. The tumour measured 2.0 cm in greatest dimension and was brown when unfixed. (Courtesy of Dr Philip B. Clement.)

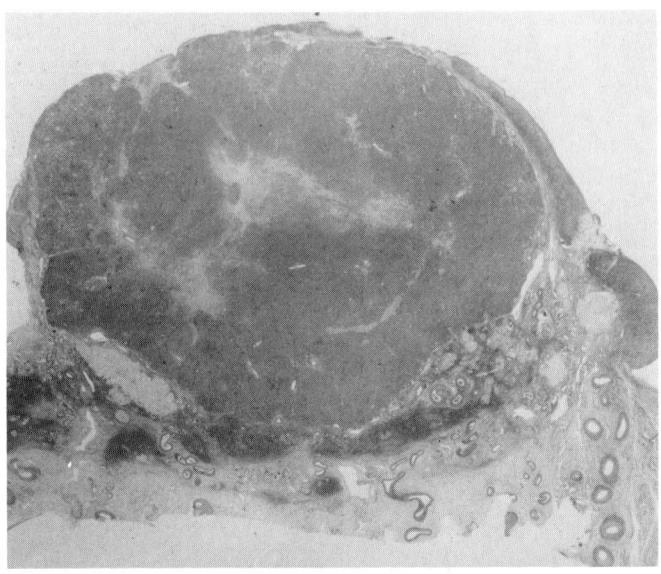

Fig. 14.2   Stromal luteoma. The tumour is confined to the ovarian stroma (H & E, × 10).

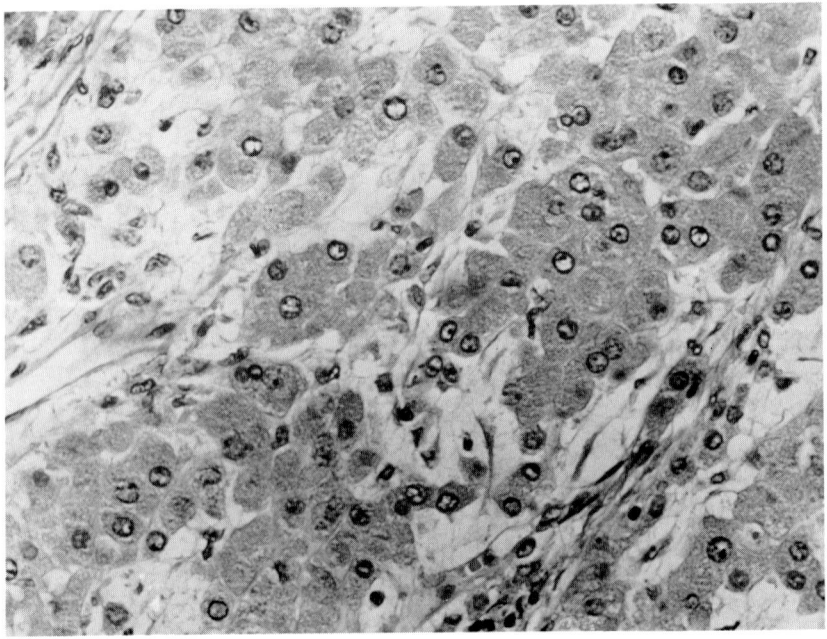

Fig. 14.3   Stromal luteoma. The cells have abundant cytoplasm that is granular and eosinophilic. The nuclei are round and regular; some of them have a prominent nucleolus (H & E, × 313).

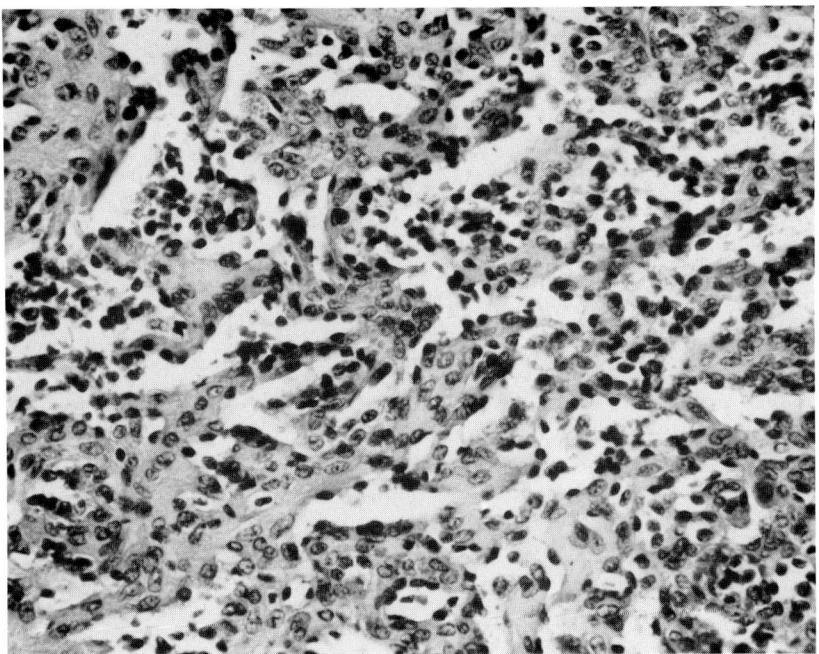

Fig. 14.4   Stromal luteoma. Degenerative changes have produced irregular spaces containing red blood cells that simulate vascular spaces (H & E, × 400). (Reproduced with permission from Young & Scully 1987b.)

20% of cases, resulting in the presence of spaces that vary from elongated and slit-like (Fig. 14.4) to rounded and cystically dilated. The spaces may contain, or be surrounded by, lipid-laden cells and chronic inflammatory cells and may be associated with fibrosis. In some cases they contain red blood cells (Fig. 14.4). The stroma is typically sparse and consists of delicate connective tissue, but in about 20% of the cases it is more prominent and fibrous or hyalinized. The cytoplasm of the neoplastic cells is abundant and usually eosinophilic and slightly granular, but occasionally it is pale or foamy; it often contains lipochrome granules. The nuclei are typically small and round with single prominent nucleoli; mitotic figures are rare. As noted above, stromal hyperthecosis is present in the stroma of one or both ovaries in almost all cases, and hilus cell hyperplasia is also seen in 25% of cases (Hayes & Scully 1987a).

LEYDIG CELL TUMOURS

Leydig cells cannot be distinguished from lutein or adrenocortical cells unless they contain cytoplasmic Reinke crystals, and a steroid cell tumour cannot be demonstrated conclusively to be of Leydig cell nature unless these inclusions are found on either light microscopic or electron microscopic examination. As only 35–40% of Leydig cell tumours of the testis contain crystals on light microscopic examination (Kim et al 1985), it is probable that many steroid cell tumours NOS are crystal-negative Leydig cell tumours that can not specifically be identified as such. Almost all ovarian Leydig cell tumours arise in the hilus from hilar Leydig cells (hilus cells); these can be identified in over 80% of normal adult ovaries that are sampled extensively for microscopic examination (Sternberg 1949). The very rare category of small Leydig cell tumours located in the ovarian stroma away from the hilus is referred to as Leydig cell tumour non-hilar type.

Hilus cell tumours and tumours designated as probable (crystal-negative) hilus cell tumours account for about 20% of steroid cell tumours (Paraskevas & Scully 1980) and, like stromal luteomas, usually occur in postmenopausal patients (Table 14.1). They are only rarely palpable (Dunnihoo et al 1966, Salm 1974, Motlik et al 1988, Ichinohasawa et al 1989, Paraskevas & Scully 1989). Androgenic manifestations are present in about 80% of patients (Paraskevas & Scully 1989), and in some have been present for many years before the tumour was detected; the androgenic changes are typically less abrupt in onset and milder than those associated with Sertoli–Leydig cell tumours (Young & Scully 1987), though the patients usually have a high serum concentration of testosterone. Virilizing changes regress, but may not disappear, after removal of the tumour. Oestrogenic changes may also be present and can be attributed to secretion of oestrogens by the tumour, peripheral conversion of androgens produced by the tumour, associated stromal hyperthecosis, or a combination of these factors. Almost all the hilus cell tumours that have been reported have been benign; only one purportedly malignant case in the literature merits serious consideration (Echt & Hadd 1968), but Reinke crystals were not convincingly documented in the illustrations of that neoplasm.

Hilus cell tumours are typically reddish-brown to yellow but can be dark brown or almost black (Fig. 14.5). They are characteristically small (mean

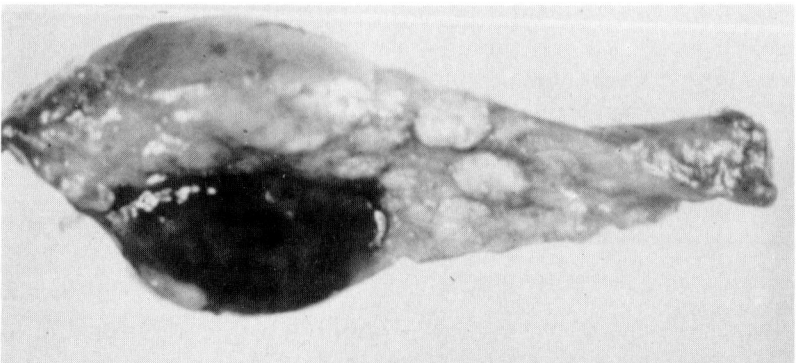

Fig. 14.5   Leydig cell tumour (hilus cell type). The small tumour is located in the hilus and was black.

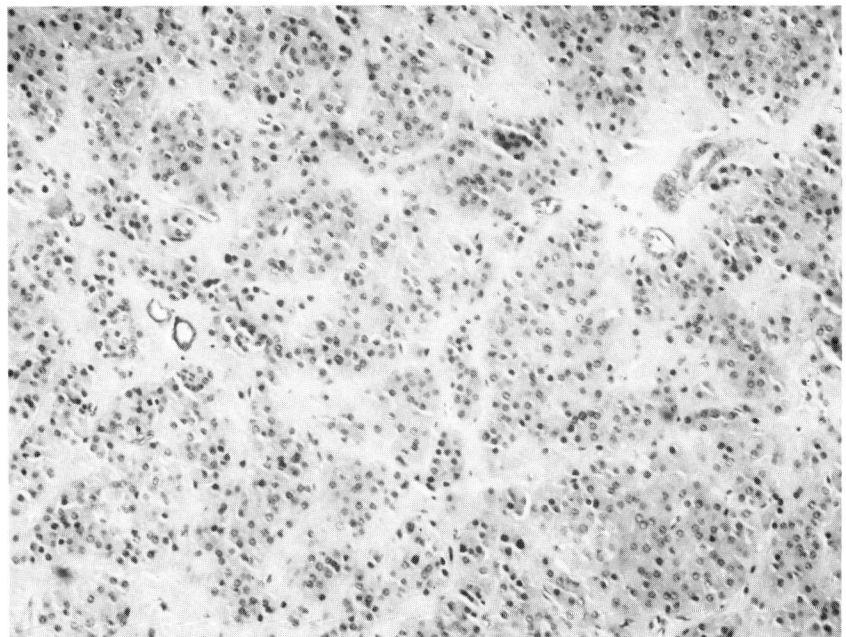

Fig. 14.6   Hilus cell tumour. The Leydig cells are aggregated and separated by acellular tissue (H & E, × 125).

diameter 2.4 cm), circumscribed nodules centered in the ovarian hilus (Fig. 14.5) but may extend for varying distances into the ovarian stroma (Paraskevas & Scully 1989). Rarely they are bilateral (Baramki et al 1983). Microscopic examination reveals an unencapsulated nodule composed of steroid cells typically growing diffusely but occasionally growing as nests (Fig. 14.6) or nodules separated by fibrous stroma. Perivascular nuclear clustering with pooling of cytoplasm or hyalinized stroma is present in half the cases (Fig. 14.6). An unusual feature in one-third of cases is fibrinoid replacement of the walls of moderate-sized vessels unaccompanied by an inflammatory cell infiltrate (Fig. 14.7). Degenerative spaces similar to those seen in stromal luteomas may be present (Fig. 14.8). The tumour cells typically contain abundant granular eosinophilic cytoplasm (Fig. 14.9); occasional cells have spongy cytoplasm indicating the presence of lipid. Cytoplasmic lipochrome pigment, which is usually sparse, is present in most cases. The typically round nuclei are often hyperchromatic and contain single small nucleoli. There may be a slight to moderate variation in nuclear size and shape; occasional bizarre nuclei (Fig. 14.10) and multi-nucleated cells may be found. Pseudoinclusions of cytoplasm into the nucleus may be apparent. Rarely, mitotic figures are present. Elongated eosinophilic Reinke crystals of varying sizes are present in varying numbers in the cytoplasm (Fig. 14.9) or sometimes in the nucleus, but are often found

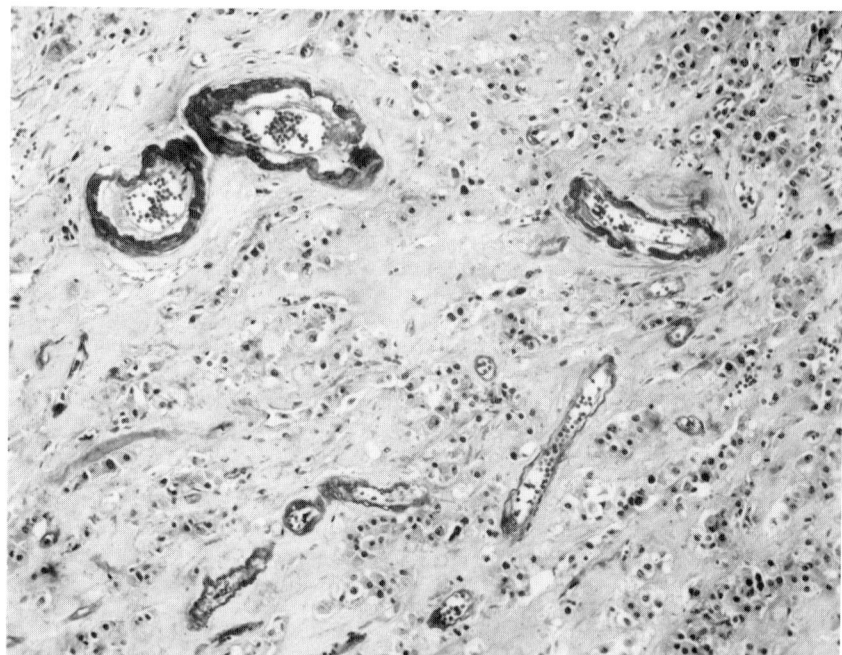

Fig. 14.7 Leydig cell tumour. Several blood vessels show fibrinoid change of their walls (H & E, × 125).

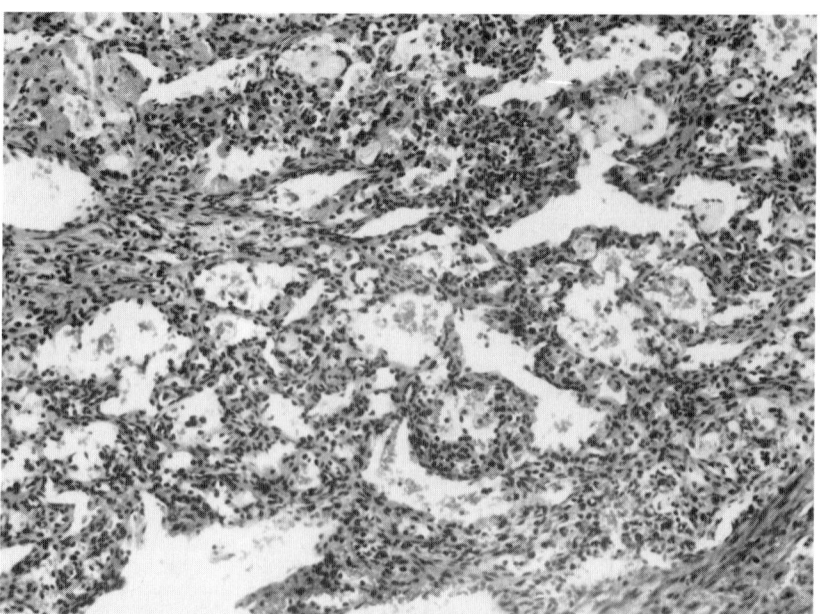

Fig. 14.8 Leydig cell tumour. Degenerative spaces, which are irregular in size and shape, are conspicuous (H & E, × 125).

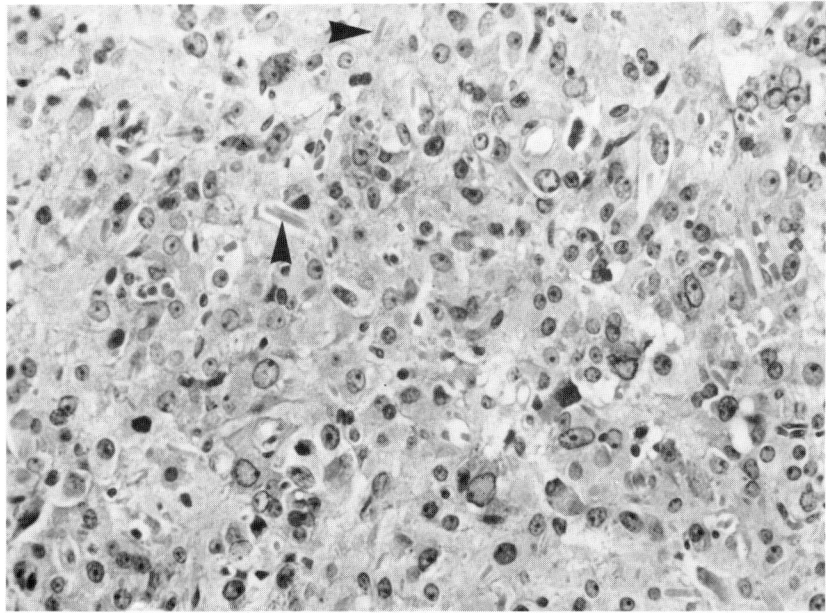

Fig. 14.9 Leydig cell tumour. The tumour cells have abundant cytoplasm that was eosinophilic and crystals of Reinke are seen in the cytoplasm of occasional cells (arrows). Many of the nuclei have a prominent nucleolus (H & E, × 313).

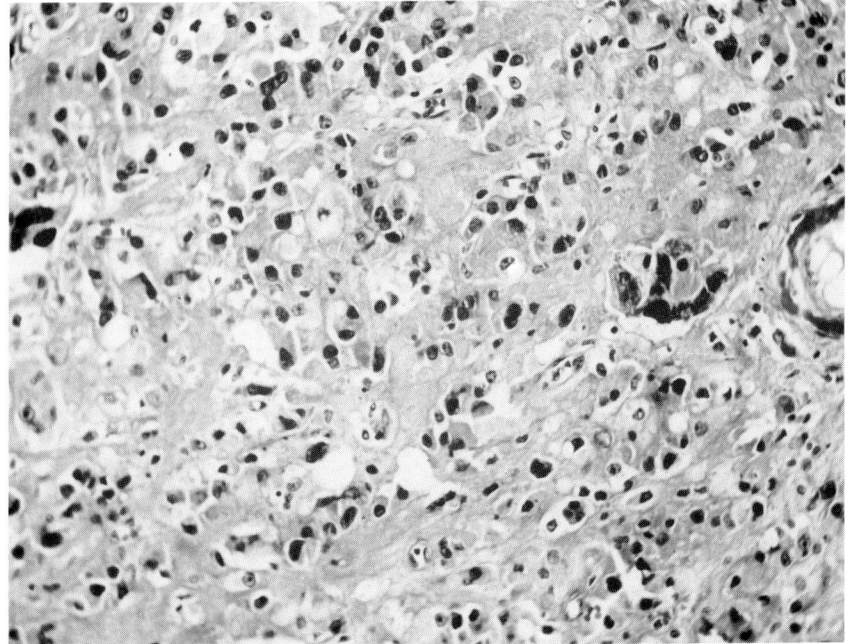

Fig. 14.10 Leydig cell tumour. The stroma between the cells is hyalinized and some of the nuclei are enlarged and bizarre (H & E, × 125).

only after prolonged search. They have tinctorial characteristics that differ slightly from those of red blood cells, which can be confused with crystals when compressed and elongated within capillaries. Special stains such as iron haematoxylin and trichrome stains may make the crystals more conspicuous. On electron microscopic examination crystals of Reinke typically appear as needle-shaped structures when cut longitudinally, or as hexagonal structures when cut in cross section (Schnoy 1982). The interior of the crystal has a cross-hatched appearance. Intracytoplasmic eosinophilic spheres, which may be crystal precursors, are also typically present but are not specific for hilus cell tumours. Stromal hyperthecosis, hilus cell hyperplasia, or both, are associated findings in occasional cases.

A diagnosis of crystal-negative or probable hilus cell tumour is occasionally made if a crystal-free steroid cell tumour has a predominant location in the hilus and one or more of the following features: a juxtaposition to non-medullated nerve fibres similar to that of normal hilus cells; a background of hilus cell hyperplasia; nuclear clustering with intervening anuclear zones; and fibrinoid change in vessel walls (Paraskevas & Scully 1989). These tumours have clinical and laboratory features similar to those of definite hilus cell tumours.

Only four non-hilar Leydig cell tumours have been reported, and their features were similar to those of hilus cell tumours except for their location (Roth & Sternberg 1973). An ovarian stromal derivation of these tumours is supported by the rare finding of stromal Leydig cells in otherwise typical cases of stromal hyperthecosis (Sternberg & Roth 1973). In some cases it may be impossible to determine whether a Leydig cell tumour is a hilus cell tumour or a Leydig cell tumour, non-hilar type; in such cases a diagnosis of Leydig cell tumour NOS is appropriate.

STEROID CELL TUMOUR, NOT OTHERWISE SPECIFIED

These tumours account for about 60% of steroid cell tumours (Taylor & Norris 1967, Hayes & Scully 1987b). They occur at any age but the patients are typically younger (mean age 43 years) than those with other types of steroid cell tumour. In contrast to stromal luteomas and Leydig cell tumours, the neoplasms occasionally occur in children, in whom they may cause heterosexual precocious puberty (Case Records of the Massachusetts General Hospital 1982) and, less commonly, isosexual precocious puberty (Campbell & Danks 1963, Hayes & Scully 1987b). Steroid cell tumours NOS are associated with androgenic changes, which may be of many years duration, in approximately half the cases; oestrogenic changes in approximately 10% of cases; and, occasionally, progestogenic changes. Four tumours have been reported that secreted cortisol and caused Cushing's syndrome (Hayes and Scully 1987b, Young & Scully 1987) and three others have been accompanied by raised serum cortisol concentrations without any clinical manifestations of Cushing's syndrome. Rare tumours have been associated with hypercalcaemia, erythrocytosis or ascites (Hayes & Scully 1987b), whilst one appeared to secrete aldosterone (Kulkarni et al 1990). The remaining cases have not been associated with endocrine or para-endocrine manifestations. Hormone studies in patients with androgenic changes, Cushing's syndrome, or both, typically show raised urinary concentrations of 17-ketosteroids and 17-hydroxycorticosteroids as well as increased serum concentrations of testosterone and androstenedione. The tumours that resulted in Cushing's syndrome were generally associated with raised concentrations of free cortisol in the blood or urine.

In 20% of cases, extraovarian spread of tumour is apparent at the time of operation; three of the four patients with Cushing's disease had extensive intra-abdominal tumour spread (Young & Scully 1987). In the two largest series in the literature, the proportion of tumours that were clinically malignant was 25% in one (Taylor & Norris 1967) and 43% in the other (Hayes & Scully 1987b); rare tumours recur as many as 19 years post-operatively. In one series, patients with clinically malignant tumours were on average 16 years older than patients with benign tumours (Hayes & Scully 1987b); no malignant steroid cell tumours have been reported in patients in the first two decades of life.

The tumours are typically solid and well circumscribed (Figs 14.11 and 14.12), are occasionally lobulated, and range in diameter from 1.2 to 45 cm (mean 8.4 cm); only about 5% are bilateral. The cut surface is typically yellow (Fig. 14.11) or orange if large amounts of cytoplasmic lipid are present, red to brown if the cells are lipid-poor, or dark brown to black (Fig. 14.12) if large quantities of cytoplasmic lipochrome pigment are present. Necrosis, haemorrhage and cystic degeneration are occasionally

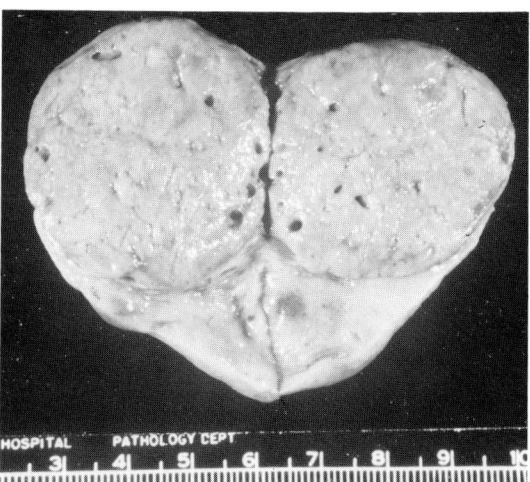

Fig. 14.11   Steroid cell tumour, not otherwise specified. The tumour, which was virilizing, is predominantly solid with occasional cysts and was yellow in the fresh state.

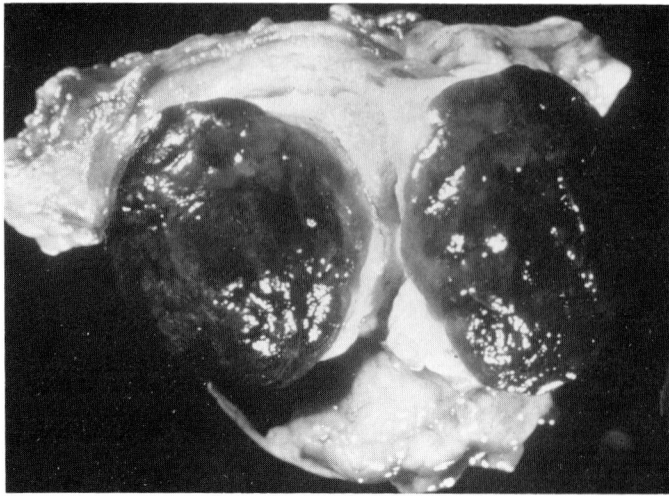

Fig. 14.12   Steroid cell tumour, not otherwise specified. The tumour, which was virilizing, is well circumscribed and was dark brown in the fresh state.

observed. On microscopic examination, the cells are characteristically arranged diffusely but occasionally they grow in large aggregates (Fig. 14.13), small nests, irregular clusters (Fig. 14.14), thin cords (Fig. 14.14) or columns. The stroma is inconspicuous in most cases but in about 15% it is

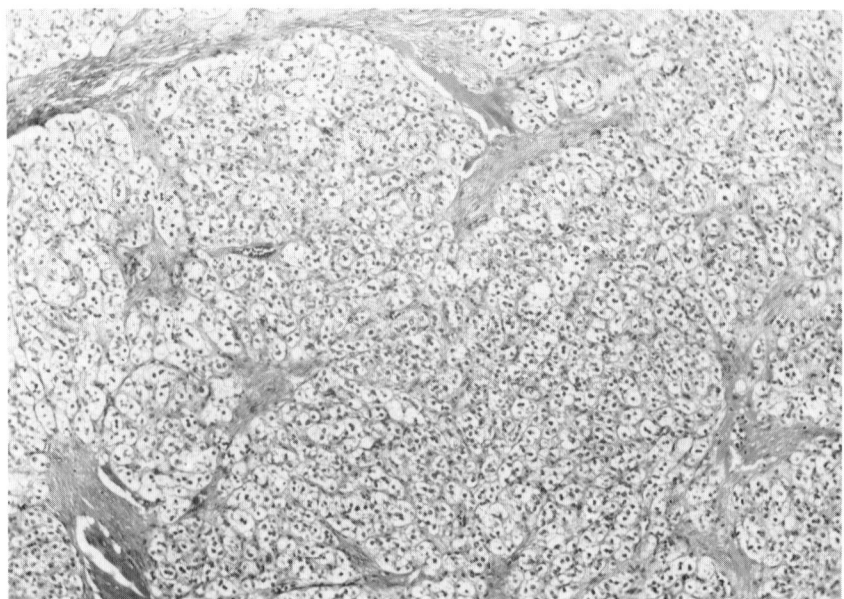

Fig. 14.13   Steroid cell tumour, not otherwise specified. Large aggregates of cells with abundant pale cytoplasm are intersected by fibrous bands (H & E, × 79).

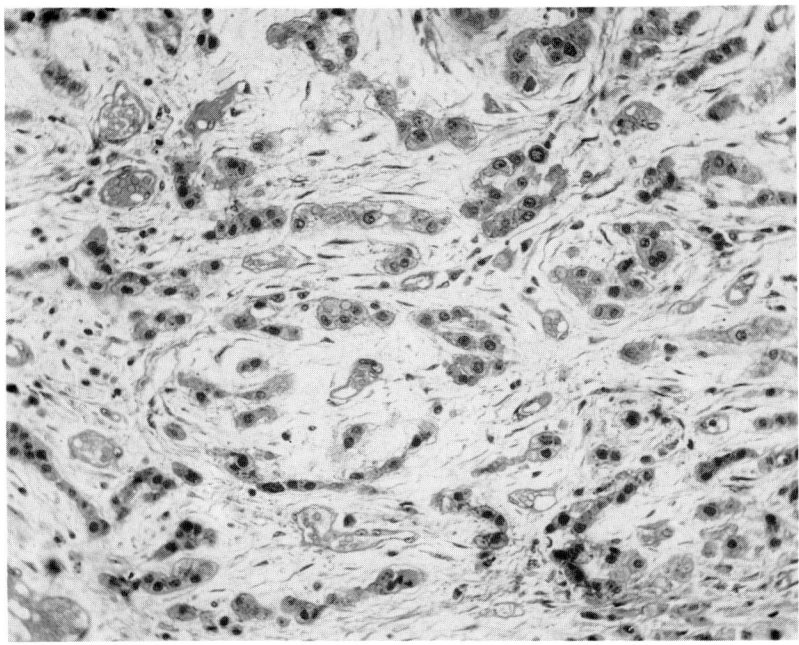

Fig. 14.14   Steroid cell tumour, not otherwise specified. The tumour cells are growing in small clusters and cords and are separated by an oedematous stroma (H & E, × 200).

relatively prominent. A minor fibromatous component may be seen indicating, as suggested by Hughesdon, that steroid cell tumours may be completely luteinized thecomas (Hughesdon 1983). Rarely the stroma is oedematous or myxoid, with tumour cells loosely dispersed in it. Exceptionally, the stroma exhibits calcification and even psammoma body formation. Necrosis and haemorrhage may be prominent, particularly in tumours that have significant cytologic atypia.

The polygonal to rounded tumour cells have distinct cell borders, central nuclei and moderate to abundant amounts of cytoplasm that varies from eosinophilic and granular (lipid-free or lipid-poor) to vacuolated and spongy (lipid-rich) (Fig. 14.15); in one series, lipid was present in 75% of the tumours stained specifically for this (Hayes & Scully 1987b). Steroid cell tumours NOS have lipid-rich cytoplasm more often than other subtypes of steroid cell tumour. Rarely, cells with large fat droplets have a signet-ring appearance. Cytoplasmic lipochrome pigment has been found in 40% of the tumours. In 60% of cases in the largest published series (Hayes & Scully 1987b), nuclear atypia was absent or slight, and mitotic activity was low (less than two mitotic figures per 10 high power fields. In the remaining cases, grade 1–3 nuclear atypia was present (Fig. 14.16), usually associated with a parallel increase in mitotic activity (up to 15 mitotic figures per 10 high-

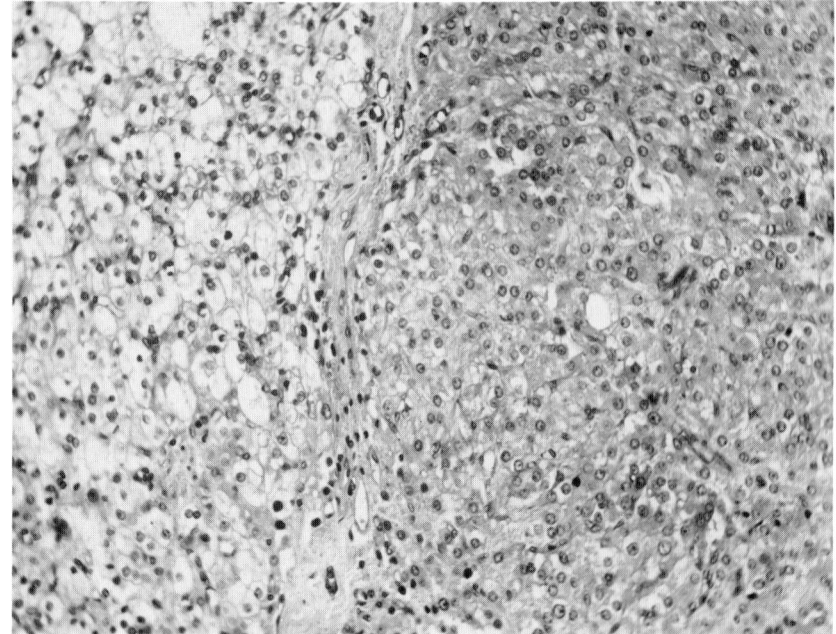

Fig. 14.15 Steroid cell tumour, not otherwise specified. This illustration shows two characteristic cell types, cells with abundant lipid-rich vacuolated cytoplasm on the left and smaller cells with abundant lipid-poor dense cytoplasm on the right (H & E, × 200).

power fields). Ultrastructural examination in some cases has demonstrated abundant smooth endoplasmic reticulum in the cytoplasm of the tumour cells (Koss et al 1969).

The best pathological correlates with malignant behaviour in one series (Hayes & Scully 1987b) were two or more mitotic figures per 10 high-power fields (92% malignant); necrosis (86% malignant); a tumour diameter of 7 cm or more (78% malignant); haemorrhage (77% malignant); and grade 2 or 3 nuclear atypia (64% malignant). Occasional tumours that appear cytologically benign, however, may behave in a malignant fashion. Metastatic tumours appear similar to the primary neoplasm in some cases (Fig. 14.17) but are more poorly differentiated in others.

Because of the high incidence of malignancy of steroid cell tumours NOS, careful staging should be performed. In a young patient with a Stage Ia tumour, unilateral oophorectomy is adequate but careful follow-up is essential and should include measurement of hormone levels. Follow-up is particularly important in those cases demonstrated to have had raised concentrations before removal of the primary tumour. In perimenopausal or postmenopausal patients, hysterectomy with bilateral salpingo-oophorectomy is the procedure of choice. In patients with high-stage disease, tumour debulking is advisable. Radiation therapy and chemotherapy have

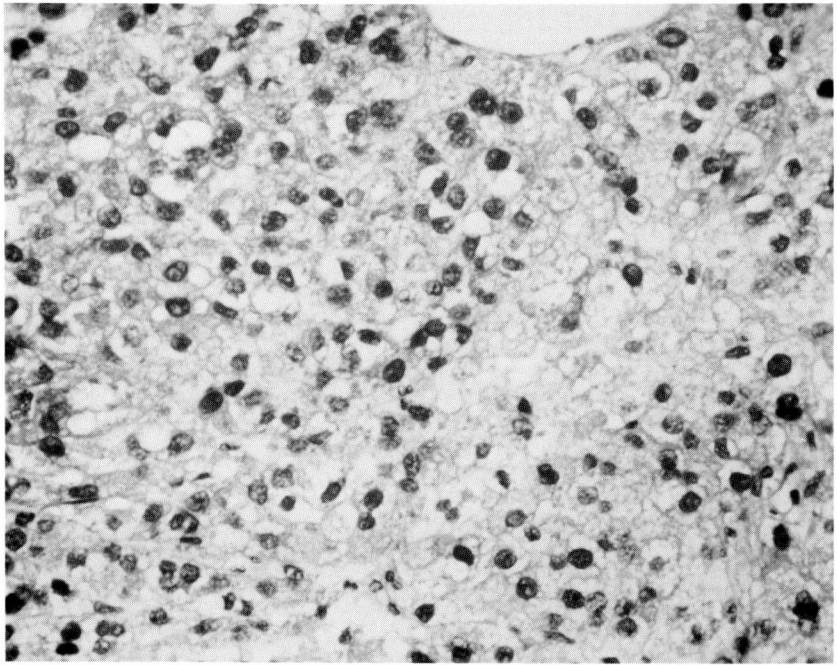

Fig. 14.16 Steroid cell tumour, not otherwise specified. The tumour cells exhibit moderate nuclear atypia. This tumour was clinically malignant and associated with Cushing's syndrome (H & E, × 256).

generally proved disappointing, but have been effective in occasional cases (Hayes & Scully 1987b).

DIFFERENTIAL DIAGNOSIS OF STEROID CELL TUMOURS

Stromal luteomas and Leydig cell tumours do not usually pose much diagnostic difficulty for the pathologist because of their characteristic locations, relatively uniform appearances and obvious composition of steroid-type cells, with those of Leydig cell tumours containing crystals of Reinke. The extensive formation of degenerative spaces in occasional tumours in these categories (see Figs 14.4 and 14.8), particularly stromal luteomas, may result in confusion with an adenocarcinoma or, more often, a vascular tumour. Awareness of this phenomenon and of its association with cellular degeneration, inflammatory cell infiltration and fibrosis, together with the finding of typical steroid cell tumour elsewhere in the specimen, should facilitate the diagnosis.

Steroid cell tumours in the NOS category vary more widely in appearance than do the stromal luteoma and Leydig cell tumour, from both architectural and cytological viewpoints, and are accordingly the cause of greater

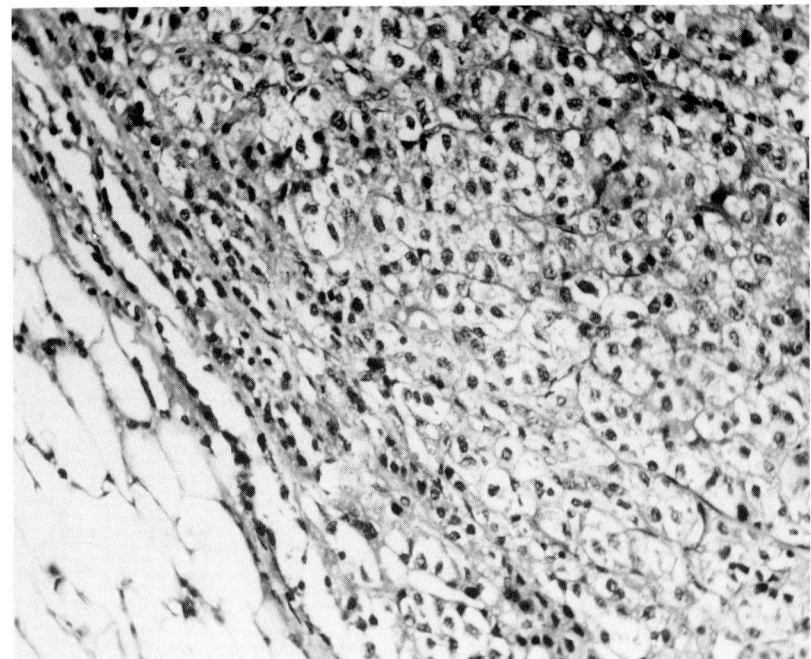

Fig. 14.17   Steroid cell tumour, not otherwise specified, metastatic in the omentum. Same case as Figure 14.16 (H & E, × 200).

diagnostic difficulty. Neoplasms that enter into the differential diagnosis in these cases include extensively luteinized granulosa cell tumour and thecoma, lipid-rich Sertoli cell tumour, clear cell carcinoma (particularly those of oxyphil type), rarely oxyphilic endometrioid carcinoma, hepatoid yolk sac tumour and hepatoid carcinoma, endocrine tumours such as oxyphilic struma ovarii, pituitary-type tumours and paragangliomas (phaeochromocytoma), metastatic renal cell carcinoma, adrenocortical carcinoma, hepatocellular carcinoma, primary melanoma and other metastatic tumours with an oxyphilic appearance, and metastatic melanoma.

The presence of characteristic non-luteinized cells in luteinized granulosa cell tumours and thecomas, the typical cytological features and patterns of these neoplasms and the finding of abundant reticulum in thecomas are of help in the identification of these tumours. Recognition of areas with a solid tubular pattern helps distinguish a usually oestrogenic lipid-rich Sertoli cell tumour with a predominantly diffuse pattern (Young & Scully 1984) from a typically androgenic steroid cell tumour. In contrast to steroid cell tumours, the clear cells of clear cell carcinomas and metastatic renal parenchymal cell carcinomas have glycogen-rich cytoplasm and eccentric nuclei. Also the presence of other growth patterns such as tubular, glandular and papillary

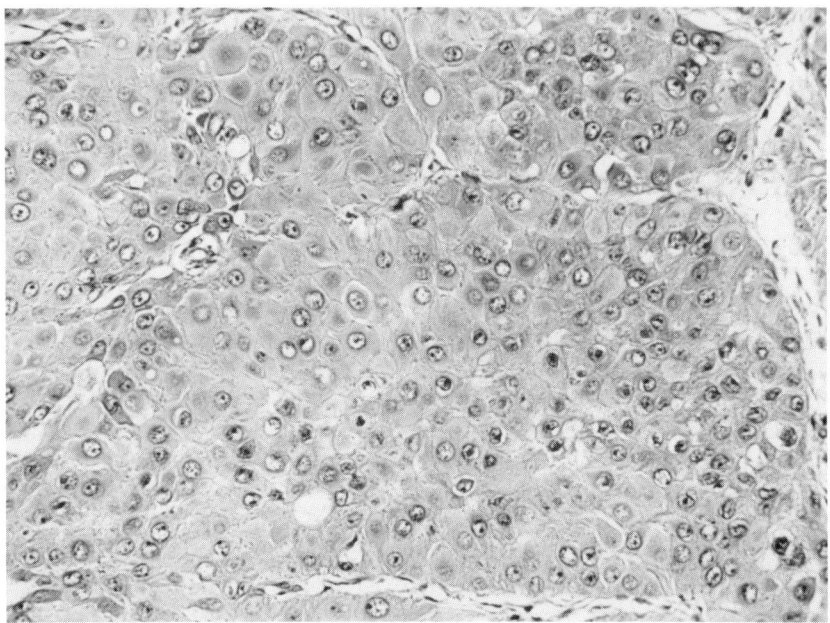

Fig. 14.18 Oxyphilic clear cell carcinoma resembling a steroid cell tumour. In this field the tumour cells have abundant cytoplasm that was eosinophilic (H & E, × 200).

arrangements, which are inconsistent with a steroid cell tumour, generally facilitate the differential diagnosis. Radiological studies to rule out a renal parenchymal cell carcinoma may be additionally helpful.

Oxyphilic clear cell (Young & Scully, 1987) (Fig. 14.18) and endometrioid carcinomas, hepatoid yolk sac tumours (Prat et al 1982) and hepatoid carcinomas (Ishikura & Scully 1987) are all characterized by the presence of neoplastic cells with abundant eosinophilic cytoplasm. The first two tumours generally exhibit epithelial patterns, may contain glandular lumens, and are almost always accompanied by more typical growth patterns. The oxyphilic clear cell carcinoma almost always has a variable component of other distinctive cell types not seen in steroid cell tumours. Hepatoid tumours also have epithelial patterns and may contain glandular lumens; they are characterized by positive immunohistochemical staining for α-fetoprotein. We are not aware of any cases of hepatocellular carcinoma or adrenocortical carcinoma that have presented in the form of a metastatic mass involving the ovary, but the possibility exists (see Addendum, p. 296).

Primary and metastatic melanomas can simulate steroid cell tumours when they are amelanotic, and if they are pigmented the pigment granules may be confused with the lipochrome granules of a steroid cell tumour. Melanomas generally have more malignant nuclear features than steroid cell tumours. Staining for melanin and lipochrome granules and immuno-histochemical staining for S100 protein and HMB-45 may be helpful in difficult cases. We have seen oxyphilic change focally in struma ovarii, but it is possible that this change might be encountered diffusely and result in a resemblance to a steroid cell tumour. An association with other terato-matous elements, the presence of thyroid colloid and positive immuno-staining for thyroglobulin are features that should enable one to distinguish these two neoplasms. A pituitary-type tumour containing cells with abundant eosinophilic cytoplasm that arose in the wall of a dermoid cyst has been described that secreted adrenocorticotrophic hormone and caused Cushing's syndrome (Axiotis et al 1987). Such a tumour could be confused with a steroid cell tumour but would immunostain positively for several pituitary hormones.

Finally, we have recently seen a case of an apparently primary phaeo-chromocytoma (paraganglioma) of the ovary (Fig. 14.19) in which the diagnosis of a steroid cell tumour was considered. Phaeochromocytoma of the ovary, though rare, has been reported (Fawcett & Kimbell 1971). In our case immunohistochemical staining of the tumour cells for chromogranin was helpful in establishing the diagnosis. Electron microscopical exam-ination of most of the neoplasms that simulate steroid cell tumours should disclose strikingly different features. Finally, the presence or absence of

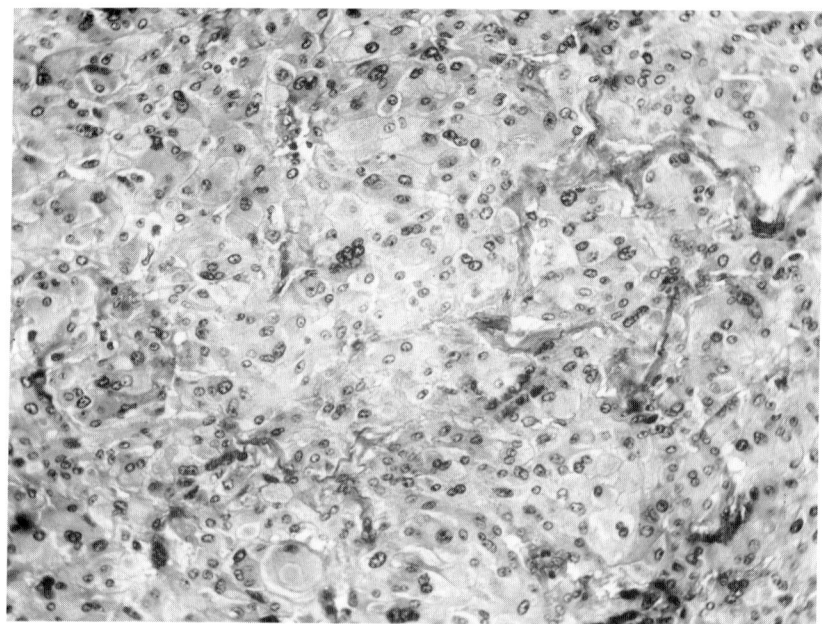

Fig. 14.19 Paraganglioma of ovary. The tumour cells have abundant cytoplasm that was eosinophilic and round regular nuclei (H & E, × 200).

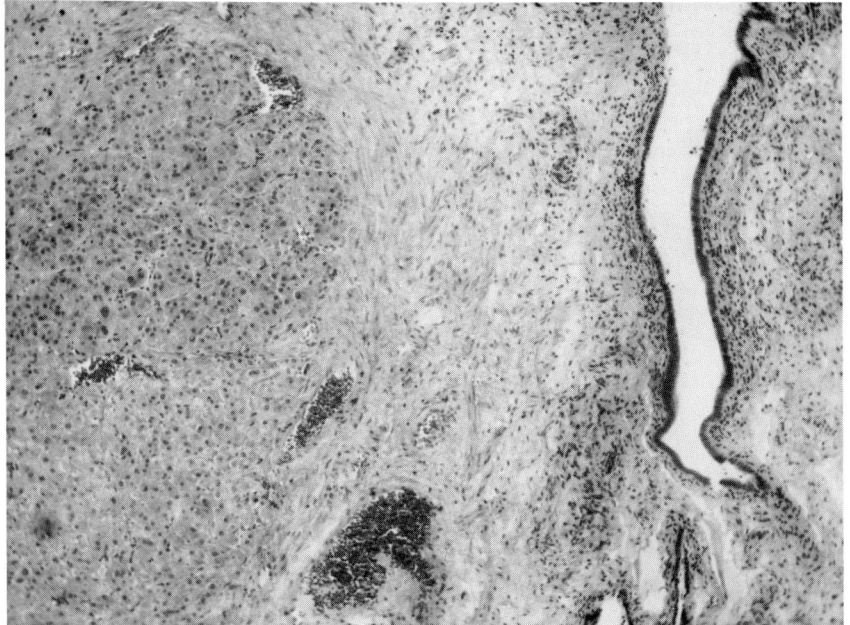

Fig. 14.20 Paratubal steroid cell nodule in patient with Nelson's syndrome. A portion of fallopian tube is seen at the right and a hyperplastic aggregate of steroid cells at the left (H & E, × 79).

endocrine manifestations and their nature may be important clinical clues to the diagnosis.

The pregnancy luteoma, a non-neoplastic lesion, can also closely resemble a steroid cell tumour (Norris & Taylor 1966, Sternberg & Barclay 1966). Pregnancy luteomas are hyperplastic nodules of lutein cells that are dependent on the human chorionic gonadotrophin stimulation of pregnancy, are discovered almost exclusively during the third trimester, and involute spontaneously after the pregnancy. They may measure up to 30 cm. They may also be associated with virilization of the mother, female infant, or both. Unlike steroid cell tumours, however, pregnancy luteomas are bilateral in about one-third of cases and multiple in almost half. On microscopical examination, the cells have abundant eosinophilic cytoplasm with little or no cytoplasmic lipid, and the nuclei often show mitotic activity, with up to 7 mitotic figures per 10 high-power fields (mean 2–3). In contrast, a steroid cell tumour with minimal cytological atypia that resembles a pregnancy luteoma rarely contains mitotic figures. It may be impossible to distinguish a lipid-poor or lipid-free steroid cell tumour NOS in a pregnant patient from a solitary pregnancy luteoma, but if the lesion is encountered during the third trimester it is usually presumed to be the latter unless clearly proven otherwise.

EXTRAOVARIAN STEROID CELL TUMOURS IN THE FEMALE GENITAL SYSTEM

Exceptionally, steroid cell tumours originate in the broad ligament. Adrenocortical rests were found in this site in 27% of hysterectomy specimens in one study (Falls 1955) and could be the source of these rare tumours. Adrenocortical rests may also undergo hyperplasia in congenital adrenal hyperplasia and thus simulate a steroid cell tumour. Multiple hyperplastic nodules in the vicinity of the ovaries, presumably of adrenal rest origin, can develop in Nelson's syndrome (development of a pituitary tumour after bilateral adrenalectomy for adrenocorticotrophic hormone-dependent adrenal hyperplasia), sometimes associated with virilization (Baranetsky et al 1979, Wild et al 1988) and resemble small steroid cell tumours on microscopic examination (Fig. 14.20). The clinical background and location of these lesions enable one to differentiate them from ovarian steroid cell tumours.

ADDENDUM

Since completing this review, we have seen two patients in whom hepatocellular carcinoma was associated with ovarian metastases at the time of presentation (Young et al 1991).

ACKNOWLEDGEMENTS

We are extremely grateful to Bernadette Vijayakanthan for outstanding secretarial assistance.

REFERENCES

Axiotis C A, Lippes H A, Merino M J, deLanerolle N C, Stewart A F, Kinder B 1987 Corticotroph cell pituitary adenoma within an ovarian teratoma. A new cause of Cushing's syndrome. American Journal of Surgical Pathology 11: 218–224

Baramki T A, Leddy A L, Woodruff J D 1983 Bilateral hilus cell tumors of the ovary. Obstetrics and Gynecology 62: 128–131

Baranetsky N G, Zipser R D, Goebelsmann U et al 1979 Adrenocorticotrophin-dependent virilizing paraovarian tumors in Nelson's syndrome. Journal of Clinical Endocrinology and Metabolism 49: 381–386

Campbell P E, Danks D M 1963 Pseudoprecocity in an infant due to a luteoma of the ovary. Archives of Disease in Childhood 38: 519–523

Case Records of the Massachusetts General Hospital (Case 22-1982) 1982. New England Journal of Medicine 306: 1348–1355

Dunaif A, Hoffman A R, Scully R E et al 1985 Clinical, biochemical, and ovarian morphologic features in women with acanthosis nigricans and masculinization. Obstetrics and Gynecology 66: 545–552

Dunnihoo D R, Grieme D L, Woolf R B 1966 Hilar cell tumors of the ovary. Report of 2 new cases and a review of the world literature. Obstetrics and Gynecology 27: 703–713

Echt C R, Hadd H E 1968 Androgen excretion patterns in a patient with a metastatic hilus cell tumor of the ovary. American Journal of Obstetrics and Gynecology 100: 1055–1061

Falls J L 1955 Accessory adrenal cortex in the broad ligament. Incidence and functional significance. Cancer 8: 143–150

Fawcett F J, Kimbell N K B 1971 Phaeochromocytoma of the ovary. Journal of Obstetrics and Gynaecology of the British Commonwealth 78: 458–459

Givens J R, Kerber I J, Wiser W L, Andersen R N, Coleman S A, Fish S A 1974 Remission of acanthosis nigricans associated with polycystic ovarian disease and a stromal luteoma. Journal of Clinical Endocrinology and Metabolism 38: 347–355

Hayes M C, Scully R E 1987a Stromal luteoma of the ovary: A clinicopathological analysis of 25 cases. International Journal of Gynecological Pathology 6: 313–321

Hayes M C, Scully R E 1987b Ovarian steroid cell tumor (not otherwise specified): a clinicopathological analysis of 63 cases. American Journal of Surgical Pathololology 11: 835–845

Hughesdon P E 1983 Lipid cell thecomas of the ovary. Histopathology 7: 681–692

Ichinohasama R, Teshima S, Kishi K et al 1989 Leydig cell tumor of the ovary associated with endometrial carcinoma and containing 17-β-hydroxysteroid dehydrogenase. International Journal of Gynecological Pathology 8: 64–71

Ishikura H, Scully R E 1987 Hepatoid carcinoma of the ovary. A newly described tumor. Cancer 60: 2775–2784

Kim I, Young R H, Scully R E 1985 Leydig cell tumors of the testis. A clinicopathological analysis of 40 cases and review of the literature. American Journal of Surgical Pathology 9: 177–192

Koss L G, Rothschild E O, Fleisher M, Francis J E Jr 1969 Masculinizing tumor of the ovary, apparently with adrenocortical activity. Cancer 23: 1245–1258

Kulkarni J N, Mistry R C, Kamat M R, Chinoy R, Lotlikar R G 1990 Case report of autonomous aldosterone-secreting ovarian tumor. Gynecologic Oncology 37: 284–289

Motlik K, Stejskalova A, Stejskal J, Kobilkova J, Starka L 1988 Hilus cell tumors of the ovary. Ceskoslovenska Patologie 24: 144–160

Norris H J, Taylor H B 1966 Nodular theca-lutein hyperplasia of pregnancy (so-called 'pregnancy luteoma'). A clinical and pathological study of 15 cases. American Journal of Clinical Pathology 47: 577–566

Paraskevas M, Scully R E 1989 Hilus cell tumor of the ovary: A clinico-pathological analysis of 12 Reinke-crystal-positive and 9 crystal-negative cases. International Journal of Gynecological Pathology 8: 299–310

Prat J, Bhan A K, Dickersin G R, Robboy S J, Scully R E 1982 Hepatoid yolk sac tumor of the ovary (endodermal sinus tumor with hepatoid differentiation). A light microscopic, ultrastructural and immunohistochemical study of seven cases. Cancer 50: 2355–2368

Roth L M, Sternberg W H 1973 Ovarian stromal tumors containing Leydig cells. II. Pure Leydig cell tumor, non-hilar type. Cancer 32: 952–960

Salm R 1974 Ovarian hilus-cell tumours: their varying presentations. J Pathol 113: 117–127

Schnoy N 1982 Ultrastructure of a virilizing ovarian Leydig-cell tumor. Hilar cell tumor. Virchows Archiv A Pathological Anatomy and Histopathology 397: 17–27

Scully R E 1964 Stromal luteoma of the ovary. A distinctive type of lipoid cell tumor. Cancer 17: 769–778

Scully R E 1979 Tumors of the ovary and maldeveloped gonads: Atlas of tumor pathology, second series, Fascicle 16. Armed Forces Institute of Pathology, Wahington, D.C., p 215

Sternberg W H 1949 The morphology, androgenic fuction, hyperplasia and tumors of the human ovarian hilus cells. American Journal of Pathology 25: 493–521

Sternberg W H, Barclay D L 1966 Luteoma of pregnancy. American Journal of Obstetrics and Gynecology 95: 165–184

Sternberg W H, Roth L M 1973 Ovarian stromal tumors containing Leydig cells. I. Stromal–Leydig cell tumor and non-neoplastic transformation of ovarian stroma to Leydig cells. Cancer 12: 940–951

Symmonds D A, Driscoll S G 1973 An adrenal cortical rest within the fetal ovary. Report of a case. American Journal of Clinical Pathology 60: 562–564

Taylor H B, Norris H J 1967 Lipid cell tumors of the ovary. Cancer 20: 1953–1962

Wild R A, Albert R D, Zaino R J, Abrams C S 1988 Virilizing paraovarian tumors: A consequence of Nelson's syndrome? Obstetrics and Gynecology 71: 1053–1056

Young R H, Scully R E 1984 Ovarian Sertoli cell tumors. A report of ten cases. International Journal of Gynecological Pathology 2: 349–363

Young R H, Scully R E 1987 Ovarian steroid cell tumors associated with Cushing's syndrome: a report of three cases. International Journal of Gynecological Pathology 60: 40–48

Young R H, Scully R E 1987a Oxyphilic clear cell carcinoma of the ovary. A report of nine cases. American Journal of Surgical Pathology 11: 661–667

Young R H, Scully R E 1987b Sex cord-stromal tumors, steroid cell tumors and other ovarian tumors with endocrine, paraendocrine and paraneoplastic manifestations. In: Kurman R J (ed) Blaustein's pathology of the female genital tract. Springer-Verlag, New York, p 607–658

Young R H, Gersell D J, Clement P B, Scully R E 1991 Hepatocellular carcinoma metastatic to the ovary: a report of three cases discovered during life with discussion of the differential diagnosis of hepatoid tumours of the ovary. Human Pathology in press

Zhang J, Young R H, Arseneau J, Scully R E 1982 Ovarian stromal tumors containing lutein or Leydig cells (luteinized thecomas and stromal Leydig cell tumors)—A clinicopathological analysis of fifty cases. International Journal of Gynecological Pathology 1: 275–285

15. Ovarian epithelial tumours with atypical proliferation

Peter Russell

Nothing in progression can rest on its original plan. We might as well think of rocking a grown man in the cradle of an infant.

Edmund Burke

INTRODUCTION

Whenever general principles or rules of biological behaviour, applied to a particular disease entity, appear to be in conflict or, indeed, totally incompatible, it is valuable to examine which of these principles or conventions prevails, and why. Historical precedent and resistance to changing the status quo are usually given as valid reasons for adhering to outmoded or untenable concepts or for dismissing newer, apparently contradictory, evidence as irrelevant. Such a conflict surrounds a group of ovarian epithelial neoplasms designated variously as 'semi-malignant', 'borderline', 'proliferating', 'of low malignant potential' or 'with atypical proliferation'. This controversy is examined here, with special reference to the two most frequently encountered subgroups of such tumours, those of serous and mucinous types.

SEROUS TUMOURS

A special, indeed unique, biological potential was initially ascribed to a group of serous epithelial tumours in women who presented with ovarian masses and apparent widespread peritoneal seeding yet regularly pursued a benign, non-progressive clinical course (Taylor 1929, 1959). 'Semi-malignant' was Taylor's way of explaining the limited biological aggressiveness of such tumours that were capable of 'metastasizing' to the peritoneum but usually progressing no further and sometimes regressed spontaneously.

Convention states that malignant neoplastic disease commences at one anatomical site and that additional ('secondary') deposits of tumour are derived by spread from this initial ('primary') lesion. It is slavish obeisance to our organ-based system of pathology teaching that has conditioned two generations of pathologists to accept unquestionably that the ovarian mass

Table 15.1   Histological distribution of ovarian Müllerian epithelial and mesenchymal tumours

Total	Non-invasive		Invasive carcinoma (%)	All types (%)
	Benign (%)	Proliferating (%)		
Serous	23.0	7.0	16.0	46.0
Mucinous	29.5	5.0	2.0	36.5
Endometrioid	rare	1.5	6.0	7.5
Müllerian mesenchymal	rare	rare	0.7	0.7
Clear cell	rare	rare	3.0	3.0
Brenner	2.0	rare	rare	2.0
Mixed epithelial	1.5	0.5	0.5	2.5
Undifferentiated carcinoma	—	—	1.5	1.5
Unclassified epithelial	rare	rare	0.3	0.3
Total	56	14	30	100

(however large or small, however active or inactive) is invariably the progenitor or primary neoplastic lesion and that the morphologically similar extraovarian lesions are manifestations of a metastatic process. With respect to the 'semi-malignant' serous tumours of Taylor, the designated primary sites were one or both ovaries. These tumours were 'ovarian' in nature (and thus in origin). The extraovarian lesions were metastases or 'implants'.

With time, these tumours were defined morphologically. A degree of cellular proliferation greater than that encountered in a benign form of the same type of tumour, and an absence of a destructive stromal invasion in the ovarian mass/masses, were declared central to the concept of 'borderline' or 'low malignant potential' ovarian epithelial tumours (Santesson & Kottmeier 1968, Kottmeier 1968, Serov et al 1973, Fox & Langley 1976, Czernobilsky 1977, 1985, Scully 1977, 1979, 1982). Applied empirically to the entire spectrum of ovarian serous tumours, these histological criteria encompass about 15% of all cases (Table 15.1). Most are confined to one or both ovaries, but 20–40% are associated with similar epithelial lesions in extraovarian (peritoneal) sites, as first observed by Taylor. The presence of these often widely distributed peritoneal lesions is associated with a non-progressive clinical course in 60–70% of cases.

Herein lies the paradox, not yet resolved (Russell 1984): how can a type of tumour that is by definition incapable of invading its own stroma nevertheless metastasize to distant sites? This is an ability not ascribed to epithelial tumours at other sites or in any other organ system in the body. A second general rule of tumour behaviour widely used to assess and manage cytologically malignant lesions has, in this instance, been subverted to preserve the original concept of 'borderline' or 'low malignant potential' ovarian epithelial tumours.

Recent questioning of the validity of this subgroup of ovarian tumours has been aimed at resolving this dilemma and reconciling these apparently conflicting principles by approaching the problem from a different point of view (Bannatyne & Russell 1981, Genadry et al 1981, Russell et al 1985, Russell & Bannatyne 1989, Lauchlan 1990). This can be summarized in the words of Lauchlan (1990): 'ovarian epithelial tumours do not behave according to a unique set of peculiar rules. In the language of the display terminal, what you see is what you get. If invasion is not demonstrated to be present, metastasis is not a real possibility.' What then is an alternative, real possibility?

Central to this issue is examination of the role of lesions such as serosal inclusions, proliferations and metaplasias in the ovaries or elsewhere in the peritoneal cavity, and of whether they represent intermediates or precursors in the genesis of Müllerian type epithelial tumours. This is accepted for such lesions in the ovaries (Scully 1977, 1979). The nature and distribution of these preneoplastic inclusions or heterotopias may dictate their anatomical distribution as well as their relative frequency and the histological range of Müllerian-type tumours seen. Collectively, inclusions or heterotopias of serous differentiation may be termed endosalpingiosis. They may be histologically benign (the term endosalpingiosis is usually reserved for such cases) or show proliferative changes up to and including locally invasive, well-differentiated serous carcinoma. They suggest pathogenetic links between ovarian Müllerian epithelial tumours and histologically indis- tinguishable extraovarian (peritoneal) neoplasms in the female pelvis and abdomen (see Ch. 16).

Peritoneal endosalpingiosis is common. It is diagnosed more frequently in our laboratory than endometriosis (usually as an incidental finding) and is often seen in association with chronic inflammatory tubal disease, sal- pingitis isthmica nodosa and endometriosis (Zinsser & Wheeler 1982, Shen et al 1983, Jansen & Russell 1986). It may be present in association with some benign serous ovarian tumours (Sinykin 1960, Russell 1979a, Tutschka & Lauchlan 1980, Zinsser & Wheeler 1982), with a very considerable proportion of atypically proliferating serous ovarian tumours (Burmeister et al 1969, Russell 1979b, McCaughey et al 1984, Bell et al 1988) and, despite the obliterative capacity of widespread peritoneal carcinomatosis, with occasional cases of frankly malignant serous tumours (Zinsser & Wheeler 1982). The generally accepted theories of pathogenesis of these morphologically benign lesions are similar to those for endometriosis; metastasis or 'implantation' from a coexisting serous ovarian tumour (absent in most cases) is neither a logical nor practical explanation.

At the other, frankly malignant end of the biological continuum, primary peritoneal serous carcinomas are well-documented and relatively common neoplasms. By definition, they occur in the absence of ovarian disease or with only minimal superficial ovarian involvement (Foyle et al 1981, Gooneratne et al 1982, White et al 1985, Lindique et al 1985, McCaughey et al 1986, Chen & Flam 1986, Austin et al 1987, Mills et al 1988, Dalrymple et al 1989), or occur many years after bilateral oophorectomy (Tobacman et al 1982, Chen et al 1985). They are further evidence of the capacity of the peritoneum or its epithelial derivatives (of which endosalpingiosis may be one) to give rise directly to Müllerian-type neoplasms without invoking the obligatory pre-existence of an ovarian neoplasm (see Ch. 16).

Between these two extremes, endosalpingiosis with atypical epithelial hyperplasia is most frequently found associated with similarly proliferating serous tumours in one or both ovaries—the pathological substrate of Taylor's original observations (Taylor 1929, 1959). They have, however, occasionally also been identified in the absence of such ovarian masses (Zinsser & Wheeler 1982, Bell & Scully 1987, Dallenbach-Hellweg 1987). The largest series, of 13 cases (Bell & Scully 1987), identified a similar profile of clinicopathological correlates to those described above for 'benign' endosalpingiosis and noted that the peritoneal lesions were identical to non-invasive 'implants' associated with borderline serous ovarian tumours. In the absence of an ovarian tumour that was, in histological terms, capable of metastasis (this series included two cases of associated benign serous ovarian tumours), such peritoneal lesions clearly must have arisen in situ. One is mystified by a logic that mandates a different pathogenesis for such lesions which depends solely on the presence or absence of a coexistent proliferating ovarian neoplasm (Bell & Scully 1989).

Returning to the problem of atypically proliferating serous ovarian tumours: in the absence of extraovarian lesions, all patients can be expected to survive without recurrence. In their presence, only 30–40% of patients will manifest progressive disease (Katzenstein et al 1978, Russell & Merkur 1979). The biological potential of an atypically proliferating serous ovarian neoplasm therefore lies not in any intrinsic property of the ovarian tumour but in the presence and nature of extraovarian lesions. In our experience (Russell & Merkur 1979, Russell 1984) and that of others (McCaughey et al 1984, Bell et al 1988), 'implants' showing a pattern of clearly defined locally invasive serous carcinoma are most likely to reflect unfavourably on the clinical outcome for the patient, though this is not universally accepted (Bostwick et al 1986, Michael & Roth 1986).

It is my contention that the great majority of the extraovarian manifestations of atypically proliferating or borderline serous tumours are a result of widespread multifocal in situ neoplasia arising directly from peritoneal serous inclusions (endosalpingiosis), as is generally accepted for their ovarian counterparts (Scully 1979, Russell 1984). Consequent to this, without implying a peculiar, limited capacity to metastasize in the absence of local stromal invasion, the general term 'proliferating common epithelial tumour' carries more the connotations of 'atypical hyperplasia', 'premalignant atypia', 'ovarian intra-epithelial neoplasia' or 'adenocarcinoma-in-situ' ('non-invasive ovarian carcinoma'; Lauchlan 1990), rather than 'semi-malignant') (Taylor 1929), 'borderline', or 'carcinoma of low malignant potential', as advocated by Scully (1982) and Zaloudek and Kurman (1983).

While I therefore agree with Bell & Scully (1989) that 'it is not possible to be certain whether extra-ovarian peritoneal serous neoplasia co-existing with ovarian serous borderline tumours is primary or secondary', the implications of taking one position or the other are very significant, both practically and theoretically. From a practical standpoint, if we assume that the extraovarian lesions are primary rather than metastatic, this stresses the importance for both surgeons and pathologists to document, biopsy and examine these lesions as thoroughly as we have been accustomed to examining the dominant ovarian masses, and not merely noting their presence at laparotomy as part of a formal staging procedure. Their assessment is an integral part of determining the biological potential of the whole neoplastic process with consequences for management (see below). From a theoretical standpoint, if one accepts that 'implants' are primary rather than metastatic, then the very *raison d'être* for this 'borderline' category of ovarian tumours has been removed and ovarian epithelial tumours can be viewed, as are those in other organ systems, as falling into two groups once more—non-invasive or benign tumours, and invasive or malignant tumours.

Histological characterization

There is no easy answer to the question of how much epithelial proliferation is required to separate atypically proliferating tumours from their nominally benign counterparts but, as outlined above, this is not an important clinicopathological distinction. Simple guidelines currently advocated for this purpose include the 'significant presence' in the same tumour of any two of the following features: epithelial budding, multilayering of epithelium, mitotic activity, and nuclear atypia (Russell & Bannatyne 1989).

There is a continuum of increasing prominence and complexity of the papillae lining most cystic spaces as well as of the distribution and/or severity of cellular proliferative features. These proliferative changes tend to run pari passu, but the two most easily quantifiable for serous lesions are stratification of the epithelial cells lining the papillae and epithelial budding or tufting (Fig. 15.1). Nuclei are rather more hyperchromatic and rounded than those in tumours considered benign and have obvious though not prominent nucleoli. Mitoses seldom exceed four per 10 high-power fields (Katzenstein et al 1978, Russell 1979b), and bizarre nuclei and tumour giant cells are not seen. Psammoma bodies and stromal inflammatory infiltrates are seen in up to half of these tumours; the latter usually consist of a mild lymphocytic infiltrate and are not directed to focal irregularities of architecture that might suggest invasive carcinoma.

If one accepts the validity of multifocal neoplasia, the histological assessment of extraovarian 'implants' becomes an integral part of pathological grading and not merely staging of atypically proliferating serous ovarian neoplasms. The surgeon should be encouraged to biopsy as many of

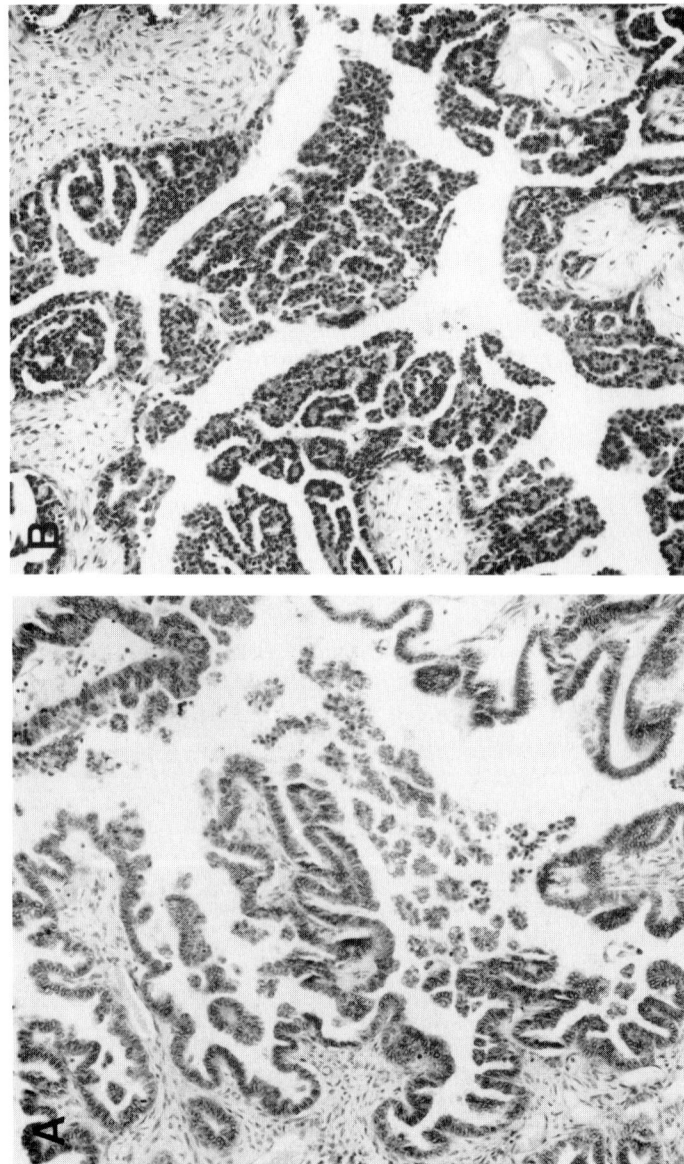

Fig. 15.1   Serous ovarian tumours showing   **A** low-grade and   **B** high-grade atypical epithelial proliferation (H & E, × 90).

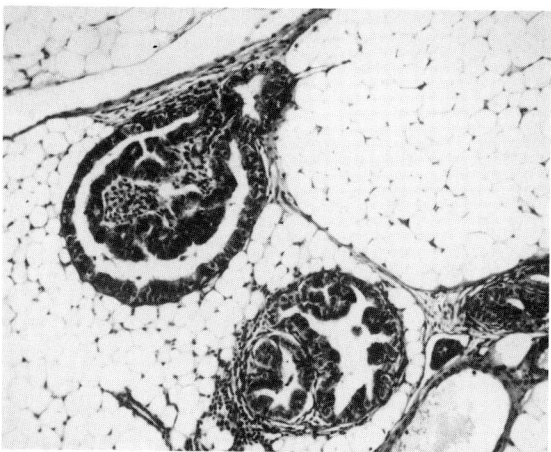

Fig. 15.2 Cytologically and architecturally benign epithelial lesions (endosalpingiosis) in omentum (H & E, × 90).

these as practicable at the time of definitive surgery. They are frequently found on or beneath the surface of pelvic viscera or the omentum, and exhibit the same cellular characteristics as the dominant ovarian mass, including papillae formation and psammoma bodies, but generally lack much of a stromal component. Most are either morphologically benign (Fig. 15.2), or proliferating but well circumscribed (Fig. 15.3), without architectural features suggesting local invasion. Some extra-ovarian lesions are associated, however, with irregular glandular structures in an immature, desmoplastic or inflamed stroma. Closer examination of such lesions

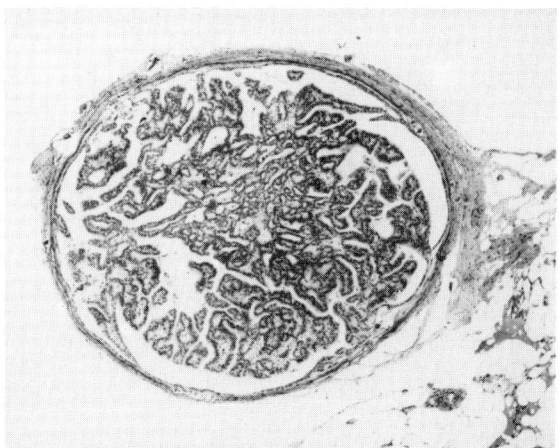

Fig. 15.3 Circumscribed non-invasive proliferating serous lesion in the greater omentum (H & E, × 35).

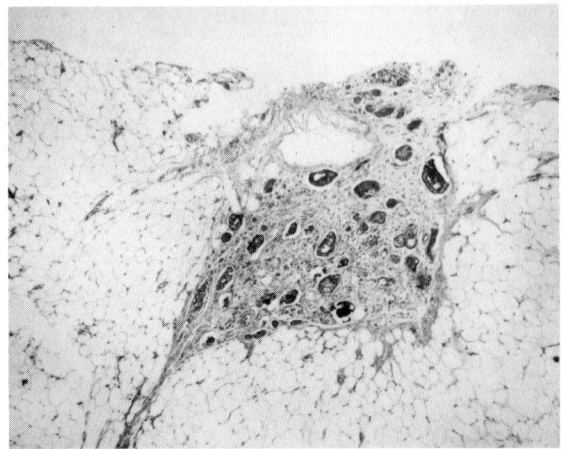

Fig. 15.4   A locally invasive omental lesion (low grade serous carcinoma) (H & E, × 25)

suggests locally invasive well-differentiated serous carcinoma in some (Fig. 15.4), while others show bland cellular components or are confined to the peritoneal surface and do not invade underlying structures (Fig. 15.5).

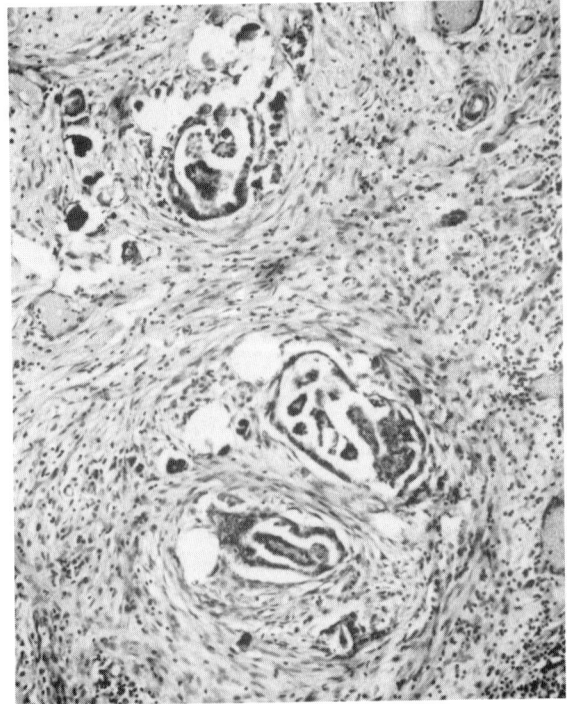

Fig. 15.5   A superficially invasive ('pseudoinvasive') omental lesion in omentum (H & E, × 90).

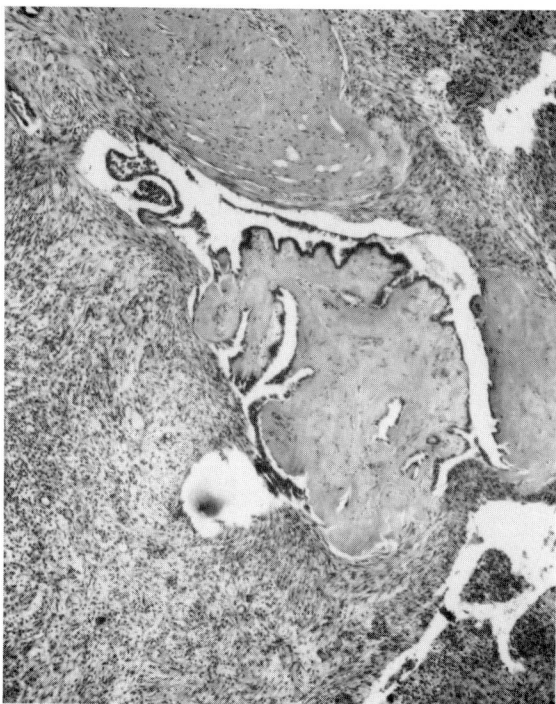

Fig. 15.6 A 'true' implant within the pelvis of a dislodged surface papillary fragment from an atypically proliferating serous ovarian tumour (H & E, × 90).

The importance of identifying these 'pseudo-invasive' lesions has been stressed by Bell & Scully (1987, 1989) as an explanation for discordant views on the relevance of subgrouping invasive and non-invasive peritoneal lesions in association with atypically proliferating serous ovarian tumours (Bostwick et al 1986, Michael & Roth 1986). The most difficult lesions to assess are those showing severe inflammation, sometimes with reactive mesothelial proliferation and scattered psammoma bodies, which can obscure the underlying presence of atypical epithelial cells (Fig. 16.3). Rarely, instances of degenerate papillary fragments associated with a local inflammatory response are encountered and these true implants add further weight to the argument for in situ genesis of the other very different lesions described above (Fig. 15.6). Cytological assessment of peritoneal washings in association with atypically proliferating serous ovarian tumours is also an integral part of staging.

Management

The aim of the preceding discussion is to stress the importance of ensuring that invasive serous carcinoma is absent from the neoplastic process in its entirety, and not merely from the ovarian mass/masses. If the tumour process is confined to one or both ovaries at thorough staging laparotomy (FIGO Stage I), it is by definition non-invasive and, essentially, all such patients can be expected to survive without recurrence. The diagnosis is assisted by intraoperative frozen section and the treatment is conservative surgery with clinical follow-up. In King George V Hospital, Camperdown, Australia, this conservative approach has included partial excision of bilaterally affected ovaries in young women desirous of pregnancies, with total hysterectomy and bilateral salpingo-oophorectomy after childbearing has been completed.

For patients with extraovarian peritoneal disease, the clinical outlook is determined by the anatomical distribution of the lesions and, more importantly, by their histological appearances. There is considerable variation in the histological features of individual peritoneal lesions, and extensive sampling and careful examination of these tumour foci is mandatory. In the presence of benign lesions (endosalpingiosis) or atypically proliferating but non-invasive lesions only, the most appropriate management again appears to be surgical excision of as much visible disease as possible with close clinical follow-up. Some such patients will have progressive disease, presumably due to missed foci of invasion at diagnosis. This risk has been estimated as about 6% by Bell & Scully (1987).

In the presence of unequivocal local invasion in any of the peritoneal lesions, upgrading such cases to the status of low grade serous carcinoma (FIGO Stage II–III) is recommended with the patients being managed accordingly. However, the experience at King George V Hospital, where about 50% of such patients survive 5 years, and of others (Bostwick et al 1986, Kliman et al 1986, Bell et al 1988), has shown equivocal results with adjuvant chemotherapy, considering the low-grade nature of the invasive malignant process.

MUCINOUS TUMOURS

In the 1960s the concept of atypically proliferating ovarian tumours ('borderline', low malignant potential') was developed, defined, and towards the end of that decade, incorporated into the FIGO classification of ovarian epithelial tumours (Santesson & Kottmeier 1968, Kottmeier 1968). Five years later, the imprimatur of the WHO was also given to this category of neoplasms in its histological classification of ovarian tumours (Serov et al 1973). During the evolution of these classifications, it was arbitrarily determined that the category of 'low malignant potential' tumours be extended beyond merely serous tumours to the other common epithelial subtypes (mucinous, endometrioid, clear cell and Brenner), despite there being no clinical parallel to Taylor's 'semi-malignant' serous tumours with widespread peritoneal 'implants' defined at that time (one has since emerged—see below). The analogy was to be purely morphological. With

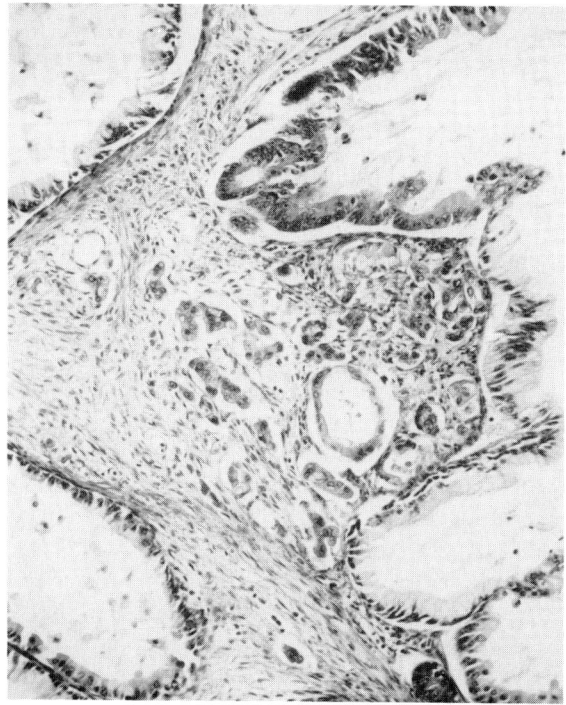

Fig. 15.7 An atypically proliferating mucinous ovarian tumour with a central area of early invasion (H & E, × 90).

regard to mucinous lesions, which are the second most frequently encountered atypically proliferating ovarian tumours (accounting for about 15% of all ovarian mucinous neoplasms) (Table 15.1), the problems this attitude gave rise to were far more complex than for their serous counterparts.

Firstly, the distinction between frankly malignant (invasive) and non-invasive but atypically proliferating mucinous tumours is not as clear-cut as in serous tumours. Their growth patterns, with ever more complex and crowded cystic and glandular structures and great variability from area to area, make it difficult to observe destructive stromal invasion as a definable change in morphology (Fig. 15.7). This was reflected in the early literature (Santesson & Kottmeier 1968, Aure et al 1971) which showed a poorer survival rate for patients with mucinous 'carcinomas of low malignant potential' compared with those with the equivalent serous tumours. Attempts were then made to optimize the discrimination between atypically proliferating and frankly malignant mucinous tumours by adding histological criteria which, in the absence of obvious stromal invasion, nevertheless would predict progressive disease. The most important of these criteria were by Hart & Norris (1973) and included significant epithelial multi-

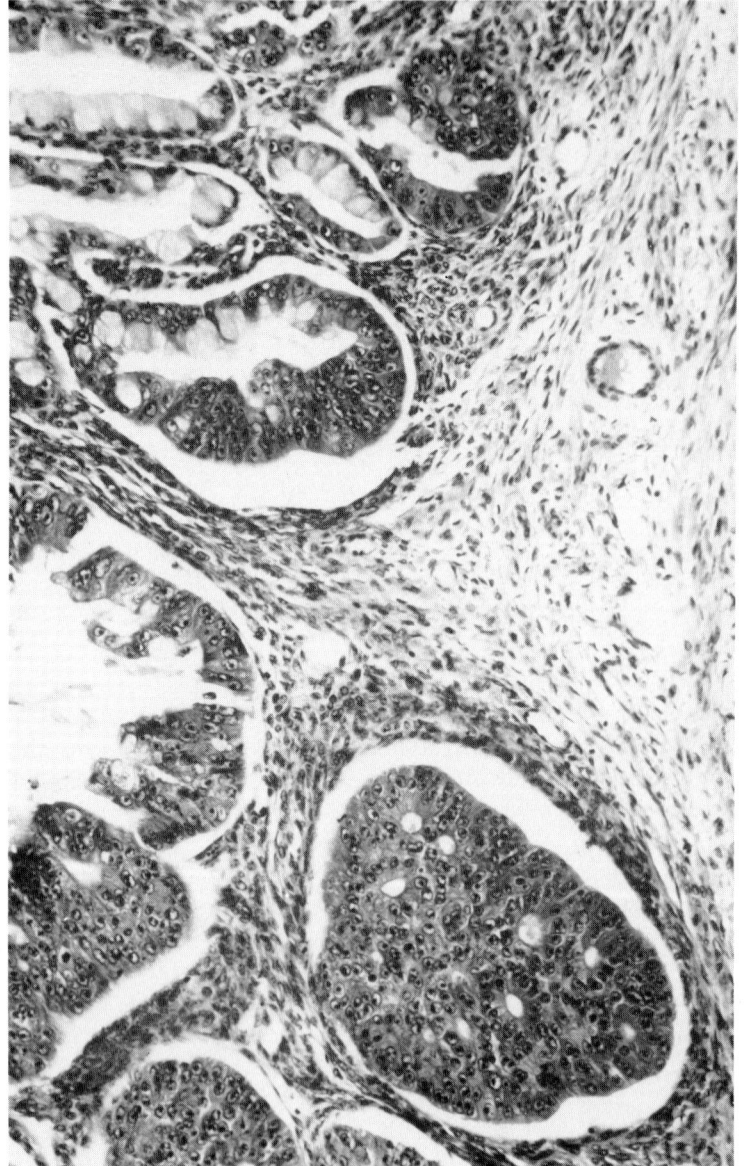

Fig. 15.8 High grade atypically proliferating mucinous ovarian tumour showing obvious intestinal differentiation and marked multilayering of the epithelium (H & E, × 125).

Table 15.2 Analysis of clinical outcome of patients with FIGO Stage I atypically proliferating mucinous ovarian neoplasms as defined by FIGO/WHO and Hart & Norris (1973)

	FIGO/WHO			Hart & Norris		
	Total cases	Clinical recurrences	Fatal outcome	Total cases	Clinical recurrences	Fatal outcome
Hart & Norris (1973)				97	5	3
Russell & Merkur (1979)	44	4	2			
Tasker & Langley (1985)	29	0	0			
Chaitin et al (1985)				21	2	2
Barnhill et al (1985)	11	0	0			
Bostwick et al (1986)				30	0	0
Nation & Krepart (1986)	34	0	0			
Kliman et al (1986)	30	0	0			
Total	148	4	2	148	7	5

layering (more than three cells thick) and 'large sheets of glands with back-to-back arrangements and no intervening stroma' (Fig. 15.8). Many reported series of atypically proliferating mucinous tumours have since employed either the Hart & Norris criteria or the original FIGO/WHO formula of absence of destructive stromal invasion (Russell & Merkur 1979, Barnhill et al 1985, Chaitin et al 1985, Tasker & Langley 1985, Nation & Krepart 1986, Bostwick et al 1986, Kliman et al 1986). Comparing data for Stage I cases from all these series reveals no increased discriminatory value in the Hart & Norris criteria. There appears to be an approximately 2–4% risk of recurrence and/or tumour-associated death, regardless of inclusion or exclusion of such cases (Table 15.2).

Given the perceptual difficulties associated with their assessment, this small recurrence rate is probably explicable on the basis of missed foci of stromal invasion. It is the present view of the International Society of Gynecological Pathologists that the original WHO criteria should be retained, and that this position should be reflected in the current revision of the WHO Histological Classification of Ovarian Tumours.

Secondly, mucinous tumours are not a single group. Many benign, most atypically proliferating, and all frankly malignant ovarian mucinous tumours are intestinal rather than Müllerian (endocervical) in type (De Boer et al 1981, Louwerens et al 1983, Szymanska et al 1983, Aguirre et al 1984, Pant et al 1986) and origin from lesions other than serosal Müllerian inclusions of mucinous type (e.g. teratomas) have been proposed for some of these neoplasms. Only the minor, endocervical, subgroup of atypically proliferating mucinous neoplasms shares clinicopathological correlates with other Müllerian-type ovarian epithelial tumours (e.g. serous, endometrioid) in being commonly bilateral, showing foci of mixed epithelial differentiation, being frequently associated with pelvic endometriosis and, in 15% of cases, with discrete extraovarian lesions or 'implants' (Rutgers & Scully 1988a).

As with most of their serous counterparts, the presence of these rare 'implants' does not necessarily bode ill for the patients, none of whom have demonstrated progressive disease so far. The major, intestinal, subtype of atypically proliferating mucinous tumours have significantly different clinicopathological correlates, in particular their extraovarian manifestations (occurring in 15% of cases) which take the form of pseudomyxoma peritonei.

Pseudomyxoma peritonei is in no way the mucinous equivalent of serous peritoneal 'implants'. It has not been reported in the absence of a preceding or notional primary lesion (whether in the ovary, appendix, colon or gall bladder). It is a poorly understood condition related to spread of mucin and cells from a small subgroup of mucinous ovarian neoplasms into the peritoneal cavity and is generally a slowly progressive ('malignant') process with the patients dying of inanition or bowel complications. The associated tumour always seems to show an insidious penetration of its stroma by pools and tracts of mucin, a pattern analogously referred to as 'pseudomyxoma ovarii', owing to breakdown in the integrity of the epithelium of cysts or smaller acini in the tumour with little or no stromal reaction to the mucins released. This appearance may complicate mucinous ovarian neoplasms at any point in their proliferative spectrum, but is found mostly in 'borderline' or atypically proliferating lesions. Pseudomyxoma peritonei is almost invariably present at the time of initial surgery (whether or not an obvious rupture can be shown in the tumour capsule) and does not seem to follow accidental intraoperative rupture. The associated ovarian tumours are bilateral in about 65% of cases (Campbell et al 1973) compared with 6–8% overall for atypically proliferating mucinous neoplasms, and appendiceal mucoceles are commonly also present. Of patients with mucinous ovarian tumours, those with pseudomyxoma are considerably older than those without (Russell 1987a, b).

Pseudomyxoma ovarii is generally regarded as a special process and not as destructive stromal invasion (Hart & Norris 1973), and such atypically proliferating mucinous neoplasms are not reclassified as carcinomas. This may merely be a question of semantics, however, and a more pragmatic approach, given the prognosis of patients with abdominal spread of pseudomyxomatous type, could well change this point of view (Radi et al 1988). Precisely the same histological spectrum can be seen in appendiceal mucoceles that may or may not progress to generalized pseudomyxoma (Higa et al 1973). This circumstantial evidence suggests that a small but specific subgroup of ovarian mucinous tumours (included in the 'intestinal' group showing colonic epithelial differentiation) is responsible for development of pseudomyxoma pertonei (Russell 1979a, b), and its genesis appears to have more to do with the intestinal nature of the epithelial element than the proliferative or 'semi-malignant' potential of the tumour.

An analysis of relations between the more recently observed (and rarely observed) peritoneal 'implants' and atypically proliferating mucinous ovarian neoplasms of Müllerian (endocervical) type (Rutgers & Scully 1988a) discloses a clear analogy with those of serous differentiation described above. Logically, the pathogenetic argument applied to the extraovarian serous lesions could well be extended to cover the origin of these mucinous lesion from the peritoneum or subperitoneum mesenchyme, although such a concept has yet to be tested. Like their serous counterparts, mucinous tumours have been described as benign, atypical but non-invasive, or 'superficially invasive' ('pseudo-invasive'). Peritoneal and lymph node lesions ('implants') have been identified, but no patient has demonstrated progressive disease over an average follow-up period of 3.7 years. Thus, the presence of mucinous tumours should not be seen as de facto evidence of metastatic spread from tumours that are by definition non-invasive.

Histological characterization

Mucinous tumours showing mildly atypical proliferation (Fig. 15.9) differ

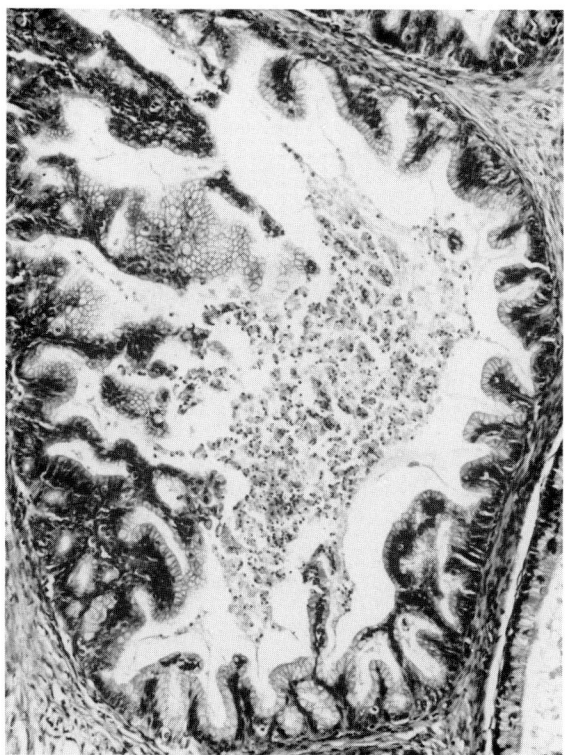

Fig. 15.9 Mucinous ovarian tumour with mild atypical epithelial proliferation (H & E, × 90).

from nominally benign lesions only in the exuberant growth of the epithelial component at the relative expense of the stroma. Glandular buds and a microscopic filigree pattern similar to the tufting of atypically proliferating serous tumours are noted. Increasingly atypical hyperplasia leads to more complex glandulopapillary patterns with epithelial multilayering and bridging (luminal reduplication). Variability from field to field in the same tumour is a hallmark of these mucinous neoplasms, and it is common to find all grades of proliferation as well as benign areas in the same section. Extensive sampling is thus vital in assessment. The epithelium also demonstrates variable atypia, with irregular, hyperchromatic nuclei, large nucleoli and decreased cytoplasmic mucin. Mitotic figures may be numerous; they are diffusely distributed, tend to be confined to the periphery of benign mucinous tumours, and may be atypical. In most tumours, the epithelium is recognizably intestinal or enteroid in character with goblet cells present (see Fig. 15.8), but in some such lesions (particularly with a papillary pattern of growth) Müllerian endocervical features are present (Fig. 15.10).

The stroma of these neoplasms does not differ significantly from that in

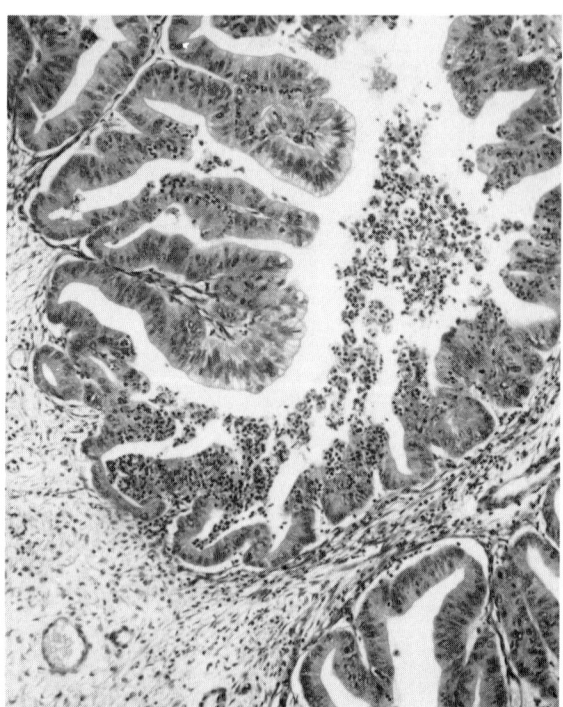

Fig. 15.10 Mucinous tumour with moderate atypical epithelial proliferation of Müllerian (endocervical) type and a florid acute inflammatory infiltrate typical of these lesions (H & E, × 90).

the architecturally benign tumours. This similarity has been of value in assessing the presence or absence of invasive cancer and identifying the various patterns of pseudo-invasion or benign intrusion of the stroma in cystic tumours and the increasingly complex proliferative pattern of glands in solid tumours, a difficult perceptual problem in mucinous lesions. The following histological features have proved useful in identifying areas of invasion: (1) changes in the architectural contour at the epithelial/stromal interface (see Fig. 15.7); (2) alteration in the character of the tumour stroma; (3) presence of a chronic inflammatory cell infiltrate, particularly when focal.

Management

Occasional patients (2–4%) with atypically proliferating mucinous tumours confined to the ovaries (Stage I) develop recurrent or metastatic disease. They are often patients who have had removal of the tumour only, and the first recurrence is frequently in the contralateral ovary or elsewhere in the pelvis: it is a reasonable assumption that small focal areas of invasion were missed during histological assessment of the primary neoplasm. Close clinical follow-up is justifiable in young women desirous of retained fertility who have a neoplasm of this type confined to one ovary. Pelvic clearance is recommended when childbearing has finished. Hysterectomy and bilateral salpingo-oophorectomy is suggested in all other cases.

For patients with the rare extraovarian lesions of focal type ('implants' as defined by Rutgers & Scully 1988a), careful examination of these lesions is mandatory. To date, these have not shown destructive tissue invasion, and no further active therapy appears indicated. For patients with pseudo-myxoma peritonei, standard protocols of repeated surgery, paracenteses, and occasionally chemotherapy have little modified the natural history of the condition to date.

ENDOMETRIOID, CLEAR CELL, BRENNER AND MIXED EPITHELIAL TUMOURS

Collectively, other ovarian epithelial tumour types showing atypical epithelial proliferation are extremely uncommon, have almost always pursued a benign clinical course, and offer little to our understanding of the group as a whole.

Many ovarian endometrioid tumours are thought to be derived from the surface epithelium of the ovary without the interposition of pre-existing endometriosis, although up to 31% of such tumours are found in patients with endometriosis in the same ovary or elsewhere in the pelvis (Russell 1979a, Roth et al 1981). With regard to our overall understanding of the nature of atypically proliferating epithelial ovarian neoplasms and with particular reference to their histogenesis, it is an interesting casual observation that no one has suggested that pelvic or abdominal endometriosis represents metastatic 'implants' from an ovarian endometrioid neoplasm. Ovarian endometrioid tumours showing atypical proliferation are rare, and the criteria for defining them are less well established than for their serous or mucinous counterparts, particularly the criteria for distinguishing between atypically proliferating endometrioid tumours and invasive endometrioid carcinomas (Fox & Langley 1976). Both of these may be associated with synchronous or metachronous hyperplasia, or adenocarcinoma, of the uterine endometrium (Russell 1979b, Bell & Scully 1985a).

Infrequent examples of atypically proliferating clear cell ovarian tumours have been reported (Russell 1979b, Roth et al 1984, Bell & Scully 1985b). Extraovarian lesions have not been recorded in association with such tumours and only one case of possible distant (lung) metastasis is to be found in the literature (Bell & Scully 1985b).

Since the original description (Roth & Sternberg 1971) of 'proliferating' Brenner tumour, other authors have also preferred the term proliferating (Miles & Norris 1972, Russell 1979b, Woodruff et al 1981) to 'borderline' (Hallgrimsson & Scully 1972) implying a benign clinical course. Roth et al (1985) have more recently expanded the spectrum by differentiating between proliferating Brenner tumours and those 'of low malignant potential'. Rarely, such Brenner tumours are associated with synchronous or metachronous transitional cell carcinoma of the urinary bladder (Colgan & Norris 1983, Kunze et al 1983, Svenes & Eide 1984) but, of the 50 or so cases in the literature (Roth & Sternberg 1971, Miles & Norris 1972, Hallgrimsson & Scully 1972, McKenna & Ansford 1976, Pratt-Thomas et al 1976, Chang et al 1977, Klemi & Nevalainen 1977, Russell 1979b, Woodruff et al 1981, Genton 1984, Roth et al 1985), only one can be considered not to have behaved in an entirely benign fashion (McKenna & Ansford 1976), leading to local recurrence.

Atypically proliferating ovarian tumours of mixed epithelial differentiation are defined by the presence of two or more of the epithelial elements described in the preceding sections; these can be present in variable proportions, intimately mixed, or as discrete areas. By convention, minor components (isolated fields or cellular aggregates amounting to less than 10% of the total) of a second or third epithelial tissue type should be disregarded in Müllerian tumours for the purposes of tumour classification (Serov et al 1973, Russell 1979a), and such neoplasms are best categorized according to the differentiation of the dominant epithelial element. There is some evidence to suggest that these tumours behave like the 'pure' counterpart of their dominant epithelial element with respect to patterns of pathogenesis and clinical outcome. For example, a predominantly serous tumour is more likely to have extraovarian manifestations at laparotomy, and a predominantly endometrioid tumour to be associated with pelvic endometriosis. All have behaved in a benign fashion (Russell & Merkur 1979, Rutgers & Scully 1988b).

REFERENCES

Aguirre P, Daval Y, Scully R E, De Lellis R A 1984 Mucinous tumors of the ovary with argyrophil cells. An immunohistochemical analysis. American Journal of Surgical Pathology 8: 345–356

Aure J C, Hoeg K, Kolstad P 1971 Clinical and histological studies of ovarian carcinoma. Obstetrics and Gynecology 31: 1–9

Austin M B, Mills S E, Fechner R E, Anderson W A 1987 Serous surface carcinoma (SCC) of the peritoneum (Abstract). Laboratory Investigation 56: 3a

Bannatyne P M, Russell P 1981 Early adenocarcinoma of the fallopian tubes. A case for multifocal tumorigenesis. Diagnostic Gynecology and Obstetrics 3: 49–60

Barnhill D, Heller P, Brzozowski P, Advani H, Gallup D, Park R 1985 Epithelial ovarian carcinoma of low malignant potential. Obstetrics and Gynecology 65: 53–59

Bell D A, Scully R E 1985a Atypical and borderline endometrioid adenofibromas of the ovary. American Journal of Surgical Pathology 9: 205–214

Bell D A, Scully R E 1985b Benign and borderline clear cell adenofibromas of the ovary. Cancer 56: 2911–2931

Bell D A, Scully R E 1987 Serous borderline tumors of the peritoneum (Abstract). Laboratory Investigation 56: 5a

Bell D A, Scully R E 1989 Benign and borderline serous lesions of the peritoneum in women. Pathology Annual 24 (pt 2): 1–21

Bell D A, Weinstock M A, Scully R E 1988 Peritoneal implants of ovarian serous borderline tumors: Histologic features and prognosis. Cancer 62: 2212–2222

Bostwick D G, Tazelaar H D, Ballon S C, Hendrickson M R, Kempson R L 1986 Ovarian epithelial tumors of borderline malignancy. A clinical and pathologic study of 109 cases. Cancer 58: 2052–2065

Burmeister R E, Fechner R E, Franklin R R 1969 Endosalpingiosis of the peritoneum. Obstetrics and Gynecology 34: 310–318

Campbell J S, Lou P, Ferguson J P, Kemeny T, Mitton D, Allen N 1973 Pseudomyxoma peritonei et ovarii with occult neoplasms of the appendix. Obstetrics and Gynecology 42: 897–902

Chaitin B A, Gershenson D M, Evans H L 1985 Mucinous tumours of the ovary: a clinicopathologic study of 70 cases. Cancer 55: 1958–1962

Chang S H, Roberts J M, Homesley H D 1977 Proliferating Brenner tumor. Obstetrics and Gynecology 49: 489–493

Chen K T K, Flam M S 1986 Peritoneal papillary serous carcinoma with long-term survival. Cancer 58: 1371–1373

Chen K T K, Schooley J L, Flam M S 1985 Peritoneal carcinomatosis after prophylactic oophorectomy in familial ovarian cancer syndrome. Obstetrics and Gynecology 66: 93s–94s

Colgan T J, Norris H J 1983 Ovarian epithelial tumors of low malignant potential: a review. International Journal of Gynecological Pathology 2: 367–382

Czernobilsky B 1977 Primary epithelial tumors of the ovary. In: Blaustein A (ed) Pathology of the female genital tract, 2nd ed. Springer-Verlag, New York, p 453–504

Czernobilsky B 1985 Common epithelial tumours of the ovary. In: Roth L M, Czernobilsky B (eds) Tumors and tumorlike conditions of the ovary. Churchill Livingstone, New York, p 11–43

Dalrymple J C, Bannatyne P, Russell P et al 1989 Extraovarian peritoneal serous papillary carcinoma. A clinicopathologic study of 31 cases. Cancer 64: 110–115

Dallenbach-Hellweg G 1987 Atypical endosalpingiosis. A case report with consideration of the differential diagnosis of glandular subperitoneal inclusions. Pathology Research and Practice 182: 180–182

De Boer W G R M, Ma J, Nayman J 1981 Intestine associated antigens in ovarian tumours: an immunohistological study. Pathology 13: 547–555

Fox H, Langley F A 1976 Tumours of the ovary. Heinemann, London, p 74–118

Foyle A, Al-Jabi M, McCaughey W T E 1981 Papillary peritoneal tumors in women. American Journal of Surgical Pathology 5: 241–249

Genadry R, Poliakoff S, Rotmensch J, Rosenhein N B, Parmley T H, Woodruff J D 1981 Primary papillary peritoneal neoplasia. Obstetrics and Gynecology 58: 730–734

Genton C Y 1984 An unusual tumor of the ovary. Pathology Research and Practice 179: 110–112

Gooneratne S, Sassone M, Blaustein A, Talerman A 1982 Serous surface papillary carcinoma of the ovary: a clinicopathologic study of 16 cases. International Journal of Gynecological Pathology 1: 258–269

Hallgrimsson J, Scully R E 1972 Borderline and malignant Brenner tumours of the ovary. A report of 15 cases. Acta Pathologica Microbiologica et Immunologica Scandinavica (A) 80 (suppl 233): 56–66

Hart W R, Norris H J 1973 Borderline and malignant mucinous tumors of the ovary. Cancer 31: 1031–1045

Higa E, Rosai J, Pizzimbono C A, Wise L 1973 Mucosal hyperplasia, mucinous cystadenoma, and mucinous cystadenocarcinoma of the appendix. Cancer 32: 1525–1541

Jansen R P S, Russell P 1986 Nonpigmented endometriosis: clinical, laparoscopic, and pathologic definition. American Journal of Obstetrics and Gynecology 155: 1154–1159

Katzenstein A-L A, Mazur M T, Morgan T E, Kao M-S 1978 Proliferative serous tumors of the ovary. Histologic features and prognosis. American Journal of Surgical Pathology 2: 339–355

Klemi P J, Nevalainen T J 1977 Ultrastructure of the benign and borderline Brenner tumors. Acta Pathologica et Microbiologica Scandinavica (A) 85: 826–835

Kliman L, Rome R M, Fortune D W 1986 Low malignant potential tumors of the ovary: a study of 76 cases. Obstetrics and Gynecology 68: 338–344

Kottmeier H L 1968 Surgical management—conservative surgery. Indications according to the type of tumour. In: Gentils F, Junqueira A C (eds) Ovarian cancer (UICC Monograph Series, Vol 11). Springer-Verlag, New York, p157–164

Kunze E, Schauer A, Schmitt M 1983 Histology and histogenesis of two different types of inverted urothelial papillomas. Cancer 51: 348–358

Lauchlan S C 1990 Non-invasive ovarian carcinoma. International Journal of Gynecological Pathology 9: 158–169

Lindeque B G, Cronje H S, Deale C J C 1985 Prevalence of primary papillary peritoneal neoplasia in patients with ovarian carcinoma. South African Medical Journal 67: 1005–1007

Louwerens J K, Schaberg A, Bosman F T 1983 Neuroendocrine cells in cystic mucinous tumours of the ovary. Histopathology 7: 389–396

McCaughey W T E, Kirk M E, Lester W, Dardick I 1984 Peritoneal epithelial lesions associated with proliferative serous tumours of ovary. Histopathology 8: 195–208

McCaughey W T E, Schryer M J P, Lin X-S, Al-Jabi M 1986 Extraovarian pelvic serous tumor with marked calcification. Archives of Pathology and Laboratory Medicine 110: 78–80

McKenna H, Ansford A 1976 Malignant Brenner tumour. Australian and New Zealand Journal of Obstetrics and Gynaecology 16: 244–248

Michael H, Roth L M 1986 Invasive and non-invasive implants in ovarian serous tumors of low malignant potential. Cancer 57: 1240–1247

Miles P A, Norris H J 1972 Proliferative and malignant Brenner tumors of the ovary. Cancer 30: 174–186

Mills S E, Anderson W A, Fechner R E, Austin M B 1988 Serous surface papillary carcinoma. A clinicopathologic study of 10 cases and comparison with Stage III–IV ovarian serous carcinoma. American Journal of Surgical Pathology 12: 827–834

Nation J G, Krepart G V 1986 Ovarian carcinomas of low malignant potential: staging and treatment. American Journal of Obstetrics and Gynecology 154: 290–293

Pant K D, Fenoglio-Preiser C M, Berry C O A et al 1986 COTA (colon-ovarian tumor antigen). An immunohistochemical study. American Journal of Clinical Pathology 86: 1–9

Pratt-Thomas H R, Kreutner A Jr, Underwood P B, Dowdeswell R H 1976 Proliferative and malignant Brenner tumors of the ovary. Report of 2 cases, one with Meig's syndrome, review of the literature and ultrastructural comparisons. Gynecologic Oncology 4: 176–193

Radi M, Tazelaar H, Kempson R L, Hendrickson M R 1988 Mucinous neoplasms of the ovary: a clinicopathologic study of 270 cases and a proposed clinicopathologic re-definition of the LMP category (abstract). Laboratory Investigation 57: 74a

Roth L M, Sternberg W H 1971 Proliferating Brenner tumors. Cancer 27: 687–693

Roth L M, Czernobilsky B, Langley F A 1981 Ovarian endometrioid adenofibromatous and cystadenofibromatous tumors: benign, proliferating and malignant. Cancer 48: 1838–1845

Roth L M, Langley F A, Fox H, Wheeler J E, Czernobilsky B 1984 Ovarian clear cell adenofibromatous tumors: benign, of low malignant potential, and associated with invasive clear cell carcinoma. Cancer 53: 1156–1163

Roth L M, Dallenbach-Hellweg G, Czernobilsky B 1985 Ovarian Brenner tumors. I: Metaplastic, proliferating and of low malignant potential. Cancer 56: 582–591

Russell P 1979a The pathological assessment of ovarian neoplasms. I: Introduction to the common 'epithelial' tumours and analysis of benign 'epithelial' tumours. Pathology 11: 5–26

Russell P 1979b The pathological assessment of ovarian neoplasms. II: The proliferating 'epithelial' tumours. Pathology 11: 251–282

Russell P 1984 Borderline epithelial tumours of the ovary: a conceptual dilemma. Clinics in Obstetrics and Gynaecology 11: 259–277

Russell P, Bannatyne P 1989 Surgical pathology of the ovaries. Churchill Livingstone, Edinburgh, ch 22

Russell P, Merkur H 1979 Proliferating ovarian 'epithelial' tumours: a clinicopathological analysis of 144 cases. Australian and New Zealand Journal of Obstetrics and Gynaecology 19: 45–51

Russell P, Bannatyne P M, Solomon H J, Stoddard L D, Tattersall M H N 1985 Multifocal tumorigenesis in the upper female genital tract—implications for staging and management. International Journal of Gynecological Pathology 4: 192–210

Rutgers J L, Scully R E 1988a Ovarian Müllerian mucinous papillary cystadenomas of borderline malignancy. A clinicopathologic analysis. Cancer 61: 340–348

Rutgers J L, Scully R E 1988b Ovarian mixed-epithelial papillary cystadenomas of borderline malignancy. A clinicopathologic analysis. Cancer 61: 546–554

Santesson L, Kottmeier H L 1968 General classification of ovarian tumour. In: Gentil F, Junqueira A C (eds) Ovarian cancer (UICC Monograph Series, Vol 11). Springer-Verlag, New York, p 1–8

Scully R E 1977 Ovarian tumors. A review. American Journal of Pathology 87: 686–720

Scully R E 1979 Tumors of the ovary and maldeveloped gonads (AFIP Fascicle 16, Second Series). Armed Forces Institute of Pathology, Washington, p 53–151

Scully R E 1982 Common epithelial tumors of borderline malignancy (carcinomas of low malignant potential). Bulletin du Cancer (Paris) 69: 228–238

Serov S F, Scully R E, Sobin L H 1973 Histological typing of ovarian tumours (International histological classification of tumours no. 9). World Health Organization, Geneva, p 17–54

Shen S C, Bansal M, Purrazzella R, Malviya V, Strauss L 1983 Benign glandular inclusions in lymph nodes, endosalpingiosis, and salpingitis isthmica nodosa in a young girl with clear cell adenocarcinoma of the cervix. American Journal of Surgical Pathology 7: 293–300

Sinykin M B 1960 Endosalpingiosis. Minnesota Medicine 43: 759–762

Svenes K B, Eide J 1984 Proliferative Brenner tumor or ovarian metastases? A case report. Cancer 53: 2692–2697

Szymanska K, Szamborski J, Miechowiecka N, Czerwinski W 1983 Malignant transformation of mucinous ovarian cystadenomas of intestinal type. Histopathology 7: 497–509

Tasker M, Langley F A 1985 The outlook for women with borderline epithelial tumours of the ovary. British Journal of Obstetrics and Gynaecology 92: 969–973

Taylor H C Jr 1929 Malignant and semimalignant tumours of the ovary. Surgery Gynecology and Obstetrics 48: 204–230

Taylor H C Jr 1959 Studies in the clinical and biological evolution of adenocarcinoma of the ovary. Journal of Obstetrics and Gynaecology of the British Commonwealth 66: 827–842

Tobacman J K, Greene M H, Tucker M A, Costa J, Kase R, Fraumeni J F Jr 1982 Intra-abdominal carcinomatosis after prophylactic oophorectomy in ovarian cancer-prone families. Lancet 2: 795–797

Tutschka B G, Lauchlan S C 1980 Endosalpingiosis. Obstetrics and Gynecology 55: 57s–60s

White P F, Merino M J, Barwick K W 1985 Serous surface papillary carcinoma of the ovary. A clinical, pathologic, ultrastructural, and immunohistochemical study of 11 cases. Pathology Annual 20 (pt 1): 403–418

Woodruff J D, Dietrich D, Genadry R, Parmley T H 1981 Proliferative and malignant Brenner tumors. Review of 47 cases. American Journal of Obstetrics and Gynecology 141: 118–125

Zaloudek C, Kurman R J 1983 Recent advances in the pathology of ovarian cancer. Clinics in Obstetrics and Gynaecology 10 (2): 155–185

Zinsser K R, Wheeler J E 1982 Endosalpingiosis in the omentum. A study of autopsy and surgical material. American Journal of Surgical Pathology 6: 109–117

16. Extraovarian tumours of Müllerian type

Annabelle Farnsworth   Peter Russell

INTRODUCTION

The well-documented occurrence of non-neoplastic and neoplastic lesions normally considered to be of Müllerian differentiation that are found outside structures derived from the Müllerian ducts has led to the concept of a 'secondary' Müllerian system (Lauchlan 1968, 1972). These lesions typically occur in the pelvis and lower abdomen, involving the peritoneum, the subjacent tissues (including retroperitoneum) and lymph nodes. It has been suggested that, given the embryological origin of the Müllerian duct system from the coelomic epithelium and subcoelomic mesenchyme (which eventually forms the mature peritoneal lining and adjacent connective tissue), the latter may retain their ability to differentiate towards Müllerian epithelial and stromal structures (Kannerstein & Churg 1977). This differentiation can be full spectrum and both normal and neoplastic, from tumour-like or metaplastic lesions through benign and atypically pro-liferating (borderline) tumours to frankly malignant neoplasms.

This concept is, however, a little confused by the rare occurrence of similar lesions in the peritoneal cavity of men and in the pleural cavity in women; these presumably arise from the mesothelial lining of these structures (Henrix 1972). In view of this, the question has been raised as to whether some of these Müllerian-differentiated neoplasms in the female pelvis and abdominal cavity should be designated as mesotheliomas rather than as Müllerian carcinomas (Kannerstein & Churg 1977, Foyle et al 1981). It has been argued that certain epithelial tumours of ovary should also be classified as *mesotheliomas*, as they are thought to arise from the surface cells covering the ovary (Parmley & Woodruff 1974), which are modified mesothelial cells. Though one cannot argue with the logic of this suggestion from an embryonic point of view, from a practical viewpoint the suggestion is nonsense. The Müllerian and Wolffian ducts are also ultimately derived from the coelomic epithelium and subcoelomic mes-enchyme and so are the sex cords of the gonads, yet there is a manifest absurdity in classifying a cervical squamous cell carcinoma, an adeno-carcinoma of Gartner's duct, or a Sertoli cell tumour of the testis as mesothelioma, and the same applies to coelomic derivatives within the

321

Table 16.1   Classification of extraovarian Müllerian tumours[1]

A. SEROUS LESIONS
    1. *Tumour-like*
        Endosalpingiosis
    2. *Benign*
        Serous cystadenoma
        Serous cystadenofibroma
    3. *Atypically proliferating (borderline)*
        Serous tumour of low malignant potential
    4. *Malignant*
        Serous papillary carcinoma

B. MUCINOUS
    1. *Tumour-like*
        Endocervicosis
    2. *Benign*
        Mucinous cystadenoma
    3. *Atypically proliferating (borderline)*
        Mucinous tumours of low malignant potential
    4. *Malignant*
        Mucinous cystadenocarcinoma

C. ENDOMETRIOID
    1. *Tumour-like*
        Endometriosis
    2. *Benign*
        Endometrioid cystadenofibroma
    3. *Atypically proliferating (borderline)*
        Endometrioid tumour of low malignant potential
    4. *Malignant*
        Endometrioid adenocarcinoma
        —with squamous differentiation

D. CLEAR CELL
    1. *Tumour-like*
    2. *Benign*
    3. *Atypically proliferating (borderline)*
    4. *Malignant*
        Clear cell carcinoma of peritoneum

E. TRANSITIONAL (BRENNER, UROTHELIAL)
    1. *Tumour-like*
        Walthard's rest
    2. *Benign*
        Brenner tumour
    3. *Atypically proliferating (borderline)*
    4. *Malignant*

F. MESENCHYMAL AND MIXED
    1. *Tumour-like*
        Deciduosis
        Stromal endometriosis (stromatosis)
        Leiomyomatosis peritonealis disseminata
    2. *Benign*
        Leiomyoma
    3. *Atypically proliferating (borderline)*
        Leiomyoma of uncertain malignant potential
    4. *Malignant*
        Stromal sarcoma
        Leiomyosarcoma
        Adenosarcoma
        Malignant mixed Müllerian tumour

[1]Extraovarian Müllerian tumours may be classified along similar lines
to ovarian lesions. In some of the categories we could find no reference
to such lesions having been reported nor do we have personal
experience of such lesions. Such lesions may potentially arise as
primary lesions in the peritoneum and are included for completeness.

peritoneal cavity. There is merit in establishing histogenetic relationships between various neoplastic entities only when it leads to an improved understanding of behaviour and management. There is a much greater value in histological classification, and we believe this should, where necessary, be pursued beyond the arbitrary constraints of conventional systemic pathology (Russell 1985).

The purpose of this chapter is to describe the clinical presentation and histological appearances of the group of neoplastic and tumourlike entities that arise in the peritoneal cavity and retroperitoneal tissues and have morphological homology with lesions of the ovaries and Müllerian duct derivatives (Table 16.1). We will also discuss some of the unique features of these lesions that justify their separation as distinct pathological entities.

Though we acknowledge that one of the most common of these lesions is endometriosis, we do not propose to discuss this extensively documented entity here. Rather, we will discuss the less frequently reported non-neoplastic or tumour-like lesions and neoplasms, the great majority of which are epithelial and show endosalpingeal (serous) differentiation. Far less frequently seen are lesions of extraovarian origin that have endocervical (mucinous), endometrioid, clear cell or transitional differentiation; extra-ovarian endometrioid, stromal and mixed Müllerian sarcomas and smooth muscle lesions are extremely rare.

MÜLLERIANOSIS

The term 'Müllerianosis' was originally coined by Bassis in 1960, but recently we have suggested its reintroduction as a genetic term for the various manifestations of Müllerian metaplasias and tumour-like proliferations (whether epithelial, mesenchymal or mixed) that can be identified on and immediately beneath the ovarian surface, the pelvic peritoneum and omentum, and in pelvic lymph nodes. Endometriosis, endosalpingiosis, deciduosis and the rare condition of leiomyomatosis are all terms in common usage that fall within our concept of Müllerianosis (Russell & Bannatyne 1989).

A similar pathogenesis for all these lesions would seem logical. They most probably arise by differentiation of undifferentiated cells in the subcoelomic mesenchyme. It is these cells that contribute to the development of the Müllerian ducts embryologically but which are inapparent in postnatal life. The pelvic and abdominal peritoneum seems to retain a potential for Müllerian differentiation conditioned by its embryonic origin. The potential appears greatest in or near the ovaries, uterus and Fallopian tubes, and decreases proportional to the distance from these structures.

The lesions of Müllerianosis are considered to be acquired, for they have not been described in premenarchal girls (Blaustein et al 1982). This suggests that they are induced by the changes in the normal milieu that follow puberty. They show varying hormonal sensitivity and most undergo atrophy after the menopause (Tutscha & Lauchlan 1980).

SEROUS LESIONS

Benign tumour-like lesions that show serous (endosalpingeal) differentiation have been termed endosalpingiosis and are most easily understood as the tubal equivalent of endometriosis. Neoplasms, (benign, atypically proliferating and frankly malignant) that have histological appearances indistinguishable from those of serous neoplasms of the ovaries have been well documented.

Tumour-like lesions — endosalpingiosis

Endosalpingiosis is defined as the presence of glandular inclusions lined by epithelium resembling the Fallopian tube mucosa (endosalpinx) located in the superficial layers of the subperitoneal tissue or in pelvic or para-aortic lymph nodes. The term is no longer used for inclusion cysts within the cortex of the ovaries, but this is by convention rather than logic (Bell & Scully 1989).

Clinical details

Endosalpingiosis occurs exclusively in girls and women in the age-range of 12–66 years. It is not found before puberty, but cases have been reported in postmenopausal women (Tutscha & Lauchlan 1980). It is a remarkably common incidental finding in gynaecological specimens and, in our experience, can be identified in most such material. If specifically sought by careful macroscopic inspection and extensive sampling, it can be identified on both the visceral and parietal pelvic peritoneum. The study of Zinsser & Wheeler (1983), who looked at a series of omenta from women and men, showed endosalpingiosis in 25.7% of women: no such lesions were identified in men.

Endosalpingiosis may be associated with disease of the Fallopian tubes and rarely may be diagnosed by identifying papillary cellular fragments or psammoma bodies in peritoneal washings or Papanicolaou smears. It is often seen in women with FIGO Stage II–III atypically proliferating serous ovarian tumours (see Ch. 15) and it is also seen less commonly in association with benign and frankly malignant serous tumours of the ovary (Fig. 16.1; see also Fig. 15.2).

Macroscopic features

At laparotomy, endosalpingiosis is typically inapparent. It may, however, appear as a fine granularity or as small blebs on the peritoneal surfaces. Larger cysts, up to 1 cm diameter, have been described. Florid cases may

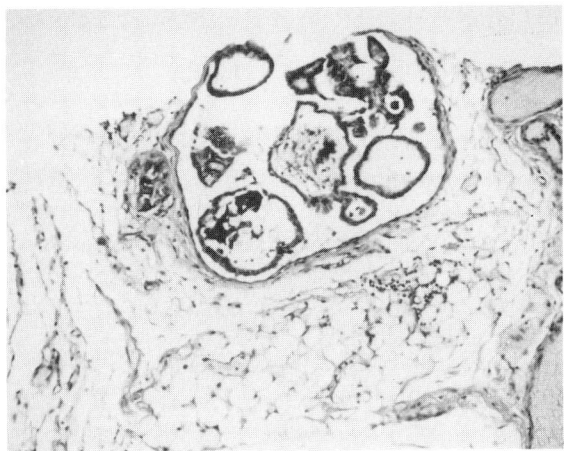

Fig. 16.1   One of multiple benign peritoneal (omental) 'implants' associated with a benign serous tumour. The patient's disease did not progress. (H & E, × 60.)

have adhesions on the serosal surfaces of pelvic viscera, and calcification is often obvious in such cases. Rarely, benign papillary structures are seen on the surfaces of the pelvic viscera and pelvic wall.

Microscopic features

The characteristic appearance is of small round or oval cystic spaces or clusters of glands lined by epithelium resembling that of the normal endosalpinx. The cells in individual lesions will vary and include differing mixtures of ciliated, non-ciliated secretory and peg-shaped intercalated cells. Endosalpingiosis is found under the serosa of the uterus or Fallopian tubes, the pelvic or abdominal visceral or parietal peritoneum. The nuclei are cytologically bland and round, oval or pencil-shaped. Blunt papillae with fibrovascular cores are often present. Psammoma bodies are often found in the stroma around the glands or unassociated with epithelial elements (so called 'burnt out' lesions). Cytological atypia is not a feature, but a mild focal inflammatory cell infiltrate may be seen.

Differential diagnosis

This includes endometriosis, reactive mesothelial hyperplasia and peritoneal inclusion cysts. Endosalpingiosis is characterized by a regular cellular arrangement and lacks any cytological atypia or mitotic activity. The absence of endometrial-like stroma or any evidence of recurrent haemorrhage usually serves to discriminate these lesions from endometriosis (though, in our experience, endometriosis and endosalpingiosis commonly occur together) and the tubal appearance of the epithelium clearly distinguishes endosalpingiosis from simple peritoneal inclusions or reactive proliferations.

Benign tumours

Serous papillary cystadenomas and serous papillary cystadenofibromas may rarely arise in extraovarian sites, especially in the pelvis attached to Fallopian tube or in the broad ligament (Honore 1976, Genadry et al 1977). They usually present as an adnexal mass, and tumours as large as 16 cm in diameter have been described. Histologically their appearances are indistinguishable from their ovarian counterparts.

In the past there has been much discussion about the origin of such neoplasms from mesonephric or Wolffian duct remnants. Given the clearly defined Müllerian differentiation of these tumours and the frequent occurrence of serous inclusions (endosalpingiosis) in the sites in which they have been reported, there seems to be little merit in considering an origin other than from such precursor lesions.

Atypically proliferating ('borderline') tumours

In the ovaries, atypically proliferating tumours are defined as neoplasms that show an unusual degree of cellular proliferation, greater than that encountered in a benign form of the same type of tumour, but with no destructive invasion of the stromal component (Scully 1979). Serous tumours that occur at extraovarian sites and have these features are also well described and fall into two main categories. In the first category are solitary atypically proliferating serous neoplasms that are characteristically large and cystic, and usually occur in the broad ligament (Chandrarathnam & Leong 1983, D'Ablaing et al 1983). Secondly, a diffuse variety arising in multiple sites in the peritoneal cavity has been recently reported (Bell et al 1988, Bell & Scully 1989). The occurrence of these lesions as part of the spectrum of serous neoplasia gives weight to the concept of multifocal tumourigenesis (see Fig. 15.3).

Clinical details

Patients with the diffuse variant of atypically proliferating tumour commonly present with infertility but a small group are diagnosed during pregnancy. Where the lesion is solitary and cystic, the most common presentation is with an abdominal mass.

Macroscopic appearance

The solitary lesions are large (usually measuring more than 10 cm in maximum dimension) and unilocular, often with obvious intracystic papillary growths. The diffuse forms, unlike their nominally benign counterparts, are usually visible at laparatomy, a common description being 'peritoneal granularity', fibrous adhesions, or a peritoneal mass or plaque. They most frequently involve the pelvic peritoneum but have also been described in the extrapelvic peritoneum.

Microscopic appearance

Large solitary tumours have histological features indistinguishable from those of their ovarian counterparts: obvious serous differentiation that is usually benign, but also papillary areas with complex branching fronds, cellular stratification and solid cellular buds detached from the lining epithelium diagnostic of atypically proliferating tumours. No invasion of underlying stroma is seen.

In the diffuse variety, unlike in endosalpingiosis, the small multifocal peritoneal lesions show cellular proliferation with tufting, stratification of cells and nuclear atypia. Mitoses are usually present. By definition no stromal invasion is present, but in all other aspects these tumours are indistinguishable from the reported range of so called 'implants' associated with atypically proliferating serous tumours of the ovaries (Bell et al 1988) (Fig. 16.2).

Differential diagnosis

The solitary lesions are usually readily diagnosable on microscopic examination, the only real difficulty being in establishing that they are truly

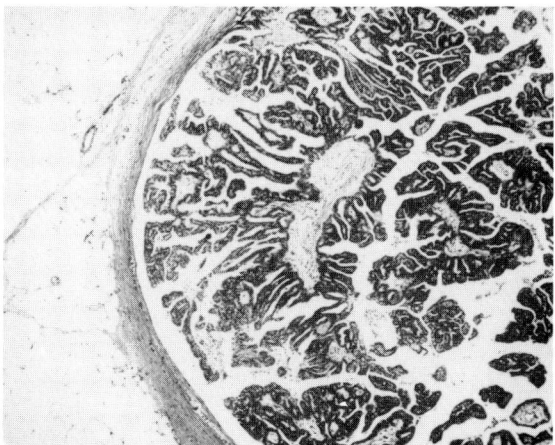

Fig. 16.2 A large circumscribed mesocolonic implant showing the same degree of atypical epithelial proliferation as the associated ovarian serous tumours but no local invasion. Similar lesions may occur in the absence of any associated ovarian lesion. (H & E, × 25.)

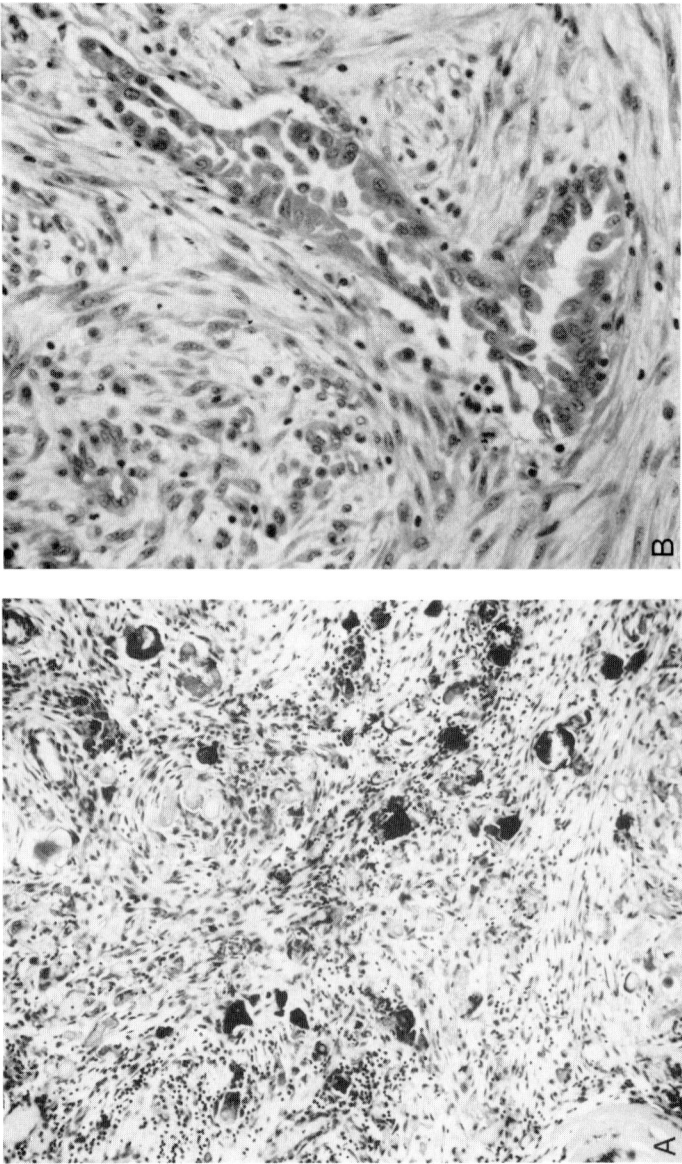

Fig. 16.3   This florid mixed inflammatory reaction was widespread in the pelvis of a woman with an atypically proliferating tumour. Similar appearances may be seen in association with other peritoneal disease. **A** Many psammoma bodies are noted. Epithelial cells if present would be difficult to identify amongst the reactive mesothelial cells and histiocytes. (H & E, × 90.) **B** Reactive mesothelial cells with eosinophilic cytoplasm and active but bland nuclei may produce small gland-like structures which must be distinguished from invasive carcinoma. (H & E, × 175.)

extraovarian. With diffuse lesions, the most important differential diagnosis is that of reactive mesothelial hyperplasia (McCaughey & Al-Jabi 1986, Bell & Scully 1990). Solid sheets of polygonal mesothelial cells or papillary aggregates with delicate or hyalinized fibrovascular cores, small irregular nests and solid cell clusters embedded in reparative stroma may all be seen in reactive hyperplasia. In atypically proliferating serous lesions the epithelial cells are usually columnar with ovoid hyperchromatic nuclei and scanty delicate, pale or amphophilic cytoplasm, whereas in mesothelial hyperplasias the cells tend to be cuboidal with uniform, round, central nuclei and glassy eosinophilic cytoplasm. Psammoma bodies may be seen in either situation but are more numerous in atypically proliferating serous lesions. Reactive mesothelial inclusions tend to be associated with reactive fibroblastic tissue and are often disposed in a linear fashion at the site of the original peritoneal surface (Fig. 16.3).

It is obviously also of great importance to distinguish these lesions from invasive serous adenocarcinoma. The definitional lack of frank invasion remains the most significant criterion. Local desmoplasia may be associated with superficial lesions, but this pseudoinvasive pattern (termed 'superficial invasion' by Bell et al 1988) is not to be mistaken for true destructive tissue invasion (see Fig. 15.5).

Behaviour

The solitary lesions should be carefully staged, optimally at the time of initial surgery, with a frozen section diagnosis of the lesion. In the absence of specific FIGO staging for these tumours, they should be staged as for a similar ovarian lesion. The diffuse atypically proliferating lesions should also be carefully staged, with multiple biopsies being taken for exclusion of invasive malignancy.

In the large series reported by Genadry et al in 1981 it was not clearly defined which cases were exclusively extraovarian lesions. In fact, most had ovarian masses with associated peritoneal lesions but the vast majority of the 154 patients were alive and well after a follow-up period varying from 24 months to 40 years.

The most recent series published by Bell & Scully (1990) also stressed the non-progressive nature of these lesions once local invasion was (by definition) excluded. After 8 years mean follow-up (range 4–13.9 years) 21 of 25 patients were alive and well with no evidence of disease. Tumours with atypical proliferation recurred in two patients, and invasive low grade carcinoma developed in one.

Malignant tumours—primary peritoneal serous papillary carcinoma

Examples of widespread intraperitoneal carcinomatosis that are morphologically indistinguishable from metastatic serous papillary carcinoma of the ovaries but in which there is no identifiable ovarian mass have been described in case reports for many years (Swerdlow 1959). The exact nature and behaviour of these lesions remains the subject of some discussion. Initially they were considered to be, and diagnosed as, mesotheliomas of the peritoneum, and some authors considered this to be an appropriate term (Parmley & Woodruff 1974). Kannerstein et al (1977) reported 15 cases of serous peritoneal carcinoma and emphasized both their homology with serous ovarian carcinomas and the need to separate such extraovarian serous papillary carcinomas from true malignant mesotheliomas in order to monitor behaviour and institute appropriate therapy.

There is no question that these primary peritoneal serous papillary carcinomas, occurring only in women, have much more in common with similar tumours originating in the Müllerian duct derivatives and ovaries than with the typical asbestos-associated mesotheliomas that arise in the pleural and peritoneal cavities of both sexes. Several authors have described the similarities between the ovarian and extraovarian serous tumours at cytological, histological and ultrastructural levels (White et al 1985, Lele et al 1988, Mills et al 1988). While their specific origin is far from certain, the very commonly observed subperitoneal epithelial nests of Müllerian (serous) differentiation noted earlier (endosalpingiosis) appear to be the most likely and acceptable explanation.

Primary peritoneal serous papillary carcinomas account for between 8 and 13% of all widespread serous carcinomas diagnosed at most large institutions and appear to occur at a comparable age and to have a similar symptomatology at presentation to their primary ovarian equivalents (Foyle et al 1981, Chen & Flam 1986, Lele et al 1988, Mills et al 1988, Dalrymple et al 1989).

Macroscopic features

The most common sites of grossly visible tumour deposits, at laparotomy, are omentum, pelvic and abdominal peritoneum and pelvic viscera (Fig. 16.4). The neoplastic lesions vary from almost microscopic deposits to large omental masses of solid carcinoma. It is important to note that while ovarian involvement is quite common, it is, when present, minimal and superficial. No tumour mass is found in the ovaries, which are usually of normal size. Surface irregularities or papillary projections may be seen.

Microscopic features

The histological features of primary peritoneal serous papillary carcinomas are indistinguishable from those of their primary ovarian equivalents. Invasion is widespread, and this distinguishes the well-differentiated lesions from serous peritoneal atypical proliferating tumours. Psammoma

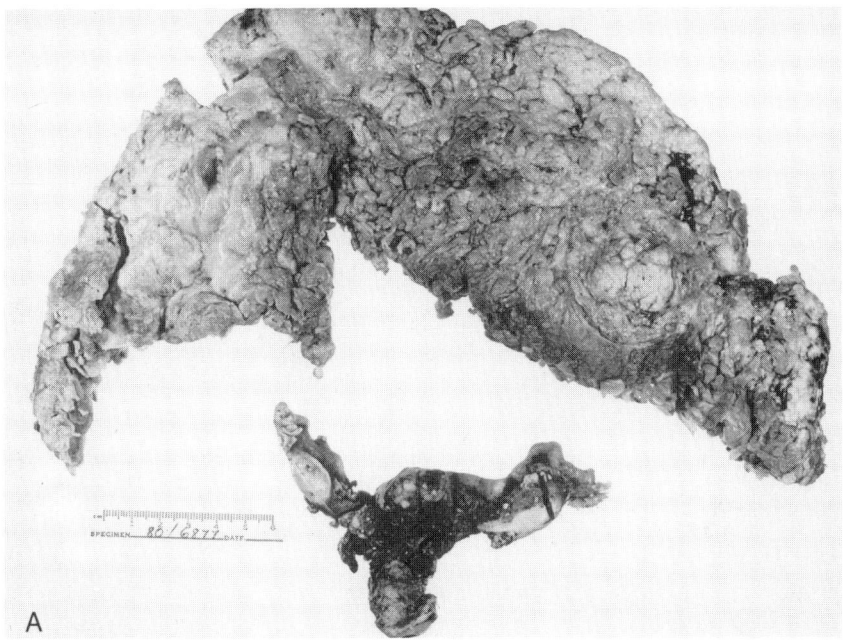

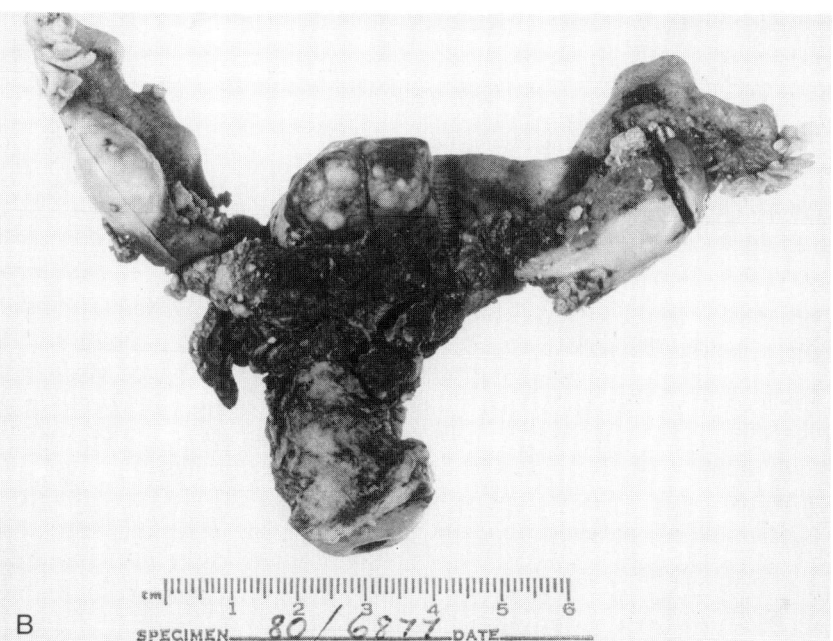

Fig. 16.4   Primary peritoneal serous papillary carcinomas.   **A** Omental 'cake' above with uterus, tubes and ovaries below. The omentum is heavily infiltrated by tumour masses.
B Closer view of tubes and ovaries showing obvious surface serosal deposits of carcinoma with no macroscopic enlargement of ovaries.

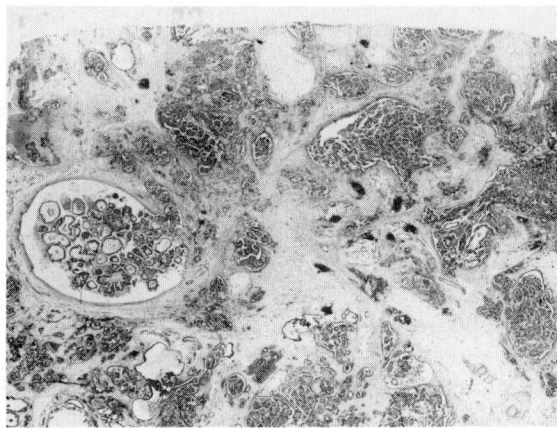

Fig. 16.5   Low power view of primary peritoneal serous papillary carcinoma. Parts of the figure show low-grade features with papillary lesions occurring in well circumscribed nodules, against a background of invasive malignancy. (H & E, × 6.)

bodies are frequently seen and are occasionally very prominent. Most cases show high-grade cellular changes equivalent to poorly differentiated serous ovarian carcinomas. However, cases do occur which show a well differentiated papillary pattern (Fig. 16.5).

Although earlier immunohistochemical studies showed no conclusive evidence of any features distinguishing between mesotheliomas, primary peritoneal serous papillary carcinomas and primary ovarian serous papillary carcinoma (White et al 1985), more recent reports have identified significant histochemical, immunohistochemical and ultrastructural similarities between papillary serous carcinomas of the ovary and non-ovarian peritoneum, and differences from typical mesotheliomas (Raju et al 1989, Wick et al 1989, Truong et al 1990). Wick et al (1989) recently published the results of an extensive immunohistochemical study which looked at general epithelial antigens (CK_1 and EMA), glycoproteinacous determinants (CA125, B72.3, Leu M1, LN1, LN2, MB2) and enzymatic markers (anti placental alkaline phophatase, amylase, S100) on primary peritoneal serous papillary carcinomas and primary ovarian serous papillary carcinomas. Statistical analysis of the staining for these markers showed no difference between these two tumour groups.

Although individually none of these cell surface or differentiation markers were specific for Müllerian epithelium, used in concert they may define a reproducible phenotype for neoplastic lesions of serous differentiation. Leu M1 was positive in 77% of primary peritoneal serous papillary carcinomas and 71% of primary ovarian serous papillary carcinomas; B72.3 was positive in 100 and 77%, S100 in 100 and 94%, carcinoembryonic antigen in 8 and 6%, respectively. Cytokeratin and epithelial membrane antigen was positive in 100% of tested cases in each group. Wick et al (1989) did not test these antigens against known mesotheliomas, but staining in residual benign mesothelial cells in their test sections was negative in all cases for Leu M1, B72.3 and S100. Truong et al (1990) also recently published an extensive light microscopic, histochemical, immunohistochemical and electron microscopic study of primary peritoneal serous papillary carcinomas. They showed that 40% stained positively for Leu M1 and 85% stained for B72.3, but that malignant mesotheliomas were negative for these antigens. They also add, and this was further confirmed by Raju et al (1989), that mesotheliomas, unlike primary peritoneal serous papillary carcinomas, rarely contain psammoma bodies (3.5%); they contain mucins which are removed by hyaluroninc acid but no others. Ultrastructurally the cells of serous tumours had slender, long microvilli of variable length with or without interspersed cilia, while the cells of mesothelioma which are not ciliated had long, wavy exuberant microvilli.

Behaviour

Recently, studies of large series have confirmed the patterns of behaviour of primary peritoneal serous papillary carcinomas and primary ovarian serous papillary carcinomas (Chen & Flam 1986, Mills et al 1988, Dalrymple et al 1989, Fromm et al 1990). The literature, however, still does not present a clear picture of the behaviour and clinical outcome of serous neoplasia in these two groups of patients, not least because of the various methods of reporting these outcomes. In our experience (Dalrymple et al 1989) there is no appreciable difference between the two groups when matched for grade and FIGO stage. Other authors have reported a worse prognosis for extraovarian serous carcinoma than for ovarian serous neoplasia (Mills et al 1988), but it cannot be determined from their reports whether the undoubted bias towards higher grade lesions amongst the extraovarian or peritoneal variants had been compensated for.

MUCINOUS LESIONS

The occurrence of lesions in the peritoneal cavity showing mucinous differentiation, although much rarer than their serous equivalents, is nevertheless well described (Roth & Ehrlich 1977, Banerjee & Gough 1988). As in the ovary and other sites in the female genital system, mucinous differentiation, in both neoplastic and non-neoplastic settings, may resemble either endocervical cells with tall, narrow columnar epithelium and basally placed nuclei, often in a single layer, or mucosa showing goblet cells suggestive of intestinal differentiation.

Tumour-like lesions—endocervicosis

Benign tumour-like epithelial lesions that are analogous to either endometriosis or endosalpingiosis but show endocervical epithelium are termed 'endocervicosis'; their significance is thought to be similar to that of endosalpingiosis (Lauchlan 1972). Mucinous metaplasia is occasionally seen in otherwise unremarkable foci of endometriosis.

Tumours

True tumours showing mucinous differentiation have also been described, in the retroperitoneum and rarely in the broad ligament (Banerjee & Gough 1988). They have shown the full neoplastic spectrum, from benign mucinous cystadenomas (Roth & Ehrlich 1977), through atypically proliferating tumours to mucinous cystadenocarcinomas. Such neoplasms usually present as large tumours mimicking the behaviour of their ovarian counterparts.

From the published reports, it appears that most of these tumours show intestinal differentiation. This poses the interesting semantic and conceptual problem of whether they should be considered as 'Müllerian' within the scope of the present discussion. Intestinal-type differentiation in the female genital tract is seen in endocervical, endometrial and ovarian neoplasms, and it is suggested that one should accept inclusion of such lesions for the sake of completeness, if not pure logic. The occurrence, however, of these extraovarian tumours, largely in the retroperitoneum and the mesocolon, raises the possibility that many have arisen in rests of intestinal epithelium rather than being primarily of Müllerian type with intestinal metaplasia. From the small number of cases available, their behaviour appears to mimic that of their biologically equivalent ovarian counterparts.

ENDOMETRIOID LESIONS

Tumour-like lesions—endometriosis

As stated in the introduction, although endometriosis fits well into the spectrum of peritoneal or extraovarian lesions of Müllerian differentiation, it has been well described and reviewed. Beyond emphasizing its place in the multidirectional spectrum of Müllerian tumour-like lesions, we will not discuss it further here.

Tumour-like lesions—deciduosis

Peritoneal deciduosis can also be placed in this category of endometrioid lesions. It is commonly seen on the ovaries and peritoneal surfaces of pelvic viscera beneath the parietal peritoneum and in lymph nodes in pregnancy, the puerperium and in unrelated high-progesterone states. It regresses spontaneously after delivery of the baby.

Tumours

Tumours showing true endometrioid differentiation are uncommon but reports in the literature have described lesions ranging from benign endometrioid cystadenofibromas (Ortega et al 1982), endometrioid atypically proliferating tumours (of low malignant potential) and probably the least rare, endometrioid adenocarcinoma (Brooks & Wheeler 1977, Mostovfizadeh & Scully 1980, Reimnitz et al 1988).

The benign tumours and atypically proliferating tumours are usually solitary well-circumscribed masses in the broad ligament. Although the numbers are very small, to date no case has pursued a progressive course. Benign tumours need to be differentiated from non-neoplastic endometriotic cysts.

Endometrioid adenocarcinomas arising in extraovarian sites are seen more frequently and have been the subject of numerous reviews. They may occur as multiple small deposits or as single tumour masses. In the most recent report (Aslani & Scully 1989), the authors discuss primary carcinomas of the broad ligament. Four of these cases were endometrioid and four clear cell in differentiation (see below).

Malignant extraovarian endometrioid neoplasms are usually seen in association with non-neoplastic endometriosis and are thought to have arisen, in most instances, from endometriotic deposits. The carcinomas have also been associated with the use of oestrogens as hormone replacement therapy or unopposed oestrogenic stimulation from another source (Mostovfizadeh & Scully 1980). They usually present in a similar fashion to intraperitoneal carcinomas and the management is similar, i.e. tumour debulking with appropriate postoperative adjuvant therapy. They may have a relatively favourable prognosis, especially if they have arisen in association with hormonal stimulation. In the cases discussed by Reimnitz et al (1988), with removal of the oestrogen source and excision of the tumour mass alone, two patients had disease free intervals of up to 5 years. Others, however, have shown that only 20% of patients were alive and free of disease after a 5-year follow-up (Ortega et al 1982).

CLEAR CELL LESIONS

Tumour-like lesions

Benign clear cell rests have been described in the ovaries, but we could find no reference to their occurrence in extraovarian tissues.

Tumours

To the best of our knowledge, neither benign nor clear cell atypically proliferating tumours lesions occurring in these sites have been reported. Rare clear cell carcinomas have, however, been described in the broad ligament and in other extraovarian sites (Reimnitz et al 1988, Aslani & Scully 1989). They are considered to reflect variations in endometrial glandular differentiation, and are the second most common type of carcinoma to arise in endometriotic foci. Their appearance, presentation and behaviour are similar to those seen in association with their ovarian equivalents.

TRANSITIONAL (UROTHELIAL) LESIONS

Tumour-like lesions—Walthard's rests

Transitional/urothelial epithelial (Walthard's) rests are some of the commonest epithelial inclusions in the peritoneum. They are frequently seen on the serosal surfaces of the Fallopian tubes, mesosalpinx and meso-ovarium but have also been described in numerous other sites. Whilst they cannot be considered to be primarily Müllerian in differentiation, they are noted here for completeness. They have also been described in men, in whom they are seen on the surfaces of the epididymis, testis and spermatic cord. They are usually incidental findings at laparotomy and may be identified as small plaques or cysts on the peritoneal surfaces.

Microscopically, they are solid or cystic rests of regular transitional type epithelium, commonly with metaplastic mucinous or serous epithelial cells lining the cystic space.

Tumours

Four Brenner tumours have been reported in extraovarian sites. These were all typical benign lesions, one in the uterus and three in the broad ligament (Wagner & Bettendorf 1980). All four were incidental findings at laparatomy.

We have not seen nor can we find reference to either an atypically proliferating Brenner tumour or malignant Brenner tumour occurring in an extraovarian site. Given the infrequency of these lesions in the ovaries, this is not surprising.

STROMAL AND MIXED LESIONS

Endometrioid stromal sarcomas

Extrauterine endometrioid stromal sarcomas are well described. They arise both in the ovaries and in extraovarian sites and have commonly been associated with endometriosis.

Recently, Baiocchi et al (1990) have reported two cases of endometrioid stromal sarcomas arising after total abdominal hysterectomy and bilateral salpingo-oophorectomy for endometriosis. They also reviewed the literature and found 12 further cases arising in extraovarian endometriosis. The tumours were present in pelvic peritoneum, colonic mesentery, omentum, broad ligament, pouch of Douglas, vagina, urinary tract and, in one instance, in the pleura. In this series, the patients' ages ranged from 22 to 64 years, and half were nulliparous. The most common presenting symptoms related to the presence of an abdominal mass. In these extraovarian sites bleeding was not uncommon. In all cases, the histological appearances were those of a typical low-grade endometrioid stromal sarcoma with fewer than 10 mitotic figures per 10 high-power fields. Management was by surgical debulking in all cases. Chemotherapy, radiotherapy and pregestational agents were used inconsistently as adjuvant therapy for disseminated disease. Four patients died of their disease within 14 months of diagnosis.

Chang et al (1990) have also recently presented data on 20 extrauterine endometrioid stromal sarcomas, of which 16 arose in extraovarian sites (pelvic cavity, abdominal cavity, Fallopian tube and retroperitoneum). In their study the histological features, including mitotic count and cytological atypia in the extrauterine lesions, were reported in greater detail. They also reviewed the clinical and morphological details from previously reported cases and could find no useful mitotic count threshhold that statistically separated those tumours that recurred from those which did not. The survival of extrauterine endometrioid stromal sarcomas was similar to that of Stage III or IV primary uterine endometrioid stromal sarcomas. The correlation between clinical behaviour and the appearances and mitotic activity of these lesions appears to be different from those seen in lesions occurring within the uterus.

Malignant mixed Müllerian tumours

Although rare, case reports do exist of mixed Müllerian tumours arising in extragenital sites. Hasiuk et al (1984) reported a case of an extragenital malignant mixed Müllerian tumour and reviewed the literature. Five cases were found in all, two arising in the posterior peritoneum and one each in the pelvic, rectovaginal and caecal peritoneum. Two of the tumours were heterologous malignant mixed Müllerian tumours, showing areas of osteosarcoma and rhabdomyosarcoma. The other three were homologous. One patient had no available follow-up but the others all died within 6 months of diagnosis.

Adenosarcoma

Rare reports of typical adenosarcomas arising in extraovarian and extra-uterine sites (Russell et al 1979) have usually documented an origin in the pelvic peritoneum and broad ligament. The histological appearances of these neoplasms are identical to those arising in the uterus or ovaries, and they appear to have a similar prognosis, i.e. they are much less malignant than malignant mixed Müllerian tumours. They may recur locally after inadequate initial excision, but no distant metastases have been reported. After short periods of follow-up (18 months) the patients were alive and well.

SMOOTH MUSCLE LESIONS

With the exception of benign leiomyomas, these lesions are extremely rare but encompass the full spectrum of disease from tumour-like conditions to malignant neoplasms.

Tumour-like lesions—disseminated peritoneal leiomyomatosis

This is a rare, tumour-like condition characterized by the presence of multiple myofibroblastic nodules on the pelvic and abdominal peritoneum. As with the Müllerian epithelial lesions and reactive deciduosis, they are thought to arise from specialized multipotential submesothelial cells, which in susceptible patients respond to a combination of hormones and proliferate along myofibromatous lines.

Clinical details

In a recent review, Dallenbach-Hellwig et al (1989) discussed the 50 cases they identified from the world literature. Of these 50 patients, 23 were pregnant and a further 17 had taken oral contraceptives for a period of 8–17 years. The patients were usually asymptomatic and the disease was often discovered incidentally at the time of caesarean section.

Macroscopic features

Disseminated peritoneal leiomyomatosis appears as multiple small (1–2 mm), grey/white nodules scattered on the surface of the intestines and omentum. The lesions rarely exceed 10 mm, and the most important differential diagnosis at laparotomy is disseminated carcinoma.

Microscopic features

The nodules are composed of smooth muscle and collagen and, given the frequent pregnant status of the patient, are not unexpectedly often associated with decidual cells. The smooth muscle cells may be plump and eosinophilic but show no evidence of any atypia, mitotic activity or other features which would suggest malignancy, either primary or secondary (i.e. metastatic leiomyosarcoma).

Benign and malignant tumours

So-called parasitic leiomyomas may arise in the uterus as subserosal lesions which become pedunculated and then present as truly extrauterine tumours. Intravascular leiomyomatosis arising in the uterus may also involve vessels in the peritoneum. True extrauterine and extraovarian leiomyomas and leiomyosarcomas have been reported (Honore 1976, Herbold et al 1983). They may arise from the smooth muscle of the uterine ligaments, metaplasia of submesothelial tissues or, as in many other sites in the body, they may arise from the ubiquitous smooth muscle cells associated with vessels (Allen 1990). Honore (1976) reported 22 cases of parauterine leiomyomas, most commonly in the broad ligaments but also in the pelvic peritoneum and retroperitoneum. They present as mass lesions and have no malignant potential.

Similarly, there are reports of leiomyosarcomas. Again, the most common site for these tumours is in the broad ligaments. Their behaviour and prognosis are similar to those of the more common uterine lesions.

CONCLUSION

Extraovarian Müllerian tumours are uncommon. They are, however, clearly defined entities that can be considered in their pathogenesis and appearance analogous to similar tumours which occur in the ovaries or Müllerian duct derivatives. Their behaviour, however, may vary from that of tumours that occur primarily within the female genital tract. An increased recognition of these distinctive lesions by the general pathological and gynaecological community is thus important. By clearly separating them from their couterparts occurring within the organs of the female genital tract, we can observe their behaviour and devise appropriate management regimes.

REFERENCES

Allen P W 1990 Benign metastasizing Müllerian tumours and uterine sarcomas. Surgical Pathology 3: 3–14
Aslani M, Scully R E 1989 Primary carcinoma of the broad ligament. Report of four cases and review of the literature. Cancer 64: 1540–1545
Baiocchi G, Kavanagh J J, Wharton J T 1990 Endometrioid stromal sarcoma arising from ovarian and extraovarian endometriosis. Report of two cases and review of the literature. Gynecologic Oncology 36: 147–151
Banerjee R, Gough J 1988 Cystic mucinous tumours of the mesentery and retroperitoneum: report of 3 cases. Histopathology 12: 527–532
Bassis M L 1960 An embryologically derived classification of ovarian tumors. Journal of the American Medical Association 174: 1316–1319
Bell D A, Scully R E 1989 Benign and borderline serous lesions of the peritoneum in women. Pathology Annual 24: 1–21
Bell D A, Scully R E 1990 Serous borderline tumors of the peritoneum. American Journal of Surgical Pathology 14: 230–239
Bell D A, Weinstock M A, Scully R E 1988 Peritoneal implants of ovarian serous borderline tumors. Histologic features and prognosis. Cancer 62: 2212–2222
Blaustein A, Kantius M, Kaganowicz A, Pervex N, Wells J 1982 Inclusions in ovaries of females aged day 1–30 years. International Journal of Gynecological Pathology 1: 145–153

Brooks J J, Wheeler J E 1977 Malignancy arising in extra-gonadal endometriosis. A case report and summary of the world literature. Cancer 40: 3065–3073

Chandrarathnam E, Leong A S-Y 1983 Papillary serous cystadenoma of borderline malignancy arising in a parovarian paramesonephric cyst. Light microscopic and ultrastructural observations. Histopathology 7: 601–611

Chang K L, Crabtree G C, Liun-Tan S K, Kempson R L, Hendrickson M R 1990 Primary extra-uterine endometrial stromal sarcomas: A clinicopathologic study of 20 cases and a review of the literature. (Abstract). Modern Pathology 3: 18A

Chen K T K, Flam M S 1986 Peritoneal papillary serous carcinoma with long term survival. Cancer 58: 1371–1373

D'Ablaing G III, Klatt E C, DiRocco G, Hubbard L T 1983 Broad ligament serous tumour of low malignant potential. International Journal of Gynecological Pathology 2: 93–99

Dallenbach C, Muklan H, Dallenbach C D, Dallenbach-Hellweg G 1989 Disseminated peritoneal leiomyomatosis. A rare disease. Geburtshilfe und Frauenheilkinde 49: 201–204

Dalrymple J C, Bannatyne P, Russell P et al 1989 Extraovarian peritoneal serous papillary carcinoma. A clinicopathologic study of 31 cases. Cancer 64: 110–115

Di Domenico A, Strange F, Bennington J 1982 Leiomyosarcoma of the broad ligament. Gynecologic Oncology 13: 412–415

Foyle A, Al-Jabi M, McCaughey W T F 1981 Papillary peritoneal tumors in women. American Journal of Surgical Pathology 5: 241–249

Fromm G, Gershenson D M, Silva E G 1990 Papillary serous carcinoma of the peritoneum. Obstetrics and Gynecology 75: 89–95

Genadry R, Parmley T, Woodruff J D 1977 The origin and clinical behavior of the parovarian tumor. American Journal of Obstetrics and Gynecology 129: 873–879

Genadry R, Poliakoff S, Rotmensch J, Rosenshein N B, Parmley T H, Woodruff J D 1981 Primary papillary peritoneal neoplasia. American Journal of Obstetrics and Gynecology 58: 730–734

Hasiuk A S, Peterson R O, Hanjani P, Griffen T D 1984 Extragenital malignant mixed Müllerian tumor. Case report and review of the literature. American Journal of Clinical Pathology 81: 102–105

Henrix T R 1972 Peritoneal mesothelioma. Gastroenterology 63: 346–349

Herbold D R, Fu Y-S, Silbert S W 1983 Leiomyosarcoma of the broad ligament. A case report and literature review with follow-up. American Journal of Surgical Pathology 7: 285–292

Honore L H 1976 Papillary serous cystadenoma arising in a paramesonephric cyst of the parovarium. American Journal of Obstetrics and Gynecology 125: 870–871

Honore L H 1981 Para-uterine leiomyomas in women: A clinicopathologic study of 22 cases. Europe Journal of Obstetrics, Gynecology and Reproductive Biology 11: 273–279

Kannerstein M, Churg J 1977 Peritoneal mesothelioma. Human Pathology 8: 83–94

Kannerstein M, Churg J, McCaughey W T E, Hill D P 1977 Papillary tumors of the peritoneum in women: mesothelioma or papillary carcinoma. American Journal of Obstetrics and Gynecology 127: 306–313

Lauchlan S C 1968 Conceptual unity of the Müllerian tumor group. Cancer 22: 601–610

Lauchlan S C 1972 The secondary Müllerian system. Obstetrical and Gynecological Survey 27: 133–146

Lele S B, Piver M S, Matharu J, Tsukada Y 1988 Peritoneal papillary carcinoma. Gynecologic Oncology 31: 315–320

McCaughey W T E, Al-Jabi M 1986 Differentiation of serosal hyperplasia and neoplasia in biopsies. Pathology Annual 21 (pt 1): 272–293

Mills S E, Anderson W A, Fechner R E, Austin M B 1988 Serous surface papillary carcinoma. A clinicopathological study of 10 cases and comparison to Stage III–IV ovarian serous carcinoma. American Journal of Surgical Pathology 12: 827–834

Mostovfizadeh M, Scully R E 1980 Malignant tumors arising in endometriosis. Clinical Obstetrics and Gynecology 3: 951–963

Ortega I, Nogales F, Gonzalez-Campora R, Matilla A, Galera H 1982 Extragenital endometrioid cystadenofibroma. Acta Obstetrica et Gynecologia Scandinavica 61: 283–284

Parmley T H, Woodruff J D 1974 The ovarian mesothelioma. American Journal of Obstetrics and Gynecology 120: 234–241

Raju U, Fini G, Greenwalk D A, Ohorodnik J M 1989 Primary papillary serous neoplasia of the peritoneum: a clinico-pathologic and ultrastructural study of eight cases. Human Pathology 20: 426–436

Reimnitz C, Brand E, Nieberg R K, Hacker N F 1988 Malignancy arising in endometriosis associated with unopposed estrogen replacement. Obstetrics and Gynecology 71: 444–447

Roth L M, Ehrlich C E 1977 Mucinous cystadenocarcinoma of the retroperitoneum. Obstetrics and Gynecology 49: 486–488

Russell P 1985 Common epithelial tumours of the ovary—a new look. Pathology 17: 555–557

Russell P, Bannatyne P 1989 Surgical pathology of the ovaries. Churchill Livingstone, Edinburgh

Russell P, Slavutin L, Laverty C R, Cooper Booth J 1979 Extrauterine mesodermal (Müllerian) adenosarcoma. A case report. Pathology 11: 557–560

Schuldenfrie R, Janovski N A 1962 Disseminated endosalpingiosis associated with bilateral papillary serous cystadenocarcinoma of the ovaries. American Journal of Obstetrics and Gynecology 84: 382–389

Scully R E 1979 Tumours of the ovary and maldeveloped gonads. (AFIP fascicle 16, 2nd series) Armed Forces Institute of Pathology, Washington, p 53–151

Swerdlow M 1959 Mesothelioma of the pelvic peritoneum. American Journal of Obstetrics and Gynecology 77: 197–200

Truong L D, Maccato M L, Awalt H, Cagle P T, Schwartz M R, Kaplan A L 1990 Serous surface carcinoma of the peritoneum: a clinico-pathological study of 22 cases. Human Pathology 21: 99–110

Tutscha B G, Lauchlan S C 1980 Endosalpingiosis. Obstetrics and Gynecology 55: 575–605

Wagner I, Bettendorf U 1980 Extra-ovarian Brenner tumour. Case report and review. Archiv für Gynäkologie 229: 191–196

White P F, Merino M J, Barwick K W 1985 Serous surface papillary carcinoma of the ovary: a clinical, pathologic, ultrastructural and immunohistochemical study of 11 cases. Pathology Annual 20: 403–418

Wick M R, Mills S E, Dehner L P, Bollinger D J, Fechner R E 1989 Serous papillary carcinomas arising from the peritoneum and ovaries. A clinicopathologic and immunohistochemical comparison. International Journal of Gynecological Pathology 8: 179–188

Zinsser K R, Wheller J E 1983 Endosalpingiosis in the omentum: a study of autopsy and surgical material. American Journal of Surgical Pathology 6: 109–117

17. Gynaecological tumours in children

M. Anna Kelsey   Melanie J. Newbould

INTRODUCTION

In terms of oncological statistical data, childhood is considered to span an age range of 0–14 years inclusive (Parkin et al 1988). Childhood cancers comprise only 0.5–3% of all neoplasms, depending on population structure (Parkin et al 1988). In the Manchester series this gives a total incidence of 102 tumours per 10^6 child years, of which leukaemia, lymphoma and central nervous system tumours account for almost 80%. Germ cell and other gonadal neoplasms have a total incidence of only 2.3 per 10^6 child years in the same series (Birch 1990). It follows, therefore, that gynaecological tumours are uncommon in this age group: only 0.2–0.3% of ovarian neoplasms occur in girls aged less than 15 years (La Vecchia et al 1983).

Since its foundation in 1953, the Manchester Children's Tumour Registry has recorded all cases of malignant neoplasms and teratomas occurring in this age group from a defined geographical area. The child population was initially one million but boundary changes in 1974 resulted in a fall of 10% (Birch 1988). In the 36 years covered by the Registry, there have been fewer than 70 neoplasms of the female genital tract. Table 17.1 illustrates the tumour types represented and their relative frequencies. The ovary is by far the commonest site, and germ cell neoplasms are the commonest tumour type. These findings are similar to those in most other series (Breen & Maxson 1977, La Vecchia et al 1983, Piver & Patton 1986).

In the Manchester series, all children with neoplasms of the female genital system other than the ovary were less than 10 years old, and all but one were less than 2 years old. Mature teratoma was the commonest single tumour type. It is possible that the figures quoted underestimate its true incidence: all malignant tumours are collected by the Registry but benign neoplasms, which are not subject to cancer registration schemes, may be missed. All of the malignant ovarian germ cell tumours in the Registry occurred in children in the 10–14 year age group.

There are few tumours that occur exclusively in the paediatric age group. Table 17.2 illustrates the age range of the commonest tumours of the first 15 years of life. In almost all cases, the range extends into the second, third or subsequent decades.

Table 17.1   Gynaecological tumours collected by Manchester
Children's Tumour Registry, 1954–1990

	Number	%
GERM CELL TUMOURS		
Mature teratomas	32	53
Malignant germ cell tumours		
Dysgerminoma	10	17
Immature teratoma	5	8
Endodermal sinus tumour	5	8
Mixed germ cell tumour	1	2
Embryonal carcinoma	1	2
Total	22	37
Total	54	90
SEX CORD/STROMAL TUMOURS	6	10
Juvenile granulosa cell tumour	1	1.5
Sertoli–Leydig cell tumour	2	4
Sex cord tumour with annular tubules	1	1.5
Fibroma	1	1.5
Unclassified	1	1.5
Grand total	60	100
EXTRA OVARIAN NEOPLASMS (1954–1990)		
Vaginal endodermal sinus tumour	3	
Vaginal embryonal rhabdomyosarcoma	2	
Vulval small celled malignant tumour	1	
Total	6	

Tumour biology in general is currently subject to intense experimental
investigation. Whilst extensive work has been carried out on epithelial
neoplasms of the ovary, cervix and endometrium there is a relative paucity
of information on the neoplasms discussed here, with the exception of
mature teratoma.

Table 17.2   Age range in and median age at which tumours common in
children occur

Tumour	Range (years)	Median (years)
Dysgerminoma	6–45	23
Immature teratoma (ovary)	1–40	18
Endodermal sinus tumour (ovary)	1–45	19
Embryonal carcinoma (ovary)	4–28	15
Mixed germ cell tumour (ovary)	5–33	15
Juvenile granulosa cell tumour	1–30	13
Sertoli–Leydig cell tumour	2–75	25
Sex cord tumour with annular tubules	4–76	34
Small cell carcinoma of ovary	9–45	22
Rhabdomyosarcoma (vaginal)	0–2	
Endodermal sinus tumour (vaginal)	1st decade	
Clear cell adenocarcinoma (cervical/vaginal, DES-associated)	9–35	19

GERM CELL TUMOURS

Epidemiology

Over the past 30 years the incidence of germ cell tumours has risen (Birch et al 1982, Walker et al 1984, Senturia 1987). This is due particularly to a rising incidence of testicular cancer, which accounts for 90% of malignant gonadal germ cell tumours (Walker et al 1984, Senturia 1987), but there is evidence that the incidence of ovarian neoplasms may have a similar trend (Walker et al 1984). In a study based on the entries of patients in the records of the Childhood Cancer Research Group over the period 1962–1978, however, La Vecchia found that the total incidence of malignant ovarian germ cell neoplasms remained static, though the incidence of endodermal sinus tumour had risen (La Vecchia 1983). Recently, it has been suggested that there is an increased, though very low, risk of a germ cell tumour arising in both male and female offspring after maternal exposure to oestrogens, including oral contraceptives, in early pregnancy (Senturia 1987, Walker et al 1988).

There are reported cases of germ cell neoplasms occurring in several members of a family (La Vecchia et al 1983, Dahl et al 1990). The Li–Fraumeni Cancer Family syndrome, in which soft tissue sarcomas and other cancers (including early onset breast cancer) occur in different members of one family, may be associated with an increased incidence of germ cell tumours (Hartley et al 1989).

Ovarian germ cell tumours

The ovary is considered to be the second commonest site of origin of germ cell tumours in the paediatric age group after sacrococcygeal neoplasms (Dehner 1983), though in one population based study (Marsden et al 1981) and in one large series from a children's hospital (Malogolowkin et al 1990), germ cell tumours of the ovary were found to be the most common.

Mature teratomas

At least 90% of ovarian germ cell tumours are mature teratomas. Two distinct types are described: the mature cystic teratoma (dermoid cyst) and the mature solid teratoma. The former accounts for over 20% of all ovarian neoplasms, affects women in all age groups from childhood to old age, and comprises over half of all ovarian tumours removed in the first two decades of life (Scully 1979).

Mature solid teratoma is a tumour of the first two decades. The diagnosis should be made only after careful sampling to exclude the presence of immature tissues or other malignant germ cell elements. Sampling of at least one block of tissue per centimetre of tumour diameter is the usual recommendation (Norris et al 1976).

Cytogenetic studies have most frequently addressed the relatively common mature cystic teratoma of the ovary. Most tumours have a 46,XX karotype, though there are reported cases with chromosomal anomalies such as trisomy 8 (Dahl et al 1990). Markers that are heterozygous in the patient can be studied in the tumour to determine whether they are heterozygous in the cells of the tumour as well. This provides a clue to the cell of origin. If it is a somatic cell, the pattern of heterozygosity would be identical with that of other cells in the patient, but if the tumour is of germ cell origin the pattern may be different because of cross-over during meiosis, depending on the stage attained. The use of enzyme markers (Parrington et al 1984) and DNA probes recognizing restriction fragment length polymorphisms (Dahl et al 1990) has indicated that a tumour may develop from germ cells at any one of several stages of meiosis. Multiple tumours in a single patient may originate from different germ cells, each of which has attained a different stage in the meiotic process (Carritt et al 1982).

Immature teratoma

This is the third most common malignant germ cell neoplasm and accounts for 8% of all ovarian tumours in patients less than 15 years old in Manchester. Grading is determined by the proportion of immature tissue present (Fig. 17.1) though the exact criteria used have varied among series (Table 17.3). It should be noted that this applies only to ovarian teratomas.

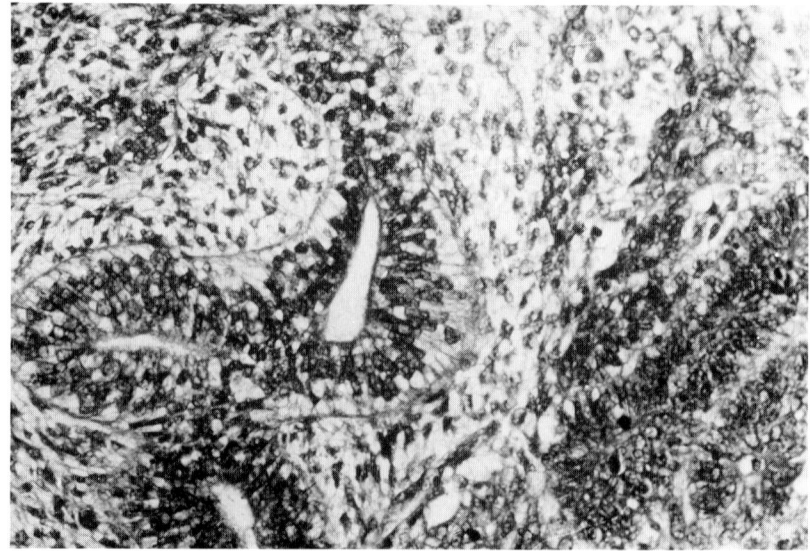

Fig. 17.1 Ovarian immature teratoma (H & E, × 250).

Table 17.3   Criteria for grading immature teratoma

Grade	Thurlbeck & Scully (1960)	Robboy & Scully (1970)	Norris et al (1976)
0	All cells well differentiated	No mitotic activity	All tissues mature
1	Rare small foci of embryonal tissue	Minor foci of embryonal tissue. Rare mitoses	Neuroepithelium limited to a rare × 40 field. Not more than 1 focus per slide
2	Moderate quantity of embryonal tissue	Moderate quantities of embryonal tissue. Moderate mitotic activity	Neuroepithelium does not exceed 3 × 40 fields in any one slide
3	Large quantity of embryonal tissue cells show mitotic activity and atypicality	Large quantity of embryonal tissue	Neuroepithelium 4 or more × 40 fields per slide

Tumours at other sites, such as the sacrococcygeal region and the mediastinum, frequently contain immature elements and these are of no prognostic significance in children of 3 months or younger (Dehner 1983, Carter et al 1982). In older children, they may indicate malignancy.

Some immature and mature solid ovarian teratomas are associated with extraovarian disease (Robboy & Scully 1970). This group accounted for a third in one series (Norris et al 1976). The factors determining prognosis are the grade of the primary tumour and the grade of the tumour deposits in extraovarian sites, rather than simply the stage. The presence of fully mature glial implants on the peritoneum increases the stage, but is not an adverse prognostic factor (Nogales et al 1976, Truong et al 1982). It therefore follows that pathological assessment requires adequate sampling of the primary tumour and extraovarian deposits to establish the extent of immature tissues and the presence of other malignant germ cell elements. Patients with grade 1 tumours have an excellent prognosis; conversely only 30% of patients with grade 3 neoplasms survive 10 years (Norris et al 1976). Modern chemotherapy has, however, resulted in considerable improvement (Taylor et al 1985). Low-grade tumours are more likely to have a 46,XX karyotype, whereas grade 3 tumours may be aneuploid (Ihara et al 1984).

Dysgerminoma

Germinoma is the general designation for the neoplasm that is called seminoma in the testis and dysgerminoma in the ovary. It is the commonest malignant germ cell tumour of the ovary and comprised almost half of those in the Manchester Registry. In contrast to other malignant germ cell tumours, a relatively high proportion (10–15%) are bilateral, but involvement of the contralateral ovary may be discovered only on microscopic examination. A quarter of patients have metastases at the time of diagnosis (Björkholm et al 1990); local spread to the pelvis and lymphatic involvement of the para-aortic region is particularly common.

As in classical seminoma, in 95% of cases the tumour cells are accompanied by abundant lymphocytes and 3% of tumours have giant cells that produce human chorionic gonadotrophin (Zaloudek et al 1981). In 5% the tumour cells are anaplastic with nuclear pleomorphism and frequent mitoses (Nogales 1987). Histological parameters are, however, of no predictive value (Björkholm et al 1990). Recently, studies involving flow cytometry have also failed to define factors of prognostic value (Oud et al 1988).

The overall 5-year survival, 96%, is high for tumours confined to the ovary but is only 63% in patients with extensive extraovarian disease (Kurman & Norris 1977). Important prognostic factors are tumour stage and the presence of capsular rupture or penetration (Nogales et al 1977). In one recently published series, no patient was found to have died of dysgerminoma since the introduction of megavoltage radiotherapy in 1963 (Björkholm et al 1990).

On the basis of results of karyotypic analysis of testicular seminomas, it has been suggested that a specific chromosomal anomaly, an isochromosome of the short arm of chromosome 12 (i(12p)), may be a marker for tumours of germ cell lineage (Atkin & Baker 1983). Some dysgerminomas have also had this abnormality (Jenkyn & McCartney 1987). On the other hand, several neoplasms of germ cell origin other than germinoma, such as endodermal sinus tumours, have not shown this specific abnormality on karyotypic analysis (Vos et al 1990).

Yolk sac tumour

This is the second most common type of malignant germ cell tumour of the ovary in most series (Kurman & Norris 1977). Patients present with an abdominal mass, fever and pain, rather than hormonal effects (Kurman & Norris 1976a).

At least 10 histological patterns are described, though the yolk sac tumour with an endodermal sinus pattern and characteristic Schiller–Duval bodies (Fig. 17.2) is probably the best recognized (Talerman 1987a).

The tumour was once described as a highly malignant neoplasm with a 13% 3-year survival (Kurman & Norris 1976a), but modern chemotherapy has reduced mortality considerably and now over 80% of patients have a long-term survival (Gerhenson et al 1983, Taylor et al 1985).

As yet, there have been few karyotypic analyses and ploidy studies, but aneuploidy has been demonstrated in a metastatic ovarian yolk sac tumour by chromosomal analysis (Vos et al 1990). Analysis of ploidy by static cytometry has given interesting results: one study showed that a tumour with a particular histological pattern, the intestinal variety, was diploid

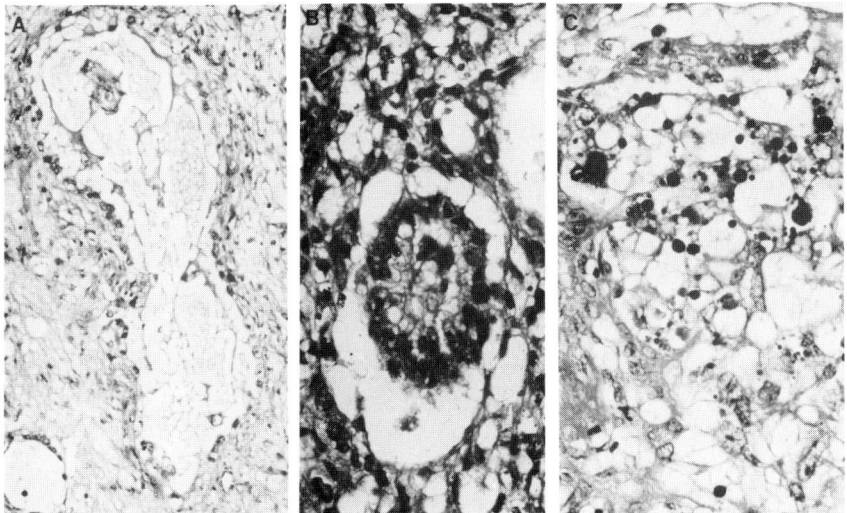

Fig. 17.2   Yolk sac tumour.   **A** Polyvesicular pattern (H & E, × 100).   **B** Endodermal sinus pattern with Schiller–Duval body. (H & E, × 250.)   **C** Hyaline globules in both intracellular and extracellular locations (H & E, × 400).

whilst the other histological variants were aneuploid (Kommoss et al 1990). The authors noted that the intestinal pattern was associated with a worse response to therapy. Other studies, however, found different results (Oosterhuis et al 1989), and clearly the number of tumours studied so far is too small to draw firm conclusions.

Other malignant germ cell tumours of the ovary

Embryonal carcinoma of the ovary resembles the tumour of the same name in the adult testis, but it is much less common. It has distinct clinico-pathological features, described by Kurman and Norris in 1976. Unlike yolk sac tumour, 60% present with hormonal manifestations. Histologically, the tumour has masses of large pleomorphic cells, and scattered multinucleate giant cells with the features of syncytiotrophoblast are a common finding (Kurman & Norris 1976b).

Mixed germ cell tumours are composed of a combination of malignant germ cell elements. Up to 40% of patients are prepubertal, and one-third have isosexual precocity, usually due to the presence of foci of chorio-carcinoma producing hCG (Kurman & Norris 1977).

In a newborn infant with multiple visceral lesions the possibility of metastases from an unrecognized intraplacental choriocarcinoma should be considered, whilst in the post pubertal female the possibility that an ovarian choriocarcinoma is, in fact, a metastasis from a uterine gestational choriocarcinoma or has developed from a primary ovarian pregnancy should be considered (Kurman & Norris 1977, Dehner 1983, Flam et al 1989).

Malignant neuroectodermal tumours resembling those of the central nervous system have been described in teenage patients (Aguirre & Scully 1982). As two of the tumours contained small areas with the features of a mature teratoma, it seems probable that these are germ cell neoplasms.

Conditions predisposing to the development of malignant germ cell tumours

Two of these, gonadoblastoma and male pseudohermaphroditism, will be discussed in detail.

Gonadoblastoma.   This is one type of mixed germ cell/sex cord–stromal neoplasm. Other tumours in the group will be addressed later in this section.

In about half of cases of gonadoblastoma, an associated malignant germ cell tumour develops in either the same or the contralateral gonad. This is most commonly a germinoma, but in some cases a highly malignant neoplasm such as a yolk sac tumour, embryonal carcinoma, chorio-carcinoma or immature teratoma may develop (Rutgers & Scully 1987).

Gonadoblastoma has a characteristic insular structure (Fig. 17.3). The tumours are frequently calcified and may be visible radiologically (Rutgers & Scully 1987). They can be microscopic in size or form a macroscopically identifiable ovarian mass.

About 95% of gonadoblastomas arise in patients with a Y chromosome or

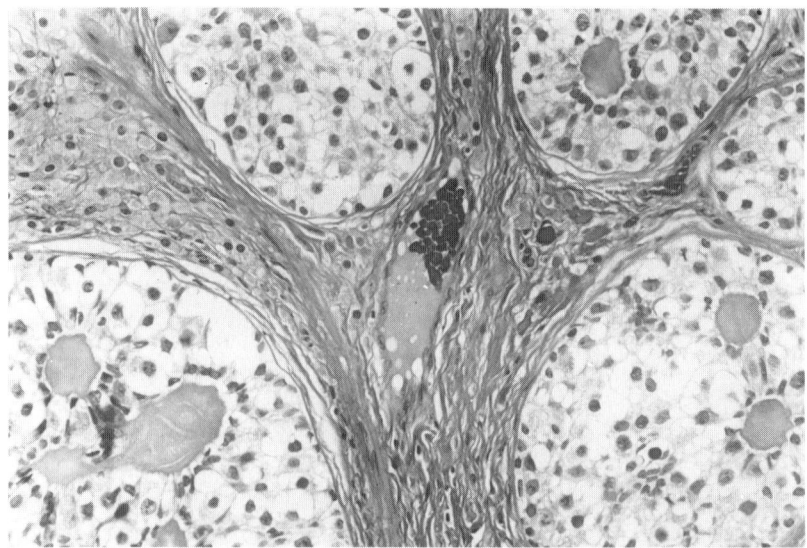

Fig. 17.3   Gonadoblastoma. Islands of cells containing both sex cord and germ cell elements. (H & E, × 250). Case provided by Dr D L Bisset.

Y chromosomal material; 80% of them are phenotypically female (Scully 1970). The tumour characteristically occurs in dysgenetic gonads of one of three syndromes: mixed gonadal dysgenesis, pure 46,XY gonadal dysgenesis, and dysgenetic male pseudohermaphroditism. One-fifth of cases occur in a streak gonad, the same proportion in a testis, and in the remaining cases the type of the underlying gonad cannot be determined because of obliteration by tumour. There are a few instances of the lesion occurring in the ovaries of apparently normal, fertile, women (Scully 1970), or in patients with 45,X Turner's syndrome (Sinisi et al 1988): one case has been reported in a 46,XX infant with autosomal recessive Fraser (cryptophthalmos) syndrome (Greenberg et al 1986). The occurrence of gonadoblastoma is recorded from infancy to the fourth decade of life (Rutgers & Scully 1987).

Mixed gonadal dysgenesis is characterized by a patient with a unilateral testis, usually abdominal, a contralateral streak gonad and persistent Müllerian structures (Davidoff & Federman 1973). Phenotypic sex is usually female (Wallace & Levin 1990) but there is always some degree of masculinization, and one-third of patients are phenotypic males. In most cases the genotype is 45,X/46,XY mosaic and stigmata of Turner's syndrome, such as congenital heart disease, may be present (Wallace & Levin 1990). In a recent series, one third of patients with mixed gonadal dysgenesis had gonadoblastoma; 60% had bilateral tumours (Wallace & Levin 1990). Other neoplasms have been reported in dysgenetic testes in mixed gonadal dysgenesis, including intratubular germ cell neoplasia (Müller et al 1985, Wallace & Levin 1990), sex cord–stromal tumour of undefined type (Wallace & Levin 1990); and juvenile granulosa cell tumour (Young et al 1985). Clear cell adenocarcinoma of the cervix and vagina has been recorded in patients with mixed gonadal dysgenesis (Resnik et al 1989), and there are a few reports of patients with endometrial adenocarcinoma (Wallace & Levin 1990), but these have been patients beyond the paediatric age group.

46,XY pure gonadal dysgenesis (Swyer syndrome) is characterized by persistent internal Müllerian structures, bilateral streak gonads and female phenotype (Olsen et al 1988, Wallace & Levin 1990). About 30% of affected people develop gonadoblastoma (Rutgers & Scully 1987).

Dysgenetic male pseudohermaphroditism is a condition in which bilateral cryptorchid testes are accompanied by persistent Müllerian structures and a 46,XY genotype (Mandell et al 1977). Again, gonadoblastoma develops in about one-third of patients. In view of the high risk of malignant germ cell neoplasms arising in childhood in mixed gonadal dysgenesis, pure gonadal dysgenesis and dysgenetic male pseudohermaphroditism, the recommended treatment is gonadectomy soon after the time of diagnosis.

In contrast to gonadoblastoma, other mixed germ cell/sex cord–stromal tumours tend to occur in normal gonads in genotypically normal people of both sexes (Talerman 1972, Bolen 1981). A mixed tumour that included epithelial elements in addition to germ cells and sex cord structures has been described in a neonatal girl (Tavassoli 1983). In contrast to gonadoblastoma, mixed tumours in prepubertal girls do not seem to be associated with malignant germ cell neoplasms, though these have been reported in girls and young women after puberty (Talerman 1987b). Mixed germ cell/sex cord–stromal tumours are usually clinically benign, but an obviously malignant tumour in this group has been described in childhood (Lacson et al 1988).

Male pseudohermaphroditism.   Male pseudohermaphroditism is rare but usually presents as a gynaecological problem. Patients have a 46,XY genotype and have testes, but due to androgen insensitivity, inherited as an X-linked trait, or due to deficiency of an enzyme involved in androgen synthesis (such as 17-α-hydroxylase deficiency), they fail to develop a male phenotype. The external genitalia are clearly female, there is breast development at puberty, Wolffian structures are poorly formed, and some vestigial Müllerian structures may be present. Fallopian tubes can be well developed (Rutgers & Scully 1987). The testes can be sited anywhere along the normal path of testicular descent.

The microscopic appearance of the testes is characteristic. There are immature seminiferous tubules with only a few germ cells but with abundant Leydig cells. There may be multiple hamartomatous nodules: these are more common in adults and consist of tightly packed seminiferous tubules containing Sertoli cells (Fig. 17.4A) and few germ cells; other elements such as Leydig cells, ovarian stroma and smooth muscle may be present (Rutgers & Scully 1987).

Of patients with male pseudohermaphroditism, 5–10% develop malignant germ cell tumours, almost always postpubertally. Seminoma is the commonest (Rutgers & Scully 1987). There may also be intratubular germ cell neoplasia (Müller & Skakkebaek 1984), (Figure 17.4B and C). Immunostains for placental alkaline phosphatase can be of great assistance in the diagnosis of this lesion; this marker can be demonstrated in normal fetal germ cells, but it is lost by 4 months of age in normal boys and in patients with testicular feminization, and so provides a specific marker in patients older than this (Armstrong et al 1991). In one series, two of 14 patients with male pseudohermaphroditism had evidence of intratubular germ cell neoplasia (Armstrong et al 1991).

Germ cell tumour of other sites in the female genital system

Endodermal sinus tumour of the vagina is the only neoplasm that occurs with any frequency in the female genital system other than the ovary. It characteristically involves a younger age group than its ovarian counterpart, and patients are often in the first decade of life (Brown & Langley 1976, Kohorn et al 1985). It is an aggressive neoplasm that metastasizes to lymph

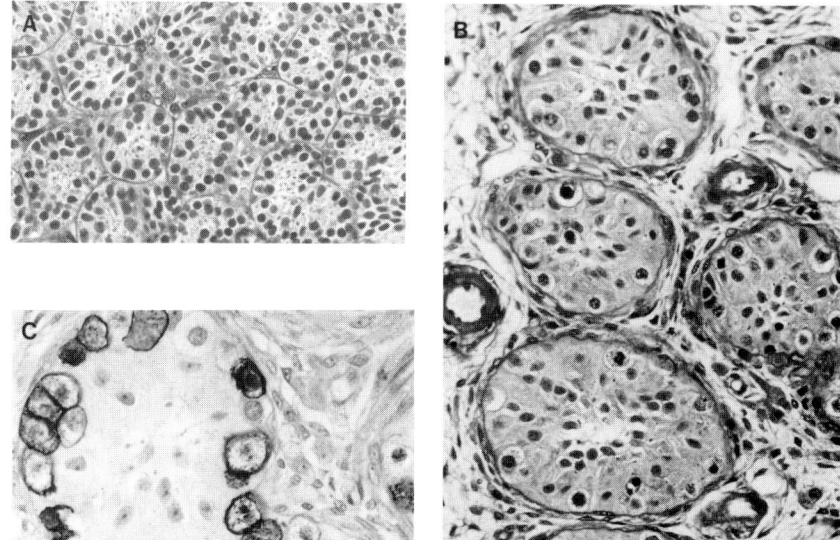

Fig. 17.4   Testis in male peudohermaphroditism. A 12-year-old phenotypic female with 17-α-hydroxylase deficiency.   **A** Tightly packed seminiferous tubules in hamartomatous nodule (H & E, × 250).   **B** Intratubular germ cell neoplasia. Characteristic large atypical germ cells within seminiferous tubules (H & E, × 250).   **C** Intratubular germ cell neoplasia. Abnormal germ cells staining positively with PLAP (× 400).

nodes, liver and lungs (Kohorn et al 1985), and has a mean survival of less than 1 year (Dehner 1987). Cases of this are rare and assessment of the impact of modern chemotherapy is therefore difficult.

Immunocytochemistry.   Table 17.4 gives a summary of the results of Niehans et al 1988; further details may be found in their account.

In germinoma, embryonal carcinoma and choriocarcinoma, the syncytio-trophoblastic giant cells and mononuclear cells with the features of

Table 17.4   Immunocytochemistry of malignant germ cell tumours using antibodies to a number of compounds[1] (from Niehans et al 1988)

Antigen	Germinoma	Embryonal carcinoma	Yolk sac tumour	Choriocarcinoma
PLAP	+	+	±	±
EMA	−	−	−	±
S100 protein	−	−	−	−
LCA	−	−	−	−
NSE	+	+	±	±
AFP	−	±	+	−
α_1AT	±	±	±	±
βhCG	+	+	−	+
Cytokeratin	−	+	+	+

[1]Abbreviations: placental alkaline phosphatase, PLAP; epithelial membrane antigen, EMA; leucocyte common antigen, LCA; neurone specific enolase, NSE; α-fetoprotein, AFP; α_1-antitrypsin, α_1AT; beta subunit of human chorionic gonadotrophin, βhCG.

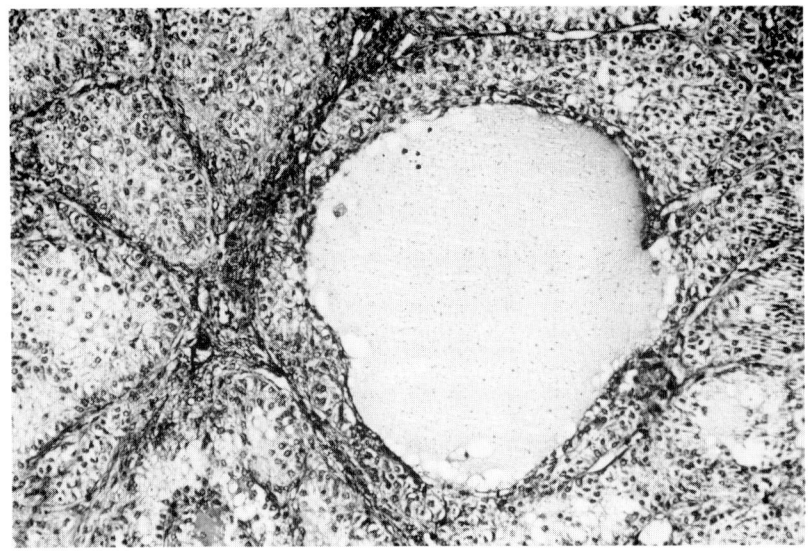

Fig. 17.5   Juvenile granulosa cell tumour. Example in a 2-year-old girl. Typical lobular pattern with follicular space and luteinized granulosa cells (H & E, × 100).

intermediate trophoblast are the source of hCG and immunostain positively for cytokeratins (Niehans et al 1988).

In yolk sac tumours, the tumour cell cytoplasm and intercellular spaces contain α-fetoprotein. The hyaline globules are often said to stain positively for this marker (Kurman & Norris 1976a) but not all workers have found this to be so (Ulbright et al 1987).

In both the ovary and vagina, clear cell carcinoma is the major differential diagnosis of yolk sac tumour. Immunostains for Leu-M1 antibody may be of some assistance (Zirker et al 1989). Most clear cell carcinomas express Leu-M1 but do not contain α-fetoprotein, and the converse applies to yolk sac tumour, but unfortunately there are exceptions.

NON-GERM CELL TUMOURS OF THE OVARY

Sex cord–stromal tumours of the ovary

Juvenile granulosa cell tumour

Fewer than 5% of granulosa cell tumours occur in premenarchal girls; about 90% of such patients have distinct clinicopathological and micro-scopical features. Typically, presentation is with isosexual precocious puberty (Lack et al 1981, Young et al 1984, Biscotti & Hart 1989). These tumours have been described in patients with multiple endochondromatosis syndromes (Ollier's and Maffucci's diseases) (Young et al 1984). Only

2–5% of ovarian sex cord–stromal tumours are bilateral, but congenital juvenile granulosa cell tumours involving both ovaries have been recorded in dysmorphic infants (Pysher et al 1981, Roth et al 1979).

Juvenile granulosa cell tumours can be solid or cystic. The microscopic appearance is characteristic and well described (Young et al 1984, Biscotti & Hart 1989) (Fig. 17.5). On immunocytochemistry, the tumour cells may be shown to express a variety of intermediate filaments, including cytokeratin, vimentin (Biscotti & Hart 1989) and desmin (Raafat et al 1990).

In one large series, survival was 92% at 5-year follow-up; extraovarian disease at diagnosis was the most significant factor in predicting adverse prognosis (Young et al 1984). Unlike adult type granulosa cell tumour, in which late recurrences occur (Young & Scully 1982), patients dying from juvenile granulosa cell tumour do so within 3 years of diagnosis (Young et al 1984).

Sertoli–Leydig cell tumours

About half of all Sertoli–Leydig cell tumours secrete hormones; patients show virilization, hirsuitism, menstrual irregularities and, occasionally, oestrogenic effects (Young & Scully 1982). Other patients present with non-specific features, such as an abdominal mass (Zaloudek & Norris 1984). In one large series, fewer than 2% were bilateral (Young & Scully 1985).

Well-differentiated neoplasms, which comprise 11% of the total, are

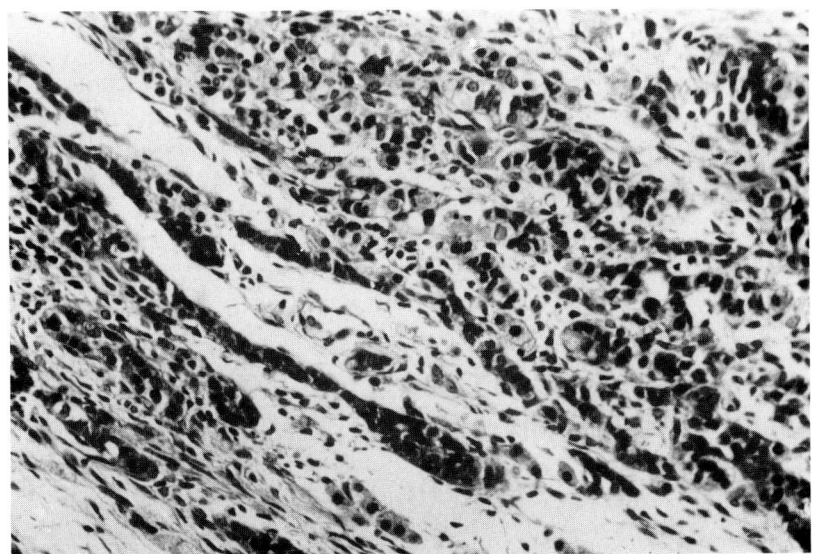

Fig. 17.6   Sertoli–Leydig cell tumour of intermediate differentiation (H & E, × 250).

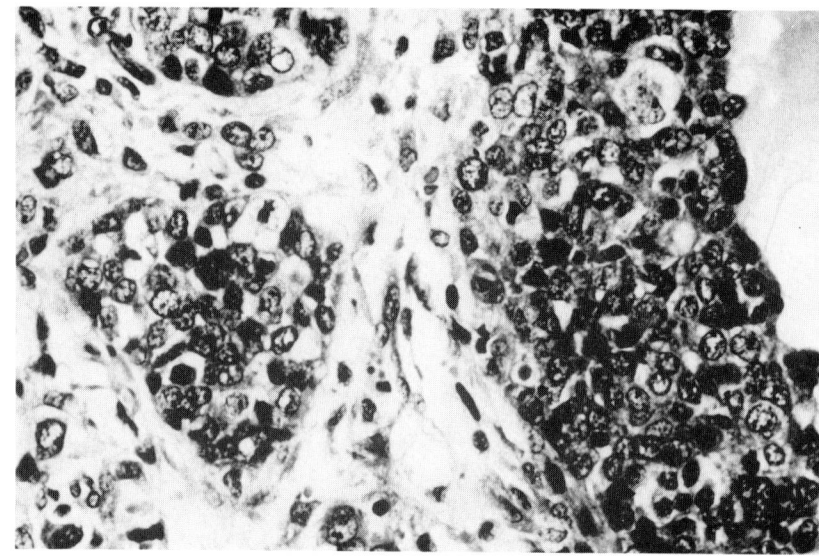

Fig. 17.7   Sertoli–Leydig cell tumour. Poorly differentiated area composed of solid cords of pleomorphic Sertoli cells and cysts lined by similar cells (H & E, × 400).

rarely seen in the paediatric years and generally found in patients aged 35 years or more. Tumours of intermediate differentiation, comprising 54% of cases, are composed of sheets, cords and aggregates of immature Sertoli cells with a stroma of mainly undifferentiated spindle cells in which there are scattered Leydig cells (Fig. 17.6). Poorly differentiated tumours, 13% of the total, are predominantly spindle cell neoplasms but rarely are pure Sertoli cell carcinomas composed of solid cords of cells showing a high degree of nuclear pleomorphism (Fig. 17.7) (Young & Scully 1982).

More than a fifth of Sertoli–Leydig cell tumours contain heterologous tissue; the most commonly encountered of these is mucinous epithelium of gastrointestinal type, usually associated with tumours of intermediate differentiation (Young et al 1982a). One in 20 cases of Sertoli–Leydig cell tumour contains immature skeletal muscle or cartilage: in these cases the associated tumour is almost always poorly differentiated (Prat et al 1982). Rarely tumours may have foci of neuroblastomatous differentiation (Prat et al 1982).

A prominent retiform component is seen in 10–15% of Sertoli–Leydig cell tumours (Young & Scully 1982, 1983, 1985) (Fig. 17.8). The mean age of patients with these tumours is 15 years, 10 years younger than the mean for Sertoli–Leydig cell tumours in general (Young & Scully 1983). The histological features of retiform androblastoma are open to misinterpretation, and may be misdiagnosed as yolk sac tumour or serous papillary tumour, particularly if it is the predominant feature in a tumour.

Important prognostic factors are stage and degree of differentiation.

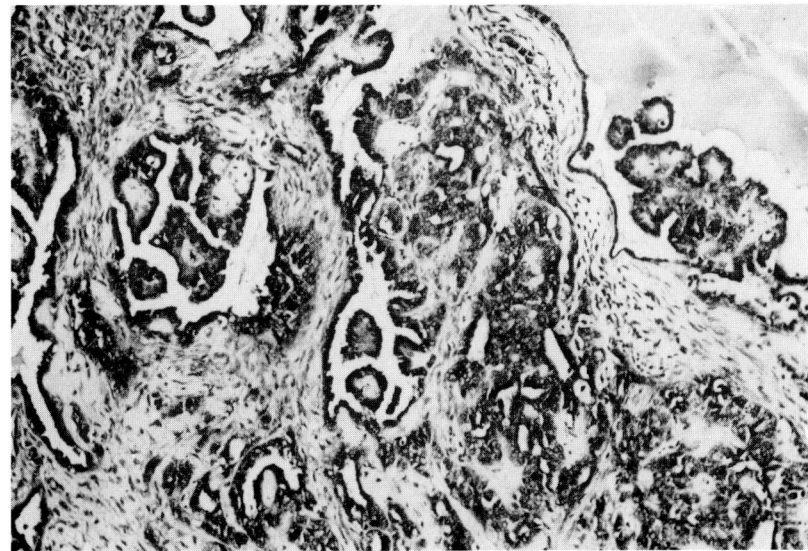

Fig. 17.8   Sertoli–Leydig cell tumour. Retiform area. Blunt papillae covered by low cuboidal epithelium (H & E, × 100).

Well-differentiated tumours are clinically benign, but in one study 11% of those showing intermediate differentiation and 59% of poorly differentiated

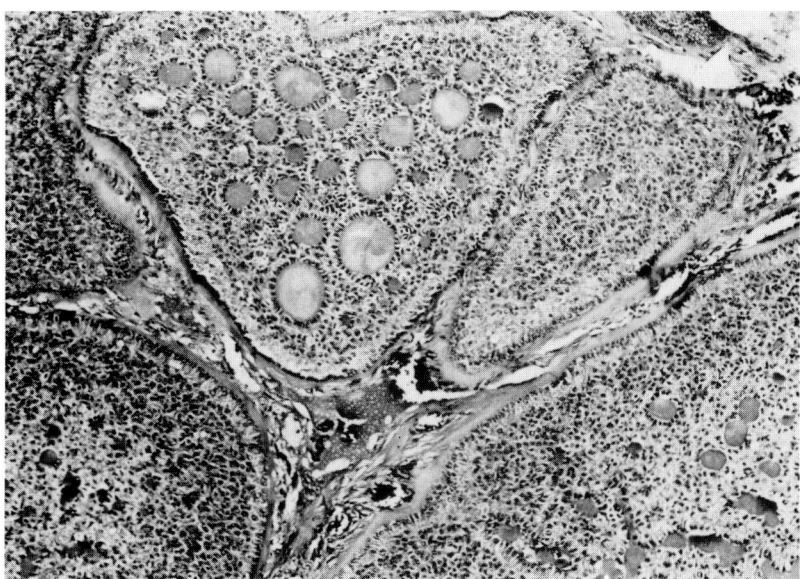

Fig. 17.9   Sex cord tumour with annular tubules. Typical appearance consisting of tubules encircling nodules of hyaline material. Example in a 12-year-old girl, not associated with Peutz–Jeghers syndrome (H & E, × 100).

tumours were clinically malignant (Young & Scully 1985). The small number (2.5%) of neoplasms in a stage higher than Stage I all behaved aggressively in the same study. Heterologous elements, in the form of immature skeletal muscle or cartilage are commonly associated with a poorly differentiated homologous component, and these tumours are usually malignant (Prat et al 1982, Young & Scully 1985). Overall, 12% of Sertoli-Leydig cell tumours behave in a malignant fashion, and about 20% of such tumours with prominent retiform areas do so; this reflects the degree of differentiation of the non-retiform component (Young & Scully 1983).

Ovarian sex cord tumour with annular tubules

This sex cord tumour has a distinctive microscopic appearance (Fig. 17.9) and as many as 40% can present with symptoms of oestrogen excess (Young & Scully 1982).

One-third of cases are associated with the rare autosomal dominant Peutz–Jeghers syndrome. It is possible that all girls and women with the syndrome have this lesion; the tumours are characteristically small (often microscopic), multifocal, bilateral, calcified and benign (Young et al 1982b). A separate, distinct type of sex cord–stromal tumour, otherwise un-classified, has been described in prepubertal girls with Peutz–Jeghers syndrome who presented with sexual precocity (Young et al 1983). All reported cases have been clinically benign.

The remaining two-thirds of patients with sex cord tumour with annular tubules do not have Peutz–Jeghers syndrome, and in these patients the tumours are large and unilateral, and up to 20% are clinically malignant (Young & Scully 1982). Cases have been reported in streak gonads associated with germinoma involving the same or the contralateral gonad (Young et al 1982b).

Tumours in the thecoma–fibroma group

Fewer than 10% of fibrothecomas occur in patients under 30 years of age (Young & Scully 1982). Steroid cell tumours, predominantly a neoplasm of the reproductive years, are occasionally seen in childhood (Scully 1979). Several distinct forms of stromal tumour are seen in this age group. Young women with the basal cell naevus (Gorlin's) syndrome may have bilateral, calcified multinodular fibromas (Young & Scully 1982), and these tumours may be the first stigmata of the syndrome. Similar tumours have been recorded rarely in children showing no other evidence of Gorlin's syndrome (Howell et al 1990). Some fibromas may show metaplastic bone formation (Bosch-Banyeras et al 1989). The sclerosing stromal tumour is a non-functioning neoplasm with a characteristic pseudolobular pattern on microscopic examination. It tends to occur in women in the third and fourth decades but has been recorded in patients under 15 years (Chalvardjian & Scully 1973).

Bilateral thecomas have been reported in children taking anticonvulsant therapy. Though usually benign (Faber 1962, Schweisguth et al 1971), in one example the tumours appeared to be clinically and pathologically malignant but responded well to surgery and chemotherapy (Dudzinski et al 1989).

Mesenchymal tumours of the female genital tract

Rhabdomyosarcoma

Rhabdomyosarcoma is the most common soft tissue sarcoma of childhood (Miller 1969). About one-third of these tumours affect the genitourinary tract and pelvis in children (Clatworthy et al 1973, Kilman et al 1973).

Historically, survival has been poor but has significantly improved with combined therapy using surgery, radiotherapy and chemotherapy (Pizzo & Triche 1987). Striking variability in outcome persists between the two major forms of childhood rhabdomyosarcoma—embryonal and alveolar.

Attempts to characterize the two major groups have focused on variables such as degree of differentiation (Schmidt et al 1986) and cytogenetic or chromosomal abnormalities (Turc-Carel et al 1986, Douglass et al 1987). It

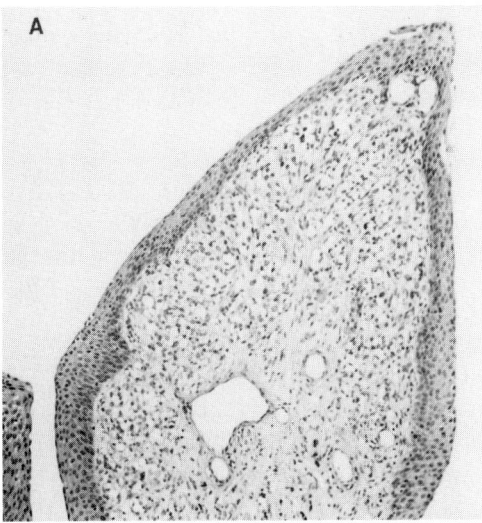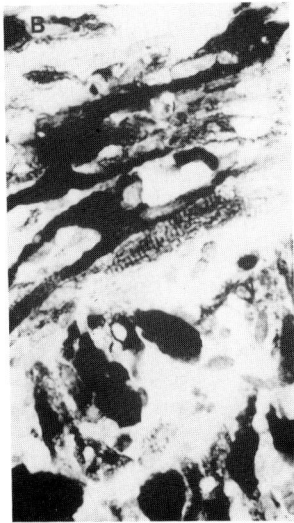

Fig. 17.10 Vaginal rhabdomyosarcoma. **A** Polypoid tumour with band of tumour cells beneath surface epithelium (H & E, × 100). **B** Tumour cells showing cross striations. Immunoperoxidase stain for desmin (× 400).

has been shown that some alveolar rhabdomyosarcomas have a translocation between chromosomes 2 and 13, t(2;13)(q37;q14), and embryonal rhabdomyosarcoma has a loss of heterozygosity on chromosome 11 (Scrable et al 1989).

Rhabdomyosarcoma in the female genital system occurs most commonly in the vagina (Hilgers et al 1970, Davos & Abell 1976). Grossly, most tumours arise in the anterior vaginal wall and may extend to the introitus and into the bladder. Histologically, there is a continuous condensed band of tumour cells below the surface epithelium (the 'cambium layer') with smaller, pleomorphic tumour cells, some of which have rhabdomyoblastic differentiation, embedded in a myxoid stroma (Fig. 17.10).

The results of the Intergroup Rhabdomyosarcoma Study were published in 1988 (Hays et al 1988). Children with primary vaginal rhabdomyosarcomas were, on average, less than 2 years old; histology was uniformly of embryonal type. In the vulva, tumours with both embryonal and alveolar patterns were seen, and these patients had a wider age range, from 1 to 19 years. Uterine sarcoma arose in patients in their teens and often, but not always, appeared as a single polyp. The number of patients studied was small (only 47 collected over 12 years) but overall survival, after a combination of surgery and chemotherapy, was over 80%; uterine tumours had a lower rate of survival than neoplasms of the vagina and vulva.

The entity called sarcoma botryoides of the uterine cervix by Daya and Scully in 1988 apears to be a different tumour from classical rhabdomyosarcoma. The patients are older with a mean of 18 years, foci of cartilage are often present within the tumour and the prognosis appears to be good (Daya & Scully 1988).

Primary rhabdomyosarcoma of the ovary is rare but cases have been described (Chan et al 1989, Akhtar et al 1989), including one case that simulated leukaemia in a 1-year-old girl (Nunez et al 1983).

Other soft tissue tumours

Occasional cases of neurofibroma of the clitoris have been described in children with neurofibromatosis (Schepel & Tolhurst 1981, Ravikumar & Lakshanan 1983, Rink & Mitchell 1983). Malignant schwannoma of the clitoris in an infant has recently been reported (Thomson 1989).

Aggressive angiomyxoma is a soft tissue tumour in which the bland histological appearance belies a tendency to form multiple local recurrences (Steeper & Rosai 1983). Cases have been reported in teenagers (Begin et al 1985). The constituent cells have ultrastructural features of myofibroblasts (Fletcher & McKee 1990) and immunostain for desmin, actin and vimentin (Manivel et al 1987).

Malignant mixed Müllerian tumours occur almost exclusively in postmenopausal women, but occasional examples have been described in children (Chumas et al 1983, Press & Scully 1985, Amr et al 1986).

Epithelial tumours

In the 36-year series from the Manchester Children's Tumour Registry there were no cases of malignant epithelial tumours at any site in the female genital system. Carcinomas did, however, account for 8% of malignant ovarian neoplasms in La Vecchia's series (La Vecchia 1983): all occurred in girls of between 10 and 15 years of age. Malignant ovarian epithelial tumours are almost unknown in prepubertal children, but there are occasional case reports (Akinola et al 1988, Blom et al 1982).

In the English-language world literature there are no undisputed examples of endometrial carcinoma occurring in girls under 15 years old. An extensive review of the period 1929–1976 identified five possible cases (Huffman et al 1981) but doubt has been cast on their veracity (Lee & Scully 1988). A recent study included 10 patients under 21 years of age with complex endometrial hyperplasia and well-differentiated adenocarcinoma, but none was aged less than 15 years (Lee & Scully 1989).

Non-diethylstilboestrol associated vaginal adenocarcinoma is primarily a disease of women in the late reproductive and perimenopausal years (Herbst et al 1970), but cases have been described in teenage patients and infants (Drogemueller et al 1970, Norris et al 1970, Kaminski & Maier 1983). In 1971, the association was reported between intrauterine exposure to diethylstilboestrol and subsequent development of adenocarcinoma of the vagina, cervix or both (Herbst et al 1971). This is an infrequent consequence of exposure to diethylstilboestrol, affecting only 0.14–1.40 per 1000 exposed daughters by the age of 24 years (Herbst 1981, Herbst & Barn 1981). These women often have developmental abnormalities of the vagina and cervix (Herbst & Barn 1981). Adenocarcinoma associated with diethylstilboestrol is predominantly a disease of patients in their late teens and twenties, but a few cases are recorded in childhood (Dehner 1987).

Spontaneous vaginal adenocarcinoma and diethylstilboestrol-associated tumours have common pathological features. Both may be seen in intimate proximity to vaginal adenosis, both are usually of clear celled type, consisting of cells with a characteristic 'hobnail' appearance and forming papillae, cysts and tubules.

Features indicative of a good prognosis are low stage, a predominantly tubulocystic pattern of growth and a low grade of nuclear atypia (Hanselaar et al 1991). Overall, between 80 and 90% of patients survive 5 years (Dehner 1987, Hanselaar et al 1991).

Cervical squamous intraepithelial neoplasia can occur in the mid teens (Sadeghi et al 1988), but there are only a few reports of teenagers with invasive squamous cell carcinoma of the cervix, vagina and vulva (Cario 1984, Dehner 1987). One vulval carcinoma in a girl under 15 years of age was associated with the presence of condylomata acuminata since infancy (Bender 1986); there is currently an epidemic of these lesions affecting children from infancy onwards (Bender 1986). In some cases the human papillomavirus types are the same as those associated with adult genital warts (types 6, 11, 16 and 18, the latter two of which may be associated with oncogenesis in adults) (Rock et al 1986, Hanson et al 1989).

OVARIAN SMALL CELL CARCINOMA

The histogenesis of this tumour is unknown and it will be considered as a separate entity. It was initially described in 1982 as a tumour frequently, though not invariably, associated with hypercalcaemia (Dickersin et al 1982). This rare neoplasm has an aggressive clinical course: in one series mortality was 88%, with most fatalities occurring in the first year; only 12% of patients were free of disease after 4 years follow-up (Young et al 1987). Extensive intra-abdominal spread is characteristic (Dickersin et al 1982). The mechanism causing the hypercalcaemia is unknown; serum levels of parathyroid hormone are not raised and surgical removal often results in restoration of normal serum concentrations of ionized calcium.

The histogenesis is a matter for speculation: origin from epithelial, neuroendocrine, germ cell and sex cord–stromal cells are obvious possibilities. In published reports, the patients range in age from 9 to 42 years, with a mean of 23 years (Dickersin et al 1982, Young et al 1987, Malfetano et al 1990). This goes against a histogenetic relation with either a common epithelial neoplasm or a small cell neuroendocrine tumour, such as pulmonary oat cell carcinoma, both of which tend to occur in older patients.

Microscopically, ovarian small cell carcinoma is a distinct entity that has little resemblance to small cell carcinoma of the lung. It consists of diffuse masses, small nests and cords of cells in a densely collagenous or myxoid stroma. Solid areas may contain follicle-like spaces lined by tumour cells (Fig. 17.11A). The constituent cell population is characteristically dimorphic (Fig. 17.11B) with a varying proportion of larger cells; in some examples cells of large or intermediate size may predominate leading to problems in differential diagnosis. Cells with abundant eosinophilic cytoplasm, intracellular mucin, clusters of periodic acid–Schiff-positive, diastase-resistant globules (Fig. 17.11C) and intercellular hyaline material may all be seen (Ulbright et al 1987, Aguirre et al 1989). The most remarkable ultrastructural finding is the presence of intracytoplasmic vesicles filled with granular material. These represent dilated segments of rough endoplasmic reticulum. Desmosome-like junctions and basal laminae are also present (Dickersin et al 1982, Ulbright et al 1987, McMahon & Hart 1988). Partly on the basis of age range and partly because of light microscopic and ultrastructural similarities to yolk sac tumour, a germ cell origin has been suggested (Ulbright et al 1987). Other than one tentative report of a testicular tumour with similar features (Ulbright et al 1987), there have been no reports of gonadal small cell carcinoma in extraovarian sites.

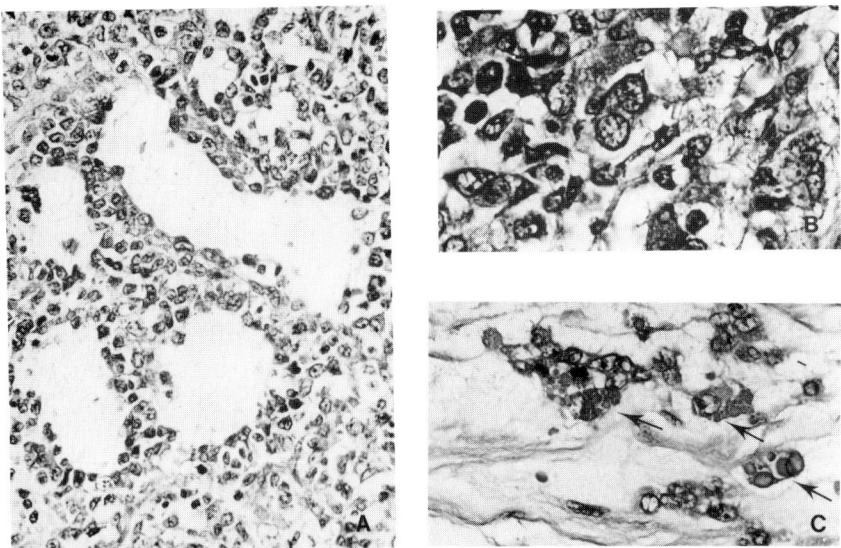

Fig. 17.11 Ovarian small cell carcinoma. Case provided by Dr R. Williams. **A** Typical pattern with follicle-like spaces. (H & E, × 250). **B** Dimorphic cell composition (H & E, × 400). **C** Intracellular hyaline eosinophillic globules (H & E, × 400).

Immunocytochemistry has so far not provided strong support for any histogenetic hypothesis. Vimentin, cytokeratin, EMA and α_1-antitrypsin have all been demonstrated in tumour cells, but none of these is sufficiently specific to be diagnostic (Aguirre et al 1989, Ulbright 1990). Neurone-specific enolase and chromogranin A have been reported in tumour cells in the same study, but the significance of this finding must be considered in the light of electron microscopy: other than in one study (Abeler et al 1988), neurosecretory granules have not been demonstrated (Ulbright 1990).

MISCELLANEOUS NEOPLASMS AND TUMOUR-LIKE LESIONS OF THE FEMALE GENITAL SYSTEM

Ovarian enlargement is very rare in infancy; a high proportion of cases are due to non-neoplastic cysts. About 36% of surgically treated ovarian lesions in children and adolescents are 'functional' cysts. Approximately half of these are follicular in origin, with corpus luteal cysts and paraovarian cysts accounting for the rest (Breen & Maxson 1977).

Although ovarian infiltration is found in 35–50% of post mortem examinations of girls who died of acute lymphoblastic leukaemia, clinically apparent ovarian disease is rare (Heaton & Duff 1989, Pais et al 1991). It can involve both ovaries (Pais et al 1991) and is most often seen as a disease that relapses some years after initial diagnosis. Treatment is with systemic chemotherapy rather than surgery; some patients have gone into remission

(Pais et al 1991). Girls with Burkitt's lymphoma often have ovarian involvement but this is rarely the presenting feature (Chorlton 1987). Primary lymphoma of the extraovarian female genital system presenting in children is rare but has been recorded (Egwuata 1989).

Müllerian papilloma is a benign neoplasm occurring exclusively in children. It involves the cervix or, more rarely, the vagina. The patients are usually 2–5 years old and present with vaginal bleeding. The tumour is a small polypoid or papillary lesion involving a cervical lip or the endocervical canal. Microscopically, it consists of oedematous fibrovascular papillae in which there may be metaplastic bone (Ulbright et al 1981), covered by a single layer of epithelium that varies from flat to columnar. Some cases may recur locally (Clement 1990).

An extrarenal Wilms' tumour occurring in the endocervix has been recorded in a teenage girl (Bell et al 1985); at this site the tumour could be of germ cell or mesonephric origin. Vaginal polyps occasionally occur in infants. They may attain a large size and clinically can be misdiagnosed as rhabdomyosarcoma (Dehner 1987).

The vulva may be the site of several diseases which present in children and which are not specific to this region, including haemangioma (Levin & Selbst 1988), granular cell tumour (Brooks 1985), and Langherhans' cell histiocytosis (Otis et al 1990).

CONCLUSION

Gynaecological tumours are rare in children, and few of those that do occur are restricted to this age group. Their behaviour appears to be similar in children and adults. The United Kingdom Children's Cancer Study Group has been conducting a study of germ cell tumours for some years, and it is hoped that this will shed more light on prognosis and response to treatment in this age group. Because of their rarity, investigation of these tumours at molecular level is in its infancy. We can expect that the next decade will bring great insights into this group of uncommon but fascinating neoplasms.

REFERENCES

Abell M R, Holtz F 1965 Ovarian neoplasms in childhood and adolescence. American Journal of Obstetrics and Gynecology 93: 850–866
Abeler V, Kjorstad K E, Nesland J M 1988 Small cell carcinoma of the ovary: a report of six cases. International Journal of Gynecological Pathology 7: 315–329
Aguirre P, Scully R E 1982 Malignant neuroectodermal tumor of the ovary. A distinctive form of monodermal teratoma. Report of five cases. American Journal of Surgical Pathology 6: 283–292
Aguirre P, Thor A D, Scully R E 1989 Ovarian small cell carcinoma. Histogenetic considerations based on immunohistochemical and other findings. American Journal of Clinical Pathology 92: 140–149
Akhtar M, Bakri Y, Rank F 1989 Dysgerminoma of the ovary with rhabdomyosarcoma. Cancer 64: 2309–2312

Akinola O, Okonofua F E, Odesanmi W O, Oshinaike A I 1988 Serous papillary
adenocarcinoma of the ovary in a Nigerian child. Tropical and Geographical Medicine 40:
251–253

Amr S S, Tavassoli F A, Hassan A A, Issa A A, Madanat F F 1986 Mixed mesodermal tumor
of the uterus in a 4 year old girl. International Journal of Gynecological Pathology 5:
371–378

Armstrong G R, Buckley C H, Kelsey A M 1991 Germ cell expression of placental alkaline
phosphatase in male pseudohermaphroditism. Histopathology 18: 541–547

Atkin N B, Baker M C 1985 i(12p): Specific chromosomal marker in seminoma and malignant
teratoma of the testis. Cancer Genetics and Cytogenetics 10: 199–204

Begin L R, Clement P B, Kirk M E, Jothy S, McMaughey W T, Ferenczy A 1985 Aggressive
angiomyxoma of pelvic soft parts: a clinicopathologic study of nine cases. Human
Pathology 16: 621–628

Bell D A, Shimm D S, Gang D L 1985 Wilms' tumor of the endocervix. Archives of
Pathology and Laboratory Medicine 109: 371–373

Bender M E 1986 New concepts of condyloma acuminata in children. Archives of
Dermatology 122: 1121–1124

Birch J M 1988 Manchester Children's Tumour Registry 1954–1970 and 1971–1983. In:
Parkin D M, Stiller C A, Draper G J, Bieber C A, Terracini B, Young J L (eds)
International incidence of childhood cancer. International Agency for Research on Cancer
Publications No 87, Lyon, p 299–304

Birch J M 1990 Epidemiology of childhood cancer. Annales Nestlé 3 (Childhood oncology).
Nestec Ltd, Vevey, Switzerland, p 105–116

Birch J M, Marsden H B, Swindell R 1982 Pre-natal factors in the origin of germ cell
tumours of children. Carcinogenesis 3: 75–80

Biscotti C V, Hart W R 1989 Juvenile granulosa cell tumors of the ovary. Archives of
Pathology and Laboratory Medicine 113: 40–46

Björkholm E, Lundell M, Gyftodimos A, Silfverswärd C 1990 Dysgerminoma. The
Radiumhemmet series 1927–1984. Cancer 65: 38–44

Blom G P, Torkildsen E M 1982 Ovarian cystadenocarcinoma in a 4-year-old girl: Report of
a case and review of the literature. Gynecologic Oncology 13: 242–246

Bolen J W 1981 Mixed germ cell–cord-stromal tumor. A gonadal tumor distinct from
gonadoblastoma. American Journal of Clinical Pathology 75: 565–573

Bosch-Banyeras J M, Lucaya X, Bernet M et al 1989 Calcified ovarian fibromas in
prepubertal girls. European Journal of Pediatrics 148: 749–750

Breen J L, Maxson W S 1977 Ovarian tumors in children and adolescents. Clinical Obstetrics
and Gynecology 20: 607–623

Brooks G G 1985 Granular cell myoblastoma of the vulva in a 6-year-old girl. American
Journal of Obstetrics and Gynecology 153: 897–898

Brown N J, Langley F A 1976 Teratomas and other genital tumours. In: Marsden H B,
Steward J K (eds) Tumours in children. Springer-Verlag, Berlin, p 362–402

Cario G M, House M J, Paradinas F J 1984 Squamous cell carcinoma of the vulva in
association with mixed vulval dystrophy in an 18-year-old girl. British Journal of
Obstetrics and Gynaecology 91: 87–90

Carritt B, Parrington J M, Welch H M, Povey S 1982 Diverse origins of multiple ovarian
teratomas in a single individual. Proceedings of the National Academy of Science USA 79:
7400–7404

Carter D, Bibro M C, Touloukian R J 1982 Benign clinical behaviour of immature
mediastinal teratoma in infancy and childhood: report of two cases and review of the
literature. Cancer 49: 398–402

Chalvardjian A, Scully R E 1973 Sclerosing stromal tumors of the ovary. Cancer 31: 664–670

Chan Y F, Leung C S, Ma L 1989 Primary embryonal rhabdomyosarcoma of the ovary in a
4-year-old girl. Histopathology 15: 211–324

Chorlton I 1987 Malignant lymphoma of the female genital tract and ovaries. In: Fox H (ed)
Haines and Taylor obstetrical and gynaecological pathology. Churchill Livingstone,
Edinburgh, p 737–762

Chumas J C, Mann W J, Tseng L 1983 Malignant mixed Müllerian tumor of the
endometrium in a young women with polycystic ovaries. Cancer 52: 1478–1481

Clatworthy H W, Braden M, Smith J P 1973 Surgery of bladder and prostatic neoplasms in
children. Cancer 32: 1157–1160

Clement R B 1990 Miscellaneous primary and metastatic tumors of the uterine cervix. Seminars in Diagnostic Pathology 7: 228–247

Dahl N, Gustavsson K-H, Rune C, Gustavsson I, Pettersson U 1990 Benign ovarian teratomas. An analysis of their cellular origin. Cancer Genetics and Cytogenetics 46: 115–123

Davidoff F, Federman D D 1973 Mixed gonadal dysgenesis. Pediatrics 52: 725–742

Davos I, Abell M R 1976 Sarcomas of the vagina. Obstetrics and Gynecology 47: 432–450

Daya D A, Scully R E 1988 Sarcoma botryoides of the uterine cervix in young women: a clinicopathological study of 13 cases. Gynecologic Oncology 29: 290–304

Dehner L P 1983 Gonadal and extragonadal germ cell neoplasia of childhood. Human Pathology 14: 493–511

Dehner L P 1987 Female Reproductive System. In: Dehner L P (ed) Pediatric surgical pathology. Williams & Wilkins, Baltimore, p 743–791

Dickersin G R, Kline I W, Scully R E 1982 Small cell carcinoma of the ovary with hypercalcaemia: a report of 11 cases. Cancer 49: 188–197

Douglass E C, Valentine M, Etcubanas E et al 1987 A specific abnormality in rhabdomyosarcoma. Cytogenetics and Cell Genetics 45: 148–155

Drogemueller W, Makowski E L, Taylor E S 1970 Vaginal mesonephric adenocarcinoma in two prepubertal children. American Journal of Diseases of Children 119: 168–170

Dudzinski M, Cohen M, Ducatman B 1989 Ovarian malignant luteinized thecoma—an unusual tumor in an adolescent. Gynecologic Oncology 35: 104–109

Egwuatu V E 1989 Non-Hodgkin's lymphoma of the uterus in a child. Journal of Pediatric Surgery 24: 220–222

Faber H K 1962 Meigs' syndrome with thecomas of both ovaries in a 4 year old girl. Journal of Pediatrics 61: 769–773

Flam F, Lundstrom V, Silfversward C 1989 Choriocarcinoma in mother and child. Case report. British Journal of Obstetrics and Gynaecology 96: 241–244

Fletcher C D M, McKeen P H 1990 Progress in benign soft tissue tumours. In: Fletcher C D M, McKee P H (eds) Pathobiology of soft tissue tumours. Churchill Livingstone, Edinburgh, p 239–264

Gershenson D M, Del Junco G, Herson J, Rutedge F N 1983 Endodermal sinus tumor of the ovary. The M D Anderson experience. Obstetrics and Gynecology 61: 194–202

Greenberg F, Keenan B, DeYanis V, Finegold M 1986 Gonadal dysgenesis and gonadoblastoma in situ in a female with Fraser (cryptophthalmos) syndrome. Journal of Pediatrics 108: 952–954

Hanselaar A G J M, Van Leusen N D M, De Wilde P C M, Vooijs G P 1991 Clear cell adenocarcinoma of the vagina and cervix. A report of the central Netherlands with emphasis on early detection and prognosis. Cancer 67: 1971–1978

Hanson R M, Glasson M, McCrossin I, Rogers M 1989 Anogenital warts in childhood. Child Abuse and Neglect 13: 225–233

Hartley A L, Birch J M, Kelsey A M, Marsden H B, Harris M, Teare M D 1989 Are germ cell tumors part of the Li–Fraumeni Cancer Family syndrome? Cancer Genetics and Cytogenetics 42: 221–226

Hays D M, Shimada H, Raney R B et al 1988 Clinical staging and treatment results in rhabdomyosarcoma of the female genital tract among children and adolescents. Cancer 61: 1893–1903

Heaton D C, Duff G B 1989 Ovarian relapse in a young woman with acute lymphoblastic leukaemia. American Journal of Hematology 30: 42–43

Herbst A L 1981 Clear cell adenocarcinoma and current status of DES exposed females. Cancer 48: 484–488

Herbst A L, Barn H A (eds) 1981 Developmental effects of diethylstilbestrol (DES) in pregnancy. Thieme Stratton, New York

Herbst A L, Green T H, Ulfelder H 1970 Primary carcinoma of the vagina: an analysis of 68 cases. American Journal of Obstetrics and Gynecology 106: 210–218

Herbst A L, Ulfelder H, Poskanzer D C 1971 Adenocarcinoma of the vagina. Association of maternal stilbestrol therapy with tumor appearance in young women. New England Journal of Medicine 284: 878–881

Hilgers R D, Malkasian G D, Soule E H 1970 Embryonal rhabdomyosarcoma (botryoid type) of the vagina. A clinicopathological review. American Journal of Obstetrics and Gynecology 107: 484–502

Howell C G, Rogers D A, Gable D S, Falls G D 1990 Bilateral ovarian fibromas in children. Journal of Pediatric Surgery 25: 690–691

Huffman J W, Dewhurst J C, Copraro V J 1981 The gynecology of childhood and adolescence, 2nd ed. W B Saunders, Philadelphia, p 270–272

Ihara T, Ohama K, Satoh H, Fujii T, Nomura K, Fujiwara A 1984 Histologic grade and karyotype of immature teratoma of the ovary. Cancer 54: 2988–2994

Jenkyn D J, McCartney A J 1987 A chromosome study of three ovarian tumours. Cancer Genetics and Cytogenetics 26: 327–337

Kaminski P F, Maier R C 1983 Clear cell adenocarcinoma of the cervix unrelated to diethylstilbestrol exposure. Obstetrics and Gynecology 62: 720–727

Kilman J W, Clatworthy H W, Newton W A, Grosfield J L 1973 Reasonable surgery for rhabdomyosarcoma. Annals of Surgery 178: 346–351

Kohorn E I, McIntosh S, Lytton B, Knowlton A H, Merino M 1985 Endodermal sinus tumor of the infant vagina. Gynecologic Oncology 20: 196–203

Kommoss F, Bibbo M, Talerman A 1990 Nuclear deoxyribonucleic acid content (ploidy) of endodermal sinus (yolk sac) tumor. Laboratory Investigation 62: 223–231

Kurman R J, Norris H J 1976a Endodermal sinus tumor of the ovary. A clinical and pathological analysis of 71 cases. Cancer 38: 2404–2419

Kurman R J, Norris H J 1976b Embryonal carcinoma of the ovary. A clinicopathologic entity distinct from endodermal sinus tumor resembling embryonal carcinoma of the adult testis. Cancer 38: 2420–2433

Kurman R J, Norris H J 1977 Malignant germ cell tumors of the ovary. Human Pathology 8: 551–562

Lack E E, Perez-Atayde A R, Murthy A S K, Goldstein D P, Crigler J F, Vawter G F 1981 Granulosa theca cell tumors in premenarchal girls: a clinical and pathological study of 10 cases. Cancer 48: 1846–1854

Lacson A G, Gillis D A, Shawwa A 1988 Malignant mixed germ cell–sex cord–stromal tumors of the ovary associated with isosexual precocious puberty. Cancer 61: 2122–2133

La Vecchia C, Morris H B, Draper G J 1983 Malignant ovarian tumours in childhood in Britain, 1962–78. British Journal of Cancer 48: 363–374

Lee K R, Scully R E 1989 Complex endometrial hyperplasia and carcinoma in adolescents and young women 15 to 20 years of age. International Journal of Gynecological Pathology 8: 201–213

Levin A V, Selbst S M 1988 Vulvar hemangioma simulating child abuse. Clinical Pediatrics 27: 213–215

McMahon J T, Hart W R 1988 Ultrastructural analysis of small cell carcinomas of the ovary. American Journal of Clinical Pathology 90: 523–529

Malfetano J H, Degnan E, Florentin R 1990 Para-endocrine hypercalaemia and ovarian small cell carcinoma. New York State Journal of Medicine 90: 206–207

Malogolowkin M H, Mahour G H, Krailo M, Ortega J A 1990 Germ cell tumours in infancy and childhood: a 45 year experience. In: Jaffe R, Dahms B B, Krous H F, Lieberman E, Triche T J (eds) Forefront of pediatric pathology. Hemishere Publishing Corporation, New York

Mandell J, Stevens P S, Fried F A 1977 Childhood gonadoblastoma and seminoma in a dysgenetic cryptorchid gonad. Journal of Urology 117: 674–675

Manivel C, Steeper T, Swanson P, Wick M 1987 Aggressive angiomyxoma of the pelvis: an immunoperoxidase study. Laboratory Investigation 56: 46A

Marsden H B, Birch J M, Swindell R 1981 Germ cell tumours of childhood: a review of 137 cases. Journal of Clinical Pathology 34: 879–883

Miller R W 1969 Fifty-two forms of childhood cancer: United States mortality experience 1960–1966. Journal of Pediatrics 75: 685–689

Müller J, Skakkebeak N E 1984 Testicular carcinoma in situ in children with the androgen insensitivity (testicular feminisation) syndrome. British Medical Journal 288: 1419–1420

Müller J, Skakkebaek N E, Ritzen M, Plöen L, Petersen K E 1985 Carcinoma in situ of the testis in children with 45X/46XY gonadal dysgenesis. Journal of Pediatrics 106: 431–436

Niehans G A, Manivel J C, Copland G T, Scheithauer B W, Wick M R 1988 Immunocytochemistry of germ cell and trophoblastic neoplasms. Cancer 62: 1113–1123

Nogales F F 1987 Germ cell tumours of the ovary. In: Fox H (ed) Haines and Taylor, obstetrical and gynecological pathology, 3rd edn. Churchill Livingstone, Edinburgh, p 623

Nogales F F, Favara B E, Major F J, Silverberg S G 1976 Immature teratoma of the ovary with a neural component ("solid" teratoma). A clinicopathologic study of 20 cases. Human Pathology 7: 625–642

Norris H J, Bagley G P, Taylor H B 1970 Carcinoma of the infant vagina: a distinctive tumor. Archives of Pathology 90: 473–479

Norris H J, Zirkin H J, Benson W L 1976 Immature (malignant) teratoma of the ovary. A clinical and pathological study of 58 cases. Cancer 37: 2359–2372

Nunez C, Abboud S L, Lemon N C, Kemp J A 1983 Ovarian rhabdomyosarcoma presenting as leukemia. Cancer 52: 297–300

Olsen M M, Caldamone A A, Jackson C L, Zinn A 1988 Gonadoblastoma in infancy: Indications for early gonadectomy in 46XY gonadal dysgenesis. Journal of Pediatric Surgery 23: 270–271

Oosterhuis J W, Castedo S M M J, DeJong B et al 1989 Ploidy of primary germ cell tumours of the testis. Pathogenetic and clinical relevance. Laboratory Investigation 60: 14–21

Otis C N, Fischer R A, Johnson N, Kelleher J F, Powell J L 1990 Histiocytosis X of the vulva: a case report and review of the literature. Obstetrics and Gynecology 75: 555–558

Oud P S, Soeters R S, Pahlplatz M M M et al 1988 DNA cytometry of pure dysgerminomas of the ovary. International Journal of Gynecological Pathology 7: 258–267

Pais R C, Kim T H, Zwiren G T, Ragab A H 1991 Ovarian tumors in relapsing acute lymphoblastic leukemia: a review of 23 cases. Journal of Pediatric Surgery 26: 70–74

Parkin D M, Stiller C A, Draper G J, Bieber C A, Terracini B, Young J L 1988 International Incidence of Childhood Cancer. International Agency for Research on Cancer Publications No 87, Lyon, p 1–2

Parrington J M, West L F, Povey S 1984 The origin of ovarian teratomas. Journal of Medical Genetics 21: 4–12

Piver M S, Patton T 1986 Ovarian cancer in children. Seminars in Surgical Oncology 2: 163–169

Pizzo P A, Triche T J 1987 Clinical staging in rhabdomyosarcoma. Current limitations and future prospects. Journal of Clinical Oncology 5: 8–9

Prat J, Young R H, Scully R E 1982 Sertoli–Leydig cell tumors with heterologous elements. Cartilage and skeletal muscle. A clinicopathologic analysis of 12 cases. Cancer 50: 2465–2475

Press M F, Scully R E 1985 Endometrial sarcoma complicating ovarian thecoma, polycystic ovarian disease and oestrogen therapy. Gynecological Oncology 21: 135–154

Pysher T J, Hitch D C, Krous H F 1981 Bilateral granulosa cell tumors in a 4 month old dysmorphic infant. American Journal of Surgical Pathology 5: 789–794

Raafat F, Klys H, Rylance G 1990 Juvenile granulosa cell tumor. Pediatric Pathology 10: 617–623

Ravikumar V R, Lakshanan D A 1983 Solitary neurofibroma of the clitoris masquerading as intersex. Journal of Pediatric Surgery 18: 617

Resnik E, Christopherson W A, Stock R 1989 Clear cell adenocarcinoma of the cervix and vagina in a woman with mixed gonadal dysgenesis. A case report. Journal of Reproductive Medicine 34: 981–984

Rink R C, Mitchell M E 1983 Genitourinary neurofibromatosis in childhood. Journal of Urology 130: 1176–1179

Robboy S J, Scully R E 1970 Ovarian teratoma with glial implants on the peritoneum. An analysis of 12 cases. Human Pathology 1: 643–653

Rock B, Naghashfar Z, Barnett N, Buscema J, Woodruff J D, Shah K 1986 Genital tract papillomavirus infection in children. Archives of Dermatology 122: 1129–1132

Roth L M, Nicholas T R, Ehrlich C E 1979 Juvenile granulosa cell tumor. A clinicopathological study of three cases with ultrastructural observations. Cancer 44: 2194–2205

Rutgers J L, Scully R E 1987 Pathology of the testis in intersex syndromes. Seminars in Diagnostic Pathology 4: 275–291

Sadeghi S B, Sadeghi A, Cosby M, Olincy A, Robboy S J 1988 Human papillomavirus infection. Frequency and association with cervical neoplasia in a young population. Acta Cytologica 33: 319–323

Schepel S J, Tolhurst D E 1981 Neurofibromata of clitoris and labium majus simulating a penis and testicle. British Journal of Plastic Surgery 34: 221–223

Schmidt D, Reimann O, Treuner J, Harms D 1986 Cellular differentiation and prognosis in embryonal rhabdomyosarcoma. Virchow's Archiv 409: 183–194

Schweisguth O, Gerard-Marchant R, Plainfosse B, Lemerle J, Watchi J M, Seringe P 1971 Bilateral non-functioning thecoma of the ovary in epileptic children under anticonvulsant therapy. Acta Paediatrica Scandinavica 60: 6–10

Scrable H, Witte D, Shimada H et al 1989 Molecular differential pathology of rhabdomyosarcoma. Genes, Chromosomes and Cancer 1: 23–35

Scully R E 1970 Gonadoblastoma. A review of 74 cases. Cancer 25: 1340–1356

Scully R E 1979 Tumors of the ovary and maldeveloped gonads. Atlas of Tumor Pathology Fascicle 16, Armed Forces Institute of Pathology, Washington DC

Senturia Y D 1987 The epidemiology of testicular cancer. British Journal of Urology 60: 285–291

Sinisis A A, Perrone L, Quarto C, Barone M, Bellastella A, Faggiano M 1988 Dysgerminoma in 45X Turner syndrome: report of a case. Clinical Endocrinology 28: 187–193

Steeper T A, Rosai J 1983 Aggressive angiomyxoma of the female pelvis and perineum. Report of nine cases of a distinctive type of gynecologic soft-tissue neoplasm. American Journal of Surgical Pathology 7: 463–475

Talerman A A 1972 A mixed germ cell–sex cord tumor of the ovary in a normal female infant. Obstetrics and Gynecology 40: 473–478

Talerman A A 1987a Germ cell tumours of the ovary. In: Kurman R J (ed) Blaustein's pathology of the female genital tract, 3rd edn. Springer-Verlag, New York, p 669–679

Talerman A 1987b Mixed germ cell sex cord-stromal tumours of the ovary. In: Fox H (ed) Haines and Taylor obstetrical and gynaecological pathology. Churchill Livingstone, Edinburgh, p 676–696

Tavassoli F A 1983 A combined germ cell–gonadal stromal–epithelial tumor of the ovary. American Journal of Surgical Pathology 7: 73–84

Taylor M H, DePetrillo A D, Turner A R 1985 Vinblastine, bleomycin and cisplatin in malignant germ cell tumours of the ovary. Cancer 56: 1341–1349

Thomas W J, Bevan H E, Hooper D G, Downey E J 1989 Malignant schwannoma of the clitoris in a 1-year-old child. Cancer 63: 2216–2219

Thurlbeck W M, Scully R E 1960 Solid teratoma of the ovary. A clinicopathological analysis of 9 cases. Cancer 13: 804–811

Turc-Carel C, Lizard-Nacol S, Justrabo E, Favrot M, Philip T, Tabone E 1986 Consistent chromosomal translocation in alveolar rhabdomyosarcoma. Cancer Genetics and Cytogenetics 19: 362–336

Truong L D, Jurco S, McGavran M H 1982 Gliomatosis peritonei. Report of two cases and review of the literature. American Journal of Surgical Pathology 6: 443–449

Ulbright T M 1990 Ovarian small cell carcinoma. New York State Journal of Medicine 90: 171–172

Ulbright T M, Alexander R W, Kraus F T 1981 Intramural papilloma of the vagina. Evidence of Müllerian histogenesis. Cancer 48: 2260–2266

Ulbright T M, Roth L M, Stehman F B, Talerman A, Senekjian E K 1987 Poorly differentiated (small cell) carcinoma of the ovary in young women: evidence supporting a germ cell origin. Human Pathology 18: 175–184

Vos A, Oosterhuis J W, DeJong B et al 1990 Karyotyping and DNA flow cytometry of metastatic ovarian yolk sac tumour. Cancer Genetics and Cytogenetics 44: 223–228

Walker A H, Ross R K, Pike M C, Henderson B E 1984 A possible rising incidence of malignant germ cell tumours in young women. British Journal of Cancer 49: 669–672

Walker A H, Ross R K, Haile R W C, Henderson B E 1988 Hormonal factors and risk of ovarian germ cell cancer in young women. British Journal of Cancer 57: 418–422

Wallace T M, Levin H S 1990 Mixed gonadal dysgenesis. A review of 15 patients reporting single cases of malignant intratubular germ cell neoplasia of the testis, endometrial adenocarcinoma and a complex vascular anomaly. Archives of Pathology and Laboratory Medicine 114: 679–688

Young R H, Scully R E 1982 Ovarian sex cord–stromal tumors: Recent progress. International Journal of Gynecological Pathology 1: 101–123

Young R H, Scully R E 1983 Sertoli–Leydig tumors with a retiform pattern. A problem in histopathologic diagnosis. American Journal of Surgical Pathology 7: 755–771

Young R H, Scully R E 1985 Ovarian Sertoli–Leydig cell tumors. A clinicopathological study of 207 cases. American Journal of Surgical Pathology 9: 543–569

Young R H, Prat J, Scully R E 1982a Ovarian Sertoli–Leydig cell tumors with heterologous elements. I. Gastrointestinal epithelium and carcinoid. A clinicopathologic analysis of 36 cases. Cancer 50: 2448–2456

Young R H, Welch W R, Dickersin G R, Scully R E 1982b Ovarian sex cord tumor with annular tubules. Review of 74 cases including 27 with Peutz–Jeghers syndrome and four with adenoma malignum of the cervix. Cancer 50: 1384–1402

Young R H, Dickersin G R, Scully R E 1983 A distinctive ovarian sex cord–stromal tumor causing sexual precocity in the Peutz–Jeghers syndrome. American Journal of Surgical Pathology 7: 233–243

Young R H, Dickersin G R, Scully R E 1984 Juvenile granulosa cell tumor of the ovary. A clinicopathological analysis of 125 cases. American Journal of Surgical Pathology 8: 575–596

Young R H, Lawrence W D, Scully R E 1985 Juvenile granulosa cell tumour: another neoplasm associated with abnormal chromosomes and ambiguous genitalia. A report of three cases. American Journal of Surgical Pathology 10: 737–743

Young R H, Dickersin G R, Scully R E 1987 Small cell carcinoma of the ovary: an analysis of 75 cases of a distinctive ovarian tumor commonly associated with hypercalcaemia. Laboratory Investigation 56: 89A

Zaloudek C, Norris H J 1984 Sertoli–Leydig tumors of the ovary. A clinicopathological study of 64 intermediate and poorly differentiated neoplasms. American Journal of Surgical Pathology 8: 405–418

Zaloudek C J, Tavassoli F A, Norris H J 1981 Dysgerminoma with syncytiotrophic giant cells. A histologically and clinically distinctive subtype of dysgerminoma. American Journal of Pathology 5: 361–367

Zirker T A, Silva E G, Morris M, Ordonez N G 1989 Immunohistochemical differentiation of clear cell carcinoma of the female genital tract and endodermal sinus tumor with the use of alpha fetoprotein and Leu-M1. American Journal of Clinical Pathology 91: 511–514

Index